# GROW HEALTHY KIDS!

A Parents' Guide to
Sound Nutrition from
Birth through Teens

# GROW HEALTHY KIDS!

## A Parents' Guide to Sound Nutrition from Birth through Teens

by Linda S. Peavy &
Andrea L. Pagenkopf, Ph.D.

*Dedication*


*To Howard, Erica Claire, and Don Sellers Peavy
and
to Gordon and Sarah Lynn Pagenkopf,
the families whose support and encouragement
helped make this book a reality
and
to all families who wish to make
optimum nutrition a way of life*

Published simultaneously in Canada
Library of Congress catalog card number: 78-67967

ISBN 0-448-16427-2
First printing 1980

Printed in the United States of America

# ACKNOWLEDGMENTS

This book, written for and about families, could not have become a reality without the patience and understanding shown by our own husbands and children throughout the long months of research, writing, and editing. Friends who became directly involved in the project also deserve acknowledgment, especially the James F. Smith family, whose seven-day dietary-intake records and family food history provided material for the concluding pages of the text.

Jean Julian, typist, deserves commendation for her struggles with dictated and hand-written early drafts. Ray and Sally Babcock and the staff at Ray Laboratories are due thanks for computer word-processing assistance. Becky Stiff contributed recipe exchanges. The staff at Montana State University's Renne Library and Vesta Anderson, Associate Professor of Home Economics, Montana State, provided research aid. Dr. George Carson, Bozeman pedodontist; Darryl Hote and Jeff Schneider, pharmacists; Paul Visscher, Eric Livers, and James Feist, pediatrics team for Medical Associates, Inc.; and Karen P. Lilly, R.D., provided editorial assistance in their respective fields.

For recipe contributions, thanks go to Phyllis Anderson, Sally Babcock, Sharon Burkhalter, Sam Cunningham, Evelyn Davis, Lillie M. Ellzey, Barbara Gunnin, Lizzie S. Hickman, Mac Hickman, Karen Leech, Sherry Lithander, Winnie H. Martin, Donna Ogle, Claribel Sellers, Dolly Smith, Mary Ullrich, and Connie van Horn.

Finally, special gratitude is due Ursula Smith for countless hours of editorial assistance, long nights of computer editing, and many months of encouragement and enthusiasm.

—Linda S. Peavy, Andrea L. Pagenkopf
Bozeman, Montana

# CONTENTS

## Foreword
By George M. Briggs, Ph.D., University of California, Berkeley..........xiii


## 1. Recognizing the Importance of Optimum Nutrition

Parental influence on lifetime eating habits . . . influence of diet on physical and mental growth and development . . . borderline nutrient deficiencies . . . diet and hyperactivity . . . infantile and childhood obesity and lifetime obesity . . . nutrition education . . . professional guidance . . . commonsense nutrition . . . establishing firm foundations............................................................................................1


## 2. Defining Optimum Nutrition

Variety is the key . . . food exchanges plan for families . . . Recommended Dietary Allowances and guidelines for other essential nutrients . . . energy . . . carbohydrates and fats . . . protein . . . protein complementarity . . . vitamins . . . minerals . . . turning nutrients into meals...................................................................................................7


## 3. Infancy—Birth to Three Months

Nutrient needs of the newborn . . . energy, protein, and water . . . vitamins and minerals . . . breast versus bottle . . . facts and fears about breast-feeding . . . the art of bottle-feeding . . . introduction of solids . . . psychological factors in breast and bottle-feeding . . . metabolic problems . . . colic . . . diarrhea . . . constipation . . . infantile obesity . . . feeding tips............................................................................................33

# 4. Infancy—Three to Six Months

Energy needs . . . carbohydrates, fats, and protein . . . vitamins and minerals . . . psychological factors . . . solid foods . . . nursing bottle syndrome . . . practical meals and snacks.....................................76

# 5. Infancy—Six to Eighteen Months

Essential nutrients . . . commercial versus homemade baby foods . . . psychological factors in feeding . . . manners . . . disliked foods . . . food jags . . . food allergies . . . diarrhea management . . . dental problems . . . infantile obesity . . . nutrition education . . . practical meals and snacks.........................................................87

# 6. Preschool—Eighteen Months to Five Years

Energy . . . carbohydrates, fats, and protein . . . vitamins and minerals . . . psychological aspects . . . food likes and dislikes . . . manners . . . television and mealtime . . . dental caries . . . between-meal snacks . . . television propaganda . . . childhood obesity . . . poor appetite . . . childhood illnesses . . . vegetarian diets . . . mealtime behavior modification techniques . . . party foods . . . kids in the kitchen . . . nutrition education . . . practical meals and snacks.............................107

# 7. Elementary School Years— Six to Ten

Energy . . . carbohydrates, fats, and protein . . . vitamins and minerals . . . vegetarian diets . . . psychological aspects . . . peer influence . . . holiday treats . . . television influence . . . allergies . . . snacks . . . dental caries . . . obesity . . . hyperactivity . . . constipation . . . hypoglycemia . . . food for young athletes . . . school lunch programs . . . vacation projects . . . practical meals and snacks....................156

# 8. Adolescent Years—Eleven to Nineteen

Physical changes . . . energy needs . . . fats, carbohydrates, and protein . . . vitamins and minerals . . . psychological aspects . . . sexual and physical changes . . . the early maturer . . . the late maturer . . . breakfast-skipping . . . obesity . . . anorexia nervosa . . . diet alterations . . . skin, teeth, hair, and nails . . . contraceptives . . . pregnancy . . . drugs . . . food for athletes . . . fast-food choices . . . college meals . . . practical meals and snacks.....................................................188

# Appendix A

Minimum Exchanges Chart; Six Exchange Lists; Recipe Conversion Chart..............................................................253

# Appendix B

Menus for Well-fed Families.....................................................267

# Appendix C

Recipes, Sack-Lunch Tips, Fun Food Ideas.....................................................271

# Appendix D

Bibliography.....................................................305

# Index..............................................................312

# Foreword

Convinced that the establishment of sound eating habits should be the highest priority of those entrusted with the feeding of infants, children, and teens, Linda Peavy and Andrea Pagenkopf have produced a book which emphasizes the importance of parental influence on lifetime eating habits. By considering psychological and social as well as physical and physiological aspects of feeding a family, the authors have made the establishment of sound nutrition habits a reasonable, attainable goal. This is an important and unique feature of *Grow Healthy Kids!*, making the book especially valuable to the reader.

Flexibility is the key to making optimum nutrition attractive to children and teens, and *Grow Healthy Kids!* offers, indeed, encourages that flexibility. For instance, if a toddler prefers six minimeals a day to three larger ones, there's no reason why his or her needs cannot be met through the program set forth in this book. If a second-grader prefers an unorthodox breakfast, such as a peanut butter sandwich and a glass of orange juice, that preference can be honored, once a parent has learned to evaluate the requested menu in light of the child's nutritional needs. The authors explain fully how, using a unit exchange system, parents—and children themselves—can keep a running tally of how family members' nutritional needs are being met, and can take action where necessary to make sure all nutritional bases are covered.

Realizing that nutrition-related problems may occur even under the best of circumstances, the authors give helpful suggestions for dealing with those problems. Infant, childhood, and adolescent obesity, nursing mouth syndrome of toddlerhood, preschooler food jags, school lunches, allergies, party foods for nutrition-conscious families, food for young athletes, teen fad diets, and many other problems which parents often encounter in feeding a child from birth through teen years are discussed in detail. The advice offered is current and reliable and is based upon the latest available information from medical and nutrition journals.

Convinced that today's consumers prefer to become well enough informed to make their own decisions on these and other nutrition-related matters, the authors of *Grow Healthy Kids!* present well-documented facts and figures but leave options open, inviting readers to adapt a basic plan for optimum nutrition to fit the specific needs of their particular family group. Colorful, pertinent examples make recall of important concepts natural and easy, and a thorough, cross-referenced index simplifies finding the answers to specific questions. A basic foods chart keyed to exchange lists simplifies the planning of varied, balanced menus. The inclusion of a full week of menus, a special section on sack lunches, and over fifty exchange-notated recipes further simplifies the meal planner's task. Development of eating habits which ensure the best possible nutrition should occur naturally for those families who follow this commonsense approach to the feeding of infants, children, and teenagers.

*Grow Healthy Kids!* bridges the gap between professional and popular approaches to nutrition education—another unique feature of this book. Indeed, the strength of this book lies in the authors' ability to translate well-researched technical facts into a meaningful, interesting form. Readers are invited to become as involved in the study of family nutrition as time and interest permit. If the discussions and conclusions drawn in the book leave questions still unanswered, an end bibliography invites further reading in the field. For those who wish to delve further into the technical aspects of specific nutrition topics or problems, the authors will provide on request a detailed, comprehensive, chapter-by-chapter bibliography, a document containing over 750 references used in the writing of *Grow Healthy Kids!*

All of this information has been brought together and made available to the public because Linda Peavy and Andrea Pagenkopf believe that families who become convinced of the importance of sound eating habits and are encouraged to find their own, unique ways of following basic nutrition guidelines will be able to help their children establish a sound foundation for a lifetime of optimum nutrition. The establishment of such a foundation has long been the goal of all professional nutrition educators, and now with this book the authors have given the American family a clear directive toward the implementation of this goal.

George M. Briggs, Ph.D.
Professor of Nutrition
University of California,
Berkeley

# 1
# Recognizing the Importance of Optimum Nutrition

From the first few moments of life, when baby's cheek touches mother's breast and the tiny mouth opens to seek the nipple that offers security, love, and life-sustaining nourishment, eating is a multidimensional activity. Throughout the early years, the pleasure children derive from eating and the nutritional patterns they develop will be dependent not only upon what foods their parents and others offer but also upon the spirit in which they present those foods.

During the kindergarten and grade-school years, these early eating habits will usually persist, despite the influence of peer pressure and persuasive television commercials. If those eating habits have been nutritionally sound, children are likely to enter the rapid-growth years of adolescence in good health and armed with a strong inclination to make proper eating a permanent part of their life structure.

If parents do, indeed, help set nutritional patterns from the earliest years, then nutrition education is a vital topic for those who wish to give their children the best possible nutritional foundation. Since few Americans have thorough, up-to-date knowledge of this important topic, conscientious parents often feel confused and frustrated by the information they do receive. Warnings against too much cholesterol, too many additives, not enough vitamins, or too little fiber frequently offer contradictory points of view. In the face of such confusion, a parent is tempted to say, "Oh, what does it matter what my kids eat? In America, they surely won't starve. Since I don't really know *what* to believe, I'll just cook what I've always cooked."

This is an understandable attitude, for parents have usually acquired deeply ingrained food habits over the years from their own parents and grandparents. Although parents of earlier generations may not have been aware of it, they were teaching nutritional patterns—both by example and by the choices they made available to other family members. From generation to generation, eating habits are passed on, often remaining basically intact. Thus, Aunt Josie's rich Southern menus—fried eggplant, deep-dish chicken pie, butter beans, fried corn and okra, sliced tomatoes, and hot biscuits and corn bread—are likely to bear a strong resemblance to those served by her great-great-grandmother.

Through the ages, those responsible for food gathering and preparation have prepared dishes according to the customs of their particular culture, assuming that these dishes contained the life-sustaining nutrients needed by family members. In many cases, the diets of even the most primitive peoples *have* proven adequate for the optimum growth and development of their children. In other cases, grossly inadequate diets have contributed greatly to high mortality and morbidity rates, especially among infants and children, whose rapid growth and development demand an adequate diet.

When is a diet "inadequate" and in what way are children affected by such diets? Basically, an inadequate diet is one that is lacking in overall calories and/or is significantly low in protein, carbohydrates, essential fatty acids, vitamins, or minerals.

A chronically undernourished child grows at a much slower rate than he or she should and is more susceptible to childhood diseases. He may suffer from deficiency disorders such as anemia, rickets, or goiter. In one study in New Delhi, India, a group of undernourished children showed lower IQ scores, smaller head circumferences, and slower visual-motor development than did well-nourished children in the same study. Such problems are often hard to trace to nutritional inadequacies, however, especially since environmental factors are also usually involved.

The severely malnourished child, on the other hand, shows such marked physical growth retardation that there can be no doubt that his problems are nutrition-related. The marasmus victim—the young child who has received inadequate calories, protein, and other nutrients, almost from birth—is particularly vulnerable to permanent damage. When severe malnutrition occurs during the first two years of life, during which time brain growth is most active, there is mounting evidence that permanent reduction of brain size and restricted intellectual development may also occur. Malnutrition begun in the prenatal stage and carried throughout the first two years has an even more devastating effect. Finally, when severe malnutrition is combined with an environment that offers the child no intellectual stimulation, negative effects on intellectual, developmental, and behavioral patterns are compounded still further. Such severe restriction of protein and calories usually means restriction of other essential nutrients as well, and these extensive multiple deficiencies contribute to the numerous mental and physical health problems of the severely malnourished child. The weight of evidence, as reported in the Department of Health, Education and Welfare (HEW) booklet *The Health of Children,* suggests that ". . . early and severe malnutrition is an input factor in later intellectual development, above and beyond the effect of social-familial influences."

While such extreme malnutrition and multiple deficiencies are relatively rare among average American children, lesser nutrition-related problems do exist among our infants and children. These problems, while often less obvious than those associated with severe malnutrition, may nonetheless lessen a child's chances for optimum physical and intellectual development. For example, one study related subtle differences in the eating behavior of infant twins to small but reliable differences in the mental development of the twins. Other studies have shown that children who consume very small amounts of milk or other calcium-rich foods may fail to reach their full height potential. There is increasing evidence that zinc deficiency causes retardation of growth and sexual development in humans as well as in animals.

Recent data suggest that iron-deficiency anemia, seen in 34 to 70 percent of low-income American children ages one through four and occurring in approximately 22 percent of all American preschoolers, has been associated with narrow attention span and marked decrease in attentiveness, lowered ability or willingness to engage in complex or purposeful behavior, less persistence, and voluntary activity. The more severe the anemia, the more severe the symptoms become. Obviously, a preschooler or a child of the lower elementary grades who exhibits the above traits is unlikely to be able to take full advantage of her opportunities for intellectual development, whether these occur at home or at school. While all children who seem to have these characteristics may not be suffering from iron deficiency, those whose attitudes and intellectual development can be improved by treatment with iron supplements or by more careful attention to iron-rich foods in the diet should certainly be given the advantage such additions may provide.

Among teenage girls, the problem of iron deficiency looms even larger, since blood loss during menstrual periods calls for a proportionate increase of iron intake, an increase not taken by 20 percent of the female teens in our country. Since the iron stores of such teens are almost completely depleted after a few years of insufficient dietary intake, these girls have no reserves with which to meet the needs of their developing babies once they become pregnant. Since iron-deficiency anemia is detrimental to the health of both mother-to-be and unborn child, young women should be informed of their need for iron and should be aided in planning meals or taking supplements which can provide this mineral in sufficient amounts.

While teens and young children often suffer from too little iron, vitamins, or minerals, some children may suffer from too *much* of a certain substance. Approximately 3 to 10 percent of U.S. children have been termed "hyperactive," with the characteristic symptoms of poor powers of concentration, short attention span, impulsive behavior, inability to delay gratification, diminished ability to experience pleasure, altered perception and cognition, altered muscular coordination, and normal IQ but underachievement in school. While doctors traditionally treat extreme cases of this hyperkinetic syndrome with drugs, mounting evidence suggests that significant alterations in the diets of these children may in some cases make medication unnecessary.

Several researchers have claimed that for some children, a diet free of artificial coloring and flavoring reduces perceived hyperactivity. In other cases, the omission of breakfast has been linked to hyperkinetic behavior during the school day. There is some evidence that hyperactive children display glucose intolerance, which would make them sensitive to concentrated sweets. While all hyperactive children may not respond to exclusion diets or to the regular consumption of a well-balanced breakfast, nutritional alternatives would seem worth investigating before a child is relegated to years of medication or years of maladjustment without medication.

Obesity is another health problem for which nutrition modification might be a safer, more effective means of control than medication. Until recently, the fat infant was considered a healthy infant, and such phrases as "Oh, what a fine fat baby!" were music to a mother's ears. Though childhood obesity usually causes more concern than baby fatness, some parents still tend to dismiss a child's weight problem with "It's just a stage she's going through" or "I'm sure he will grow out of it later." "Pretty-plus" and "chubby" sizes help parents and children minimize the problem of obesity, a problem which would be much harder to ignore were pants too tight and dresses popping buttons. While an overweight child certainly needs to feel good about himself, his parents should be aware that obesity begun in infancy probably heightens the chance for a lifetime of obesity.

New research pointing to an increase in the *number* of fat cells in obese infants and children, not just an increase in the *size* of these cells, has led researchers to examine more closely the probability that early obesity may predispose an individual to adult obesity. Though the mechanics by which this may occur are not yet clearly understood, and though the fat-cell theory has been attacked by some researchers, there are those who believe that parents should try to prevent the accumulation of an excess number of fat cells in infants and children when at all possible. *Prevention* of obesity seems much more desirable than "curing" weight problems in later life, since even the most successful diet and exercise cures are usually temporary at best.

These findings present parents with disturbing questions: Are we overfeeding our children? Is it dangerous to admonish children to clean their plates? Should we try to put children on diet programs, even though their rapidly growing bodies must have sufficient calories for growth and development?

When we consider the extreme and often dangerous weight-loss diets adolescent girls sometimes adopt in the name of "thin is beautiful," we may be understandably reluctant to begin asking children to "slim down" too early or too enthusiastically. On the other hand, given the high percentage of overweight teenagers and the psychological and physiological problems likely to be encountered as a result of a lifetime of obesity, we should not postpone nutrition education until it is too late to prevent such unhealthiness and unhappiness.

Wise eating—eating which can prevent the tragedies just described and contribute to overall health and well being—is a matter of making wise choices. In some underdeveloped countries, where a bowl of rice may be considered a good day's meal, limited resources have left parents and children no room for making such choices. All the nutrition education possible cannot alter a poor diet unless better foods are available and are within the economic reach of the malnourished individual. On the other hand, a wide range of choices and the money to take advantage of those choices do not always insure adequate nutrition.

For example, in the United States today, most families have available to them a wide variety of animal and vegetable products from which to assemble nutritionally sound meals and snacks. Nevertheless, the element of wide choice is often abused rather than used to its fullest advantage. Teens, especially those with no sound nutrition background, tend to consume empty calories, eating foods that contribute little more than unwanted pounds to their rapidly changing bodies. Young children bombarded with television commercials which sing out the virtues of high-sugar breakfast cereals and empty-calorie, sugar-laden drinks are not likely to make wise eating choices without the aid of a parent or some other adult interested in their nutritional welfare. Thus, during the years of rapid growth, the years when the nutrition foundation for good or poor lifetime health is being laid, children are too often educated only by the attractively produced propaganda of companies whose chief concern is financial gain.

How can parents offset these less-than-desirable influences and teach nutrition habits which will point the child toward a lifetime of good eating? Many parents have had no nutrition education themselves, other than a few scatter-shot programs offered during the grade- or high-school years. All too often, the doctors to whom they entrust the health of their children feel more confident prescribing multivitamins than attempting to offer counsel on balanced diets for the toddler-through-teen years.

With all other aspects of a child's health in his or her care, the physician who has not had adequate nutrition training or whose training has not kept up with nutritional innovations resulting from recent research findings is unlikely to have the time to locate and provide to families the information they need in order to plan healthful meals and snacks. Food and nutrition specialists with state or county Cooperative Extension Service, (United States Department of Agriculture) and WIC (Women, Infants, Children) programs, local health departments, and other local, state, and national organizations are willing to help families make basic decisions which will move them toward good eating habits. Still, such programs cannot reach all who want to know more about childhood and family nutrition.

Many books on this subject provide a good starting point, but unless the books have incorporated the very latest research studies, they may give well-meaning advice that contradicts new findings in the field. This book will attempt to make available the very latest information about nutrition from birth through the teen years. Further, this work will attempt to translate that information into practical suggestions which may easily be used to improve the diet patterns of the average family.

No matter how well researched and well written a book of this type may be, if it offers hard-to-follow directions for meal planning and suggests that a five-year-old, a twelve-year-old, and two adults cannot eat the same general dishes, then its advice is not likely to be followed. To avoid this pitfall, the menu ideas in this book are designed to fit the needs of the entire family. Different caloric needs and different needs for specific nutrients may be met by offering smaller or larger portions of certain foods and/or offering nutrient-rich snacks between meals. Thus, an overweight teen, an average-weight third-grader, a mother, a father, and even a diabetic grandmother can sit down to the same basic meal, yet eat items and amounts ideally suited to meet their individual needs.

Once appetizing, nutritious dishes have been prepared for the family, getting the children and teens to try them may still be a formidable task. This is especially true if family members have previously been presented with only "meat and potatoes" fare or highly processed, commercial, frozen dinners. Motivating family members to change their accustomed eating habits can be made easier through the use of simple behavior-modification techniques, nutrition education suggestions, and exciting, tasty recipes which feature the new food items. This book presents many ways by which family members may be motivated to make the desired changes in eating habits.

Basic among these techniques is giving attention to nutrition education, so that even the youngest family member can begin to sense that what one eats may, to a large extent, help determine one's immediate and future state of health. Once the whys of good nutrition are understood, making wise choices becomes easier. Thus, a junior-high daughter not only recalls that she should eat the carrots on her school lunch plate "because mama says so," but she may also recall that those carrots provide her body with the vitamin A vital to adequate night vision, healthy skin, and good bone and cartilage development. Her older brother may voluntarily forsake junk-food snacks in favor of more nutritious snack items, once he has been convinced that optimum nutrition contributes to the overall physical strength and endurance he knows is essential for top performance in his starting position on the high-school basketball team. Such changes do not occur, of course, unless a family learns why sound nutrition is important.

# 2
## Defining
## Optimum Nutrition

Most parents would gladly provide optimum nutrition for their children, if only they knew what "optimum nutrition" really means. Even nutritionists have trouble agreeing what this term means, but in this book "optimum nutrition" is assumed to be consumption of a well-balanced diet, one which provides calories, vitamins, minerals, protein, carbohydrate and fat in adequate amounts to maintain good health and ideal weight. Even the phrase "eat a well-balanced diet" may have little or no meaning for a person who has never enrolled in classes in home economics. Even those who are familiar with the phrase may have forgotten most of the precepts they learned, since one seldom retains facts not put to immediate and continuous use.

Most home economics courses of the past presented the basic four food groups—fruits and vegetables, milk and dairy products, breads and cereals, and meats. Earlier in this century, students were lectured on the seven basic food groups. Since the U.S. Department of Agriculture has devised a meal-planning guide based on five food groups, many textbooks now being written follow this alternative plan. Whatever the number of food groups, teachers have traditionally explained that by including the appropriate number of servings of food from each group in one's daily menu and snack plans, one should be fairly well assured of having a balanced diet. They are right.

The key to optimum nutrition is balance, and the key to balance is *variety*. Not only should one choose foods from all the food groups, but one should also work for variety *within* each food group. For example, if a child eats the same fruits and vegetables day after day, he will not have sufficient variety to insure that he has included all the essential nutrients in his diet. Families that are not accustomed to striving for variety may have difficulty broadening their menus beyond the most common items; Appendix A contains food lists for each of six major categories: milk and dairy products, fruits, vegetables, breads and cereals, meats, and fats.

These food lists are patterned after the exchange list developed for use by

7

diabetics, but they have been modified for use by nondiabetics. Foods are grouped into six basic lists according to generally equivalent nutritional values. All foods within a given list have approximately the same calorie, carbohydrate, protein, and fat content and contain similar vitamins and minerals. Thus, foods within any one group may be substituted for other foods within that same group.

The exchange lists used in this book are modifications of the latest Exchange List for Meal Planning of the American Diabetes Association, Inc., and the American Dietetic Association (in cooperation with the National Institute for Arthritis, Metabolism and Digestive Disease; the National Institute of Health; the Public Health Service, United States Department of Health, Education, and Welfare; and the National Heart and Lung Institute). The lists reflect current interest in modification of fat as well as carbohydrate intake and list high-, medium-, and low-fat meats separately. (Though these lists are similar to the exchange lists used by diabetics, they are **not** suitable for use by diabetics because they have been modified to include many items containing sugar in higher concentrations than diabetics normally use.)

With *variety* as the key word, planning well-balanced meals that provide excellent nutrition for all family members should be relatively easy. For those who want more exact guidelines, the chart on page 9 should be useful. This chart, which also appears in Appendix A, lists the minimum number of exchanges from each food group which should be included in any day's dietary intake. The food lists in Appendix A indicate serving sizes appropriate for adults, and serving sizes for children from birth to three years are given on the Minimum Exchanges Chart. Food lists also indicate the primary nutrients supplied by the various foods. Recipes included in this book are keyed to the exchange lists to make it easier for you to estimate whether you are meeting the recommended minimums. The recipe conversion chart given in Appendix A will enable you to determine the exchange values for other recipes.

By using recipes which include a wide variety of items from the six groups, you can plan varied meals which, over a seven-day period, should provide all your family members with adequate protein, carbohydrate, fat, vitamins, minerals, and fiber. Nevertheless, including only the minimum amounts of these foods in the diet will not allow you to meet the full calorie (energy) needs of each family member. Adding extra portions of items from the first five lists is an ideal way to increase calories to the desired level, since foods from these lists supply valuable nutrients as well as energy. As notes on the chart indicate, giving extra attention to certain fruits, vegetables, and meats will increase the likelihood of achieving a well-balanced diet. Desserts, especially high-calorie baked goods, usually add a significant number of calories to the diet of all family members. Snacks chosen from the list in Chapter 6 may be popular with children of all ages. Many teens prefer to gain calories in a "fourth meal" of hamburgers and shakes eaten after school with friends.

# Family Guide to Minimum Exchanges from Six Major Food Groups

| Age (in years) | Food Groups[1] | | | | | |
| --- | --- | --- | --- | --- | --- | --- |
| | Milk[2] | Vegetable[3] | Fruit[4] | Bread and Cereal | Meat[5] (oz) | Fat[6] |
| ½–1 | 2–3 (16–24 oz) | ½–1 (4–8 tbsp) | ½–1 (4–8 tbsp) | ½–1 (4–8 tbsp) | 2 | As |
| 1–3 | 3 (24 oz) | 1 (8 tbsp) | 1 (8 tbsp) | 2 (16 tbsp) | 3 | needed |
| 4–6 | 3 | 2 | 2 | 3 | 4 | to |
| 7–10 | 3 | 2 | 2 | 4 | 4–5 | meet |
| 11–14 | 4+ | 2 | 2 | 4 | 6 | calorie |
| 15–18 | 4+ | 2 | 2 | 4 | 6 | require-ments |

NOTE: To these minimums, one must add extra portions in order to reach recommended caloric levels each day. Once these minimums have been met, added calories may come from any of the above food groups or from the exchange lists for simple carbohydrates or prepared foods.

The recipes given in this book are exchange-keyed to make it easier to determine the exchanges gained from casseroles, breads, desserts, or other dishes. A chart for converting other recipes to exchanges is included in Appendix A.

[1]On this chart, all portions are expressed as *adult*-sized exchanges (see exchange lists). Children's portion sizes are 1 to 2 tablespoons for each year of age to age three; for children under three years of age the minimum tablespoons recommended per day are indicated in the chart, along with the equivalent number of adult-sized portions.

[2]Teens need to add more dairy products such as puddings, ice cream, and cheeses, in order to keep calcium levels high during rapid-growth years.

[3]Include two or three vitamin A vegetables each week. Do not depend on white (head) lettuce to supply vitamin A or folic acid in significant amounts; romaine, red leaf, and green leaf lettuce are all higher in these nutrients than head lettuce and contribute significant fiber.

[4]Include one vitamin C fruit or vegetable each day. Also include dried fruits to help raise iron levels.

[5]Include pork at least once a week for thiamin value. Rotate meats, including chicken, pork, beef, fish, as often as possible in the diet. This should insure iron and other mineral intake of sufficient quantity, plus intake of vitamins such as $B_6$. Peanut butter or peanuts can add $B_6$ to the diet.

[6]Include fat as a natural part of the diet in amounts suited to help meet calorie needs. If desired, polyunsaturated fats may be used to avoid excessive cholesterol intake.

# Understanding RDAs

The Minimum Exchanges chart is designed to help family members receive the Recommended Dietary Allowances (RDA) of protein, vitamins, and minerals. RDAs are the accepted standard for the intake of nutrients needed by all age groups in the United States. These recommendations are compiled by a panel of experts in the field of nutrition and published in chart form by the National Academy of Sciences in Washington, D.C., in a booklet called *Recommended Dietary Allowances.* The recommendations in this book are based on the ninth (1980) revised edition of that chart. The Minimum Exchanges chart translates the technical notations of the RDA chart into easily understood terms.

The latest edition of *Recommended Dietary Allowances* contains over a hundred pages explaining how the RDAs were determined. The RDA chart at the end of that publication is widely used by physicians, nurses, and nutritionists throughout the United States. Minicharts, adapted from the RDAs but including only the specific items being discussed, appear throughout this book.

The RDA chart is intended as a guide, not as a mandate for all individuals. Individual differences such as size and activity level must be considered before you can determine the ideal nutrition for a particular child. Once necessary adjustments have been made and RDAs have been noted for various nutrients, you should remember that all RDA listings except the one for calories provide more than the minimum daily requirement for most people, allowing for stress situations such as mild illness or emotional upset. Since most nutrients obtained from dietary sources can be tolerated in amounts far exceeding the RDA, eating foods which may provide increased amounts of nutrients is not likely to cause problems. Two exceptions must be noted: persons who have a very high intake of certain vitamins and minerals in supplement form may experience toxic effects from these substances, and excessive energy (calorie) intake will lead to obesity.

The built-in safeguards of the RDAs mean there is no need to fear that receiving slightly lesser amounts of some nutrients will cause severe deficiency symptoms. The body can store some nutrients if an overabundance exists and can conserve essential nutrients if the supply falls. Since the body makes allowances for occasional shortages, an intake below RDA standards for one day is not serious. *An average intake that meets two-thirds of the RDA over a five- to eight-day period is probably adequate for most people.* Of course, the further habitual intake falls below RDA standards for a particular nutrient—and the longer low intake continues—the greater the risk of deficiency.

For some people with unusual needs due to special circumstances, such as malabsorption problems, even strict adherence to RDA standards would not insure a high enough intake of some nutrients to prevent deficiency symptoms. In such cases, a physician can help make the needed adjustments, increasing certain nutrients and even adding supplements if necessary.

One further cautionary word is in order. There are essential nutrients for which no RDA has as yet been established. These nutrients are no less crucial to good health and optimum physical and mental development than are those which do appear on the RDA chart. They are not included only because there is not yet sufficient evidence available to allow recommendations to be made. The 1980 RDA booklet does include a special chart containing tentatively recommended ranges of several of these items, but definitive research has not yet produced enough information to allow these and other trace elements to become a part of the RDA chart itself. Thus you cannot assume that simply meeting RDAs will mean getting all essential nutrients.

As a general rule, if you meet RDAs through consumption of a variety of foods, chances are excellent that the diet you are following is diverse enough to provide you with essential nutrients for which no RDA has as yet been established. Meeting RDAs through use of highly refined, heavily fortified foods or through consumption of vitamin/mineral supplements provides no such bonus. For these reasons, families concerned with optimum nutrition should consider RDAs a starting point, not a final goal.

Since no one should be expected to place absolute faith in even such a widely accepted chart as the RDA, the following pages present a general discussion of the various nutrients given on that chart. Once one sees the role played by energy, protein, carbohydrates, fats, vitamins, and minerals, achieving RDAs should become a more meaningful goal.

A quick reading of this section, giving special attention to the vitamin and mineral overview charts, should provide the necessary background for understanding later discussions of the particular needs of various age groups. You might want to skim items which seem too technical or detailed to be interesting reading now and reconsider them later, when you desire more in-depth knowledge or when older children ask specific questions about the roles essential nutrients play in the overall health of the human body.

This material is included here because the authors believe many families will eventually enjoy learning more about the whys of good nutrition. It should be looked upon as handy reference material, not as something which must be studied and thoroughly understood before moving on to the less technical sections of this book. The bibliography offers an opportunity for reading more technical articles which space would not allow to be incorporated here. In addition, Appendix D lists several excellent books which provide in-depth discussions of the principles of nutrition.

## Energy

Energy comes from food, and, in the United States, food energy is usually expressed in *calories.* Just as weight is measured in ounces or kilograms and length is designated in inches or centimeters, so energy is expressed in terms of calories. Technically speaking, there are two kinds of calories: *small calories* and *large calories*. One thousand small calories make up 1 large calorie, or *kilocalorie*. One kilocalorie is the amount of energy required to heat up 1 kilogram (2.2 pounds) of water 1 degree Celsius. What we commonly call a calorie when speaking of food is actually a kilocalorie, and all calories referred to in this book are kilocalories.

Energy is needed for all activities that take place in the human body. Metabolic processes, physical activity or exercise, growth, tissue repair, lactation, excretory processes, physiological and psychological stress, maintenance of body temperature—all these activities require energy.

Taking as many of these factors as possible into consideration, the National Research Council has set recommended energy allowances at the lowest value thought to be consistent with good health for the average person. When calorie intake falls too far below recommended levels, weight decreases, and if caloric restriction is severe enough, health deteriorates or growth does not take place. On the other hand, calories taken in excess of need build unsightly, unhealthy fat deposits.

Although the best available methods have been used in compiling the RDA energy figures for each age group, the recommended caloric intakes might be too high or too low for certain infants, children, or teens. If a child tries the recommended calorie intake for at least two weeks and his weight remains steady, the intake is probably adequate but not excessive. If a child has been achieving desirable weight and height gains, the caloric level he is currently using is probably fairly well suited to his needs.

In most cases, a child's own appetite will probably be the best indicator of how many calories he should consume. Telling nonobese five-year-old Lucas that he cannot have another serving of carrots and potatoes because he is going to exceed his 1700-calorie limit can serve no useful purpose, since tomorrow may be a low-appetite day during which his growing body may need to depend on the few extra calories held in reserve from today.

RDA calorie levels are only a reference point by which one may gauge proper intake. For example, the calorie level suggested may not provide enough energy to allow for an under-weight child's much-needed weight gain. A mother might add nutritious, high-calorie snacks such as homemade milkshakes to this child's daily food offerings, even though eating such snacks will mean surpassing the RDA calorie level for his sex and age group. On the other hand, the obese child whose calorie intake is well above the suggested RDA level should be encouraged to move toward the recommended level by eliminating snacks low in nutrients and high in calories. Since decreasing calorie levels too drastically will not provide enough energy or nutrients for optimum growth and development, an obese youngster should be encouraged to increase his activity level to use up extra calories.

Many persons tend to underestimate the calorie-burning value of exercise. If a teenager spends a half-hour a day at the new activity of handball and continues his other accustomed daily activities, including his regular eating habits, he will probably lose sixteen pounds per year. Because the overweight person tends to burn more calories during exercise than does the slim person, owing to the extra calories required to move the heavier body, an obese teen could lose more than sixteen pounds through a year of half-hour-per-day handball sessions.

Since all calorie recommendations represent an educated guess for average individuals, and since children's energy needs are especially difficult to assess, adjustments may be necessary to arrive at the optimal calorie level. From infancy through the teen years, it is probably wise to consult a physician or a professional nutritionist if the energy figures derived from your own calculations differ greatly from those on the RDA chart. If height and weight vary sharply from that of the reference child given in the RDA standards, or if your child's activities seem more or less vigorous than those of the average child, you should make appropriate adjustments in calorie levels. Wide variations can be serious, since letting a child's calorie level fall too low is likely to interfere with her ideal growth and development, and allowing a child's calorie level to continuously exceed the RDA may mean that that child is set on the way toward a lifetime of obesity.

**Energy Sources**

Merely eating enough food to acquire the recommended number of calories is no insurance that proper nutrition is being obtained. In fact, malnutrition can often be present in grossly overweight persons who continue to eat large quantities of low-quality calories. Many American children derive a large part of their energy from highly refined sugars and fats, neither of which provides the vitamins and minerals vital to optimum growth and development. Others, especially adolescent girls, try fad diets that lead them to cut out whole categories of food, a practice likely to lead to vitamin and mineral deficiencies if it is continued for many months.

The source of a child's calories can be as important as the number of calories she consumes. Carbohydrates (4 calories/gram), fats (9 calories/gram), and protein (4 calories/gram) are the three categories which supply energy for the average child.

The body uses *carbohydrates* as a source of energy for brain function and growth and for certain other specialized processes. Between 40 and 50 percent of the total energy consumed by most American infants and children is in the form of carbohydrate foods. Enough carbohydrate  is needed each day to avoid *ketosis* (excessive body-fat breakdown) and other undesirable metabolic responses to extremely low carbohydrate intake.

Carbohydrates may be grouped into two broad classes: simple, and complex. Simple carbohydrates, including all sugars, require little digestion and are absorbed very quickly into the bloodstream. Complex carbohydrates, including starches and fiber, are digested more slowly—or not at all—and therefore do not cause a rapid rise in blood-sugar levels.

Generally speaking, Americans consume far more simple sugars than complex carbohydrates. A sixty-year survey of American eating habits showed a 25 percent decrease in total carbohydrate consumption but a 25 percent increase in sugar and syrup consumption. Since highly refined sugars give little more than pure energy, a child who fills his calorie needs through such means is likely to ignore body-building high-protein, high-vitamin/mineral foods. In addition, the child whose diet is high in sugars is likely to have a higher percentage of tooth decay than a child on a low-sugar diet.

A wide variety of carbohydrates is available to the consumer. In fact, a 1966 survey showed that 47 percent of the calories available at supermarkets were carbohydrate in nature. Making wise choices of these carbohydrates is essential. Generally, one should reduce highly refined sugar intake and concentrate on using carbohydrate foods which offer vitamins, minerals, fiber, and protein as well as energy.

*Fats,* or lipids, are the most concentrated source of energy, yielding over twice as much energy gram for gram as either protein or carbohydrates. The sixty-year decrease in overall carbohydrate consumption mentioned above has been accompanied by an increase in fat and protein consumption. The average American child now derives between 40 and 50 percent of her energy from fat.

In view of the American Heart Association's recommendation against ingesting an excess of saturated fatty acids, the trend toward increased use of fats may change. That association is recommending that the proportion of energy derived from fat should not exceed 35 percent and that less than 10 percent of total calories should come from saturated fatty acids. If the Heart Association is correct, such a diet would greatly improve the cardiac health of the American public. Since adult eating habits are harder to change than those of young children, it seems desirable to avoid diets heavy in cholesterol and saturated fats from an early age. One exception should be noted: Infants seem to need a certain amount of cholesterol in their diets; a more detailed discussion of fat intake during infancy is contained in the following chapter.

Current evidence suggests that high fat intake coupled with low fiber intake is associated with greater incidence of breast cancer and cancer of the colon. "Associated with" does not necessarily mean "caused by," and further research is needed to clarify the relationship between dietary fat intake and cancer.

All of these negatives are probably enough to make you contemplate eliminating all fats from your diet. This would be highly dangerous, for fats serve as carriers for fat-soluble nutrients, such as vitamins A, D, E, and K. They also help you feel satisfied, since the fat content of a meal helps determine the rate at which it is emptied from the stomach. Cell membranes, hormones, and other essential body components are also dependent upon adequate fat intake. Cholesterol, most often thought of in negative terms, is a component of the myelin sheath covering the brain. It is also necessary for the production of vitamin D, bile salts, and several hormones. Linoleic acid, a fat component vital to good health, may be obtained through the use of cottonseed, corn, peanut, safflower, and soybean oil, but not through the use of coconut or olive oil. Poor growth, decreased resistance to stress, and death at an early age appear in cases of extreme essential-fatty-acid deprivation.

Fat stored in the human body helps cushion the organs, insulate the body, and give protection against mechanical stresses. Fatty stores can also supply energy for certain bodily emergencies, thus sparing body-building protein for growth activity. Also, the recent trend toward reducing fats in the diet has occasionally been carried to extremes which have led to the development of chronic diarrhea in children.

## Protein

The Greek word *proteios,* which means "primary" or "holding first place," is the root from which our word *protein* was derived. Since protein forms the basic structure of all living cells and is an essential life-forming, life-sustaining element in human and animal diets, the substance is well named. Because energy takes first priority in metabolism, if a child's diet is low in carbohydrates or fat, protein will be utilized for energy and will not be available for synthesis of body tissues. Further, when energy consumption from other sources is low, protein is not as efficiently utilized for growth as when other energy sources are consumed at the same time. Using protein as an energy source is not only a wasteful use of an expensive food item, it is also a medically unsound use, since high protein loads may overwork kidneys and liver.

The need for protein is determined by a person's overall growth pattern. Recommendations for daily protein intake generally decrease from 2.2 grams per kilogram of body weight for the infant under six months of age to less than 1 gram per kilogram during adulthood. Specific protein needs of various age groups will be discussed in later chapters.

The effects of marasmus, a form of malnutrition resulting from severe protein and calorie restriction during infancy, were discussed in Chapter 1. Kwashiorkor, another severe form of malnutrition in young children, has been attributed primarily to protein deficiency. Called "the weaning disease" by some, kwashiorkor usually strikes children during the late weaning or postweaning months, as they move from human milk to a diet high in carbohydrates but low in protein. Rampant in many developing countries and seen occasionally in the United States, the disease results in extensive growth retardation, coarsened hair that is easily plucked, anemia, extreme apathy, dermatitis, irritability, water retention and swelling, loss of appetite, and enlarged liver. Death rates for children suffering from kwashiorkor are ten to forty times higher than death rates for the average child in the United States.

The intellectual growth of kwashiorkor children is apparently less likely to be permanently impaired than that of marasmus children, probably because kwashiorkor usually occurs after the critical age of brain development. Nonetheless, the apathy which accompanies the severe protein restriction of kwashiorkor, plus the laboratory-documented tendency of protein-restricted animals to adapt poorly to new surroundings, indicates that severe protein deprivation even after the age of two probably has detrimental influences on learning ability.

Most researchers agree that deciding where the effects of malnutrition end and those of depressed and deprived learning environment begin is still subject to debate. Researchers have theorized that environmental stimulation can go far toward offsetting the negative effects of protein deprivation. The question of impaired learning ability is complex and multidimensional. Diet, behavior, and environment all play important roles in the development of the brain, and often their roles are so interrelated as to make clear-cut cause-and-effect judgment nearly impossible.

The building blocks of protein are the amino acids, which are made available by hydrolysis, or digestion. Amino acids are involved in the formation and maintenance of muscle and nerve tissue, bone matrix, enzymes, hormones, lymph, plasma, and other vital elements in the human body. Those amino acids which cannot be manufactured by the body but must be obtained from food are called essential amino acids. Nine essential amino acids have been identified: threonine, leucine, isoleucine, valine, methionine, phenylalanine, tryptophan, lysine, and histidine. The remaining amino acids are termed nonessential, since the body can manufacture them.

If you use high-quality animal protein such as eggs, milk, cheese, and meat, you can be sure of getting the essential amino acids. The strict vegetarian, (vegan) who avoids these items, may have to plan meals more carefully, since there is no plant food which provides biologically complete protein. Protein from nonanimal sources such as grains, legumes, and nuts can supply all the essential amino acids if these foods are used in the right combinations. Knowing these combinations is essential for an adequate vegetarian diet. *Diet for a Small Planet,* by Frances Lappé, is an excellent sourcebook if you are interested in a vegetarian diet. The protein complementarity chart shown here follows the principles discussed by Lappé and others. By planning meals which feature the combinations needed to insure that you have a diet containing all the essential amino acids, you should be able to provide for your family a vegetarian diet containing adequate amounts of high-quality protein.

For example, grains eaten alone are deficient in two of the nine essential amino acids, isoleucine and lysine. However, certain grains, when combined with certain other vegetable items such as legumes or sesame, provide a balance of these two essential amino acids. Since absence of even one of the essential amino acids means tissue building is impaired, careful study of the principles of protein complementarity is essential for any person who wants to derive protein from nonanimal sources. These combinations should also prove useful to nonvegetarian households interested in decreasing the amount of animal protein in their diets for economical, ecological, or health reasons.

The recommended combinations must be eaten at the same meal in order to constitute a "complete" protein source. Such combinations are easy to make. For example, a whole-wheat-bread-and-peanut-butter sandwich plus one glass of milk yields protein of good quality. Combination dishes such as green peas and mushrooms or sesame rice (see Alpine Rice recipe in Appendix C) are delicious ways of meeting protein needs. A meat dish plus these two side dishes provides more than ample protein and carbohydrates, and several important vitamins and minerals as well.

## Complementary Protein Guide

To insure vegetarians a biologically complete protein intake,
the following foods should be eaten at the same meal.

| | | | |
|---|---|---|---|
| *Eat these grains* | rice, corn, or wheat | *with* | legumes |
| | wheat | " | peanuts + milk |
| | wheat | " | sesame + soybeans |
| | rice | " | sesame + Brewer's yeast |
| *Eat these nuts and seeds* | peanuts | *with* | sesame + soybeans |
| | sesame | " | beans |
| | sesame | " | soybeans + wheat |
| | peanuts | " | sunflower seeds |
| *Eat these legumes* | legumes | *with* | rice |
| | beans | " | wheat or corn |
| | soybeans | " | rice + wheat |
| | soybeans | " | corn + milk |
| | soybeans | " | wheat + sesame |
| | soybeans | " | peanuts + sesame |
| | soybeans | " | peanuts + rice + wheat |
| *Eat these vegetables* | lima beans, green peas, Brussel sprouts, cauliflower, *or* broccoli | | sesame seeds *or* Brazil nuts *or* mushrooms |
| | greens | " | millet *or* converted rice |

Since the average American diet supplies two to three times the RDA of protein, and since the American Heart Association recommends reducing saturated fat intake associated with heavy consumption of animal foods, families currently consuming unduly high levels of animal food might well consider reducing those intakes. Though such a step would probably mean parents must alter their own deep-seated habits of excessive protein consumption, the possible economic and health advantages make this step worth serious consideration.

## Vitamins

Over the years, many Americans have begun to think of vitamins as magic elements capable of preventing or curing sundry ills—if consumed in large enough quantities. The persuasive advertisements of drug manufacturers, who amass large profits from the sale of vitamin preparations, have helped to shift emphasis from vitamin-rich foods to vitamin pills or tonics.

Despite widespread advertisements to the contrary, chances are good that a person consuming a well-balanced diet needs no vitamin supplements at all. Even during the rapid-growth years of infancy, childhood, and adolescence, multivitamin preparations are probably not necessary for good health, provided family members are receiving nutritious meals and snacks. Since being sure all vitamins are included in the diet is sometimes difficult, some physicians routinely prescribe multivitamin compounds for growing children. Taken as directed, such compounds can provide extra insurance against deficiency. Taken in excess, they might well cause undesirable complications.

The attitude that *more* must mean *better* is definitely wasteful and could be dangerous where vitamins are concerned. Only in recent years has the public begun to realize that certain vitamins taken in excess are toxic. Fortunately, though concentrated vitamin tablets (both natural and synthetic) may prove toxic, you need not worry that eating too many carrots will cause vitamin A toxicity or that eating too many oranges will lead to dangerous vitamin C excesses. You should worry, however, about giving or taking overdoses of vitamin tablets, especially vitamins, A, D, K, and C.

Another danger associated with routine multivitamin consumption is that parents will develop a false sense of security, becoming so sure that the pills will avoid all problems that they make less effort to provide their children with well-balanced, vitamin-rich menus. Such an attitude will probably lead to poor overall nutrition. Eating vitamin-rich foods is not only the most natural and efficient means of gaining protection against vitamin deficiency, it is also a sure way to gain calories (energy), minerals, protein, fiber, and lesser known vitamins, all of which are just as vital to overall well-being as the elements whose names appear on the label of the vitamin pill bottle. Later chapters will discuss the specific amounts of each vitamin necessary for the maintenance of good health for various age groups and the reasons why additional amounts of certain vitamins are recommended during certain periods of growth and development.

Vitamins are usually divided into two broad groups: fat-soluble (A, D, E, K) and water-soluble (C and B-complex). RDAs for vitamin K and for biotin and pantothenic acid have not yet been set, since knowledge of these vitamins and their role in human nutrition is still relatively limited. The 1980 edition of *Recommended Dietary Allowances* features a separate chart on which ranges of recommended intakes are given. As further research yields more specific data, more exact recommendations will probably be issued. The overview charts which follow give the food sources that supply various vitamins, the role each vitamin plays in bodily functions, and the most common deficiency symptoms.

## Fat-soluble Vitamins—Overview

| Vitamin | Dietary Sources | Bodily Functions | Deficiency Symptoms | Toxicity Levels | Toxicity Symptoms |
|---|---|---|---|---|---|
| A | Liver, cream, butter, whole milk, egg yolk, fortified margarine, green vegetables, yellow fruits and vegetables | Maintenance of membranes; essential to production of visual pigment; promotes growth, reproduction, other metabolic processes | Night blindness, xerophthalmia, skin and mucous membrane infections; faulty bone and tooth development | More than 15,000 retinol equivalents or more than 75,000 IUs daily, over many months | Loss of appetite; growth failure; cracking of skin; hair loss; bone pain; headaches |
| D | Fortified milk and margarine, fish oils; lesser amounts in butter, liver, egg yolk, salmon, sardines | Increases calcium and phosphorus absorption; promotes mineralization and growth of bones | Childhood rickets (enlarged joints, bowed legs, pelvic deformities); adult osteomalacia; infant tetanic convulsions; dental caries | 20,000–50,000 IUs daily may be toxic for children, even over a short period of time; 100,000 IUs for adults (much individual variation) | Nausea, weight loss, weakness |
| E | Vegetable oils (wheat germ, rice germ, cottonseed), nuts, leafy vegetables, dried green split peas, whole grains; lesser amounts in eggs, milk, fish | Antioxidant; protects vitamins A and C and red blood cells | Possibly mild anemia; other deficiency symptoms not noted except in premature infants and people suffering from malabsorption | Some symptoms apparent after 800 IUs per day, some after only 400 IUs per day (much individual variation) | In humans: fatigue, nausea, flulike symptoms; large doses appear to interfere with activities of vitamins A and K |

| Vitamin | Dietary Sources | Bodily Functions | Deficiency Symptoms | Toxicity Levels | Toxicity Symptoms |
|---------|-----------------|------------------|---------------------|-----------------|-------------------|
| K | Green leafy vegetables (alfalfa, spinach, kale), cheese, egg yolk, liver | Aids in blood clotting | Hemorrhagic disease of newborns; prolonged blood clotting time | Excessive doses of one synthetic form (menadione and its derivatives) are potentially toxic; menadione has twice the biological activity of the natural forms of Vitamin $K_1$; the natural vitamin has not been proven toxic | Excessive doses of menadione have produced hemolytic anemia in rats and kernicterus (brain damage due to high bilirubin levels) in low-birth-weight infants (probably due to breakdown of red blood cells) |

## Water-soluble Vitamins—Overview

| Vitamin | Dietary Sources | Bodily Functions | Deficiency Symptoms | Toxicity Level | Toxicity Symptoms |
|---|---|---|---|---|---|
| C (Ascorbic Acid) | Citrus fruits, tomatoes, potatoes, cabbage, green peppers, strawberries, cantaloupes, leafy vegetables (varies with species, ripeness) | Aids in iron absorption; cements body cells together; strengthens gums | Scurvy (swelling or bleeding gums, loosening of teeth), slow wound healing, epithelial hemorrhages; loss of weight; muscular pain; loss of appetite, roughened skin | Wide individual variation | Diarrhea, formation of kidney stones in people prone to this disorder; large amounts during pregnancy may make baby vitamin-C-dependent; may cause abortion at 6 grams/day |
| Folacin | Legumes, green leafy vegetables, whole-wheat products, yeast, whole-grain cereals, lima beans, asparagus, liver, kidney, heart | Amino acid metabolism | Gastrointestinal disturbances; diarrhea; red tongue, sprue, megaloblastic anemia; fetal damage if deficiency occurs during pregnancy | No symptoms with 20 milligrams per day *but* intakes over 1 milligram may mask pernicious anemia ($B_{12}$ deficiency) | None known |
| Niacin (Nicotinic Acid) | Liver, meats, fish, poultry, yeast, dried beans and peas, whole-grain cereals, enriched cereals, peanuts | Aids in utilization of fats and proteins, aids in energy metabolism | Pellagra; dermatitis; neuritis; lesions of mucous membranes; insomnia, apprehensiveness, irritability | 3–9 grams per day | Gastrointestinal problems;elevated blood sugar; elevated blood uric acid (found in gout patients); multiple enzyme changes; liver malfunction |

**Water-Soluble Vitamins—Overview (Continued)**

| Vitamin | Dietary Sources | Bodily Functions | Deficiency Symptoms | Toxicity Levels | Toxicity Symptoms |
|---|---|---|---|---|---|
| Ribo-flavin | Milk, liver, enriched cereals, cheese, eggs, leafy vegetables, lean meat, beans | Energy metabolism | Soreness and burning of tongue; reddened lips; cracks at corners of mouth; eye irritation (itching, burning) | None known | None known |
| Thiamin | Pork, milk, lima beans, dried beans and peas, wheat germ, whole-grain and enriched breads and cereals, leafy green vegetables, nuts, bran, yeast | Aids in carbohydrate utilization | Beriberi; gastrointestinal disorders; loss of eye coordination; loss of sensation in arms; muscle weakness and paralysis; apathy, depression, irritability, moodiness, nausea, lack of appetite | Rare, unless vitamin is injected | None except when vitamin is injected |
| B₆ Pyridoxine) | Wheat, corn, meat, nuts, liver, yeast, fish, dried green split peas, whole-grain cereals, green leafy vegetables, bran, soybeans, tomatoes, white flour, white rice, pork, beef, yellow corn, barley, bananas | Aids in synthesis and utilization of amino acids | Anemia; kidney stones; central nervous system abnormalities (convulsions, irritability, muscular twitching, depression, confusion); dermatitis | 200 milligrams per day for 33 days | Pyridoxine dependency in humans; animals show behavior changes, adverse effects on blood pressure |

## Water-Soluble Vitamins—Overview (Continued)

| Vitamin | Dietary Sources | Bodily Functions | Deficiency Symptoms | Toxicity Levels | Toxicity Symptoms |
|---|---|---|---|---|---|
| B$_{12}$ (Cyano-cobala-min) | Liver, kidney, milk, muscle meats, fish, eggs, cheese, (not present in plant foods) | Constituent of bone marrow; helps form red blood cells; protein synthesis | Pernicious anemia; sprue; sore tongue; neurological disorders (degeneration of spinal cord, prickling, itching or other abnormal sensations) | None known | None known |
| Panto-thenic Acid | Widely distributed in food; best sources are liver, kidney, fresh vegetables, whole-grain cereals, yeast, egg yolk; lesser amount in fruits, vegetables, and milk | Vital to transmission of nerve impulses; important in oxidation of fatty acids; aid in energy release, synthesis of fatty acids and cholesterol | Fatigue; prickling in hands and feet; abdominal distress, nausea, sleep disturbances, headaches, leg cramps, motor impairment, flatulence | None known | None known |
| Biotin | Organ meats, egg yolk, nuts, cauliflower, legumes, mushrooms | Required in synthesis of fatty acids; coenzyme of a number of vital enzymes | Loss of appetite, vomiting, nausea, paleness, depression, dermatitis, muscle pains | None known | None known |

Though deficiency symptoms are listed on the vitamin overview charts, deficiency states are extremely rare for many of these vitamins. If a deficiency is suspected and the diet is deficient in the foods which provide that vitamin, a physician should be consulted. Various laboratory tests can usually confirm or deny vitamin-deficiency states, and these tests should be made before you assume a deficiency and begin treatment with self-prescribed doses of megavitamins. As the charts indicate, many of the vitamins are toxic in excessive amounts, and the toxicity symptoms could be far worse than the suspected deficiency symptoms.

Megavitamins can be helpful in cases in which a person's utilization of certain vitamins is impaired. Taken indiscriminately, megavitamins can be harmful or even fatal. *Since children are particularly susceptible to vitamin overdoses, they should not be given megavitamins except under a physician's supervision.*

## Minerals

Minerals seen in nature seem inert and lifeless, yet within the human body, minerals are active, performing life-sustaining functions as regulators, transmitters, controllers, activators, and builders. The National Research Council's Committee on Dietary Allowances has divided minerals into two groups: those needed in levels of 100 milligrams or more per day, and those needed in amounts no greater than a few milligrams per day.

The overview chart that follows gives dietary sources, bodily functions, deficiency symptoms, toxicity levels, and toxicity symptoms for the six minerals in the first group. Subsequent chapters will indicate the specialized mineral needs of various age groups. Except under unusual circumstances, the RDAs for these minerals can be met through dietary means. Vegetarian children who do not use dairy products may need calcium supplements, and those vegetarians who use natural sea salt and avoid all other seafoods may need iodine supplements. *Supplementation should be undertaken only under a doctor's supervision.*

The chart that follows gives a general overview of the common trace elements. These trace elements and many other micronutrients contribute to the overall health of humans, yet their exact functions remain unknown (except for iron), perhaps because no serious deficiency diseases have occurred to spur scientists into in-depth investigation of the exact roles which are played by the lesser-known trace elements. Unfortunately, dietary trace element imbalances may someday occur if the use of highly processed, highly refined foods continues to increase. Though these foods may be fortified with major vitamins and minerals, they seldom contain trace elements in significant amounts.

Ironically, many consumers feel most confident when buying such products, since government labeling mandates have forced manufacturers to let the public know what percentages of the Recommended Dietary Allowance of protein and seven vitamins and minerals are available in a portion of such

## Minerals—Group I: 100 Milligrams or More Needed Per Day

| Mineral | Dietary Sources | Bodily Functions | Deficiency Symptoms | Toxicity Levels | Toxicity Symptoms |
|---|---|---|---|---|---|
| Calcium | Milk, cheese, and other dairy products; far lesser amounts in dark green vegetables, dried legumes | Tooth and bone formation; blood clotting; nerve transmission; muscle contraction and relaxation; heart action | Rickets; stunted growth; osteoporosis; convulsions; tetany | Overdose of calcium *alone* not seen as toxic; overdoses of vitamin D in infants can cause hypercalcemia symptoms by causing superabsorption of calcium | See special instances in column at left. Vomiting, gastrointestinal bleeding, increase in blood pressure, growth retardation (in infants) |
| Phosphorus | Milk, cheese, meat, egg yolk, whole grains, legumes, nuts, poultry | Bone and tooth formation; acid-base balance; overall metabolism; buffer system; storage and release of energy | Tetany; demineralization of bone; loss of calcium; weakness; loss of appetite; bone pain (prolonged excessive use of antacids may cause deficiency symptoms) | High phosphorus intakes in cow's milk can cause toxicity symptoms in infants under one week of age | Hypocalcemic tetany seen in infants under one week of age |
| Magnesium | Whole grains, nuts, milk (dairy products), meat, legumes, green leafy vegetables (some diuretics deplete magnesium; chronic alcoholism and cirrhosis of liver may lead to magnesium deficiency) | Constituent of bones and teeth; coenzyme in carbohydrate and protein metabolism | Growth failure; behavioral disturbances; weakness, spasms; muscle tremor; convulsive seizures | 3–5 grams magnesium salts may act as a laxative, but this amount is not *toxic*; toxicity rare unless renal (kidney) function impaired; usually caused by unusual increase in absorption or marked reduction in urinary excretion | Large amounts may be cathartic (see column at left); hypermagnesemia (extreme thirst, excessive warmth, drowsiness, decrease in muscle and nerve irritability) |

| Mineral | Dietary Sources | Bodily Functions | Deficiency Symptoms | Toxicity Levels | Toxicity Symptoms |
|---|---|---|---|---|---|
| Sodium | Table salt; milk, meat, egg white, carrots, leafy vegetables, artichokes, asparagus, celery, beets, spinach, chard; preservatives such as sodium benzoate; artificial sweeteners such as sodium saccharin; acidifiers such as sodium citrate | Principal positive ion of extracellular fluid; helps maintain body's fluid and acid-base balance; controls cellular excitability, nerve-impulse conduction | Growth retardation (in animals); fluid, acid-base imbalance | None known, but excessive salt intake without sufficient water intake can be dangerous; people on low-salt diets should be aware that many commonly used preservatives are sodium-based; salt tablets should be kept out of the reach of children | Hypertension incidence in rats increases with high sodium intakes; studies indicate similar effects in susceptible humans |
| Chloride | Table salt, salt used in food processing and preparation | Principal negative ion of extracellular fluid; helps maintain fluid and electrolyte balance; vital to formation of human digestive fluids | Occur after great chloride loss (i.e., prolonged vomiting); hypochloremic alkalosis; normocalcemic tetany; digestive disturbances, fluid-electrolyte imbalance | None | None |
| Potassium | Leafy vegetables, legumes; whole grains; meats, poultry, fish; potatoes, tomatoes, carrots celery; bananas, oranges, grapefruit, and other fruits | Principal positive ion of intracellular fluid; vital to maintenance of acid-base and fluid-electrolyte balance, muscle activity, carbohydrate activity, protein syn- | Nausea, vomiting, listlessness, apprehension, muscle weakness, low blood pressure, plus tachycardia and other heart irregularities | Hyperpotassemia results in kidney failure, severe dehydration (for one infant, 3 grams of potassium chloride was a fatal dose) | Muscle weakness; breathing difficulties; heart rhythm changes; heart failure |

foods as pudding mixes and breakfast tarts. A shopper is usually favorably impressed with the information that a certain cereal features high percentages of those eight nutrients. Ironically, a natural, whole-grain product, though it is not fortified with the extra vitamins and minerals of the enriched product, may well contribute more to overall good health because it contains several micronutrients which have been refined out of most heavily fortified cereals.

The weight-conscious teen who starts her day with a highly refined, vitamin- and mineral-enriched cereal, eats a powdered, high-vitamin, low-calorie packet stirred into eight ounces of milk for lunch, then eats a processed frozen dinner in the evening will have consumed products with abundant supplies of the much-advertised nutrients appearing on package labels. Yet her diet may have been virtually devoid of the important trace elements which have been refined out of these and many other products that make up the standard American diet.

Iron, iodine, and zinc have been recognized as essential elements in the human diet for many years. Numerous research projects and population studies have yielded sufficient information to allow RDAs to be set for these vital minerals. Research efforts for other trace elements which are probably equally vital to optimum growth and development are relatively few in number. Because knowledge of these trace elements has not been exact enough to warrant the setting of recommended dietary allowances for them, RDAs are not yet available.

The 1980 RDA guidebook has a separate chart on which these trace elements appear. As that chart notes, because "there is less information on which to base allowances, these figures are not given in the main table of the RDA and are provided here in the form of ranges of recommended intakes." Furthermore, the chart warns consumers that since "the toxic levels for many trace elements may be only several times usual intakes, the upper levels for the trace elements given in the table should not be habitually exceeded."

## Turning Nutrients into Meals

The general overviews in this chapter should provide background information helpful to parents who wish to make available to their children the nutrients listed in the Recommended Dietary Allowances for various age groups. Translating the RDAs into meals and snacks could become a task which even a chemist would find frustrating, but careful attention to the Minimum Exchanges Chart on page 9 should make meeting the RDAs simple enough. By following the guidelines given early in the chapter and using the food lists in Appendix A, parents should be able to plan meals and snacks which include adequate vitamins, minerals, and protein.

Some of the nutrients available in the foods given on the exchange lists may be lost during cooking. Heating foods results in a loss of some nutrients, and the higher and longer the heating, the greater the nutrient

## Minerals—Group II: Trace Elements

| Mineral | Dietary Sources | Bodily Functions | Deficiency Symptoms | Toxicity Levels | Toxicity Symptoms |
|---|---|---|---|---|---|
| Iron | Liver, lean meats, oysters, turkey, whole grains, dark green vegetables, legumes, nuts, enriched bread and cereal, shellfish, molasses, dried fruits (apricots, dates, prunes, raisins, figs) | Hemoglobin formation; cellular oxidation | Anemia, weakness, fatigue, irritability, anxiety, depression, and restlessness | Prolonged iron therapy when *not* needed may produce toxicity; 5–10 grams equals toxic dose for two-year-old child | Iron deposited in liver cells (as in cirrhosis), lungs, pancreas, heart; may be fatal; iron poisonings now outnumber aspirin poisonings in children |
| Iodine | Saltwater fish; shellfish; seaweed; dairy products and eggs (when animals are fed iodine-rich rations); iodized salt and bread with iodates as dough conditioners | Synthesis of thyroid hormone, which regulates cell oxidation; influences physical and mental growth; functioning of nervous and muscle tissue, circulatory activity, metabolism of all nutrients | Endemic colloid goiter, endemic cretinism | Amounts greater than ten times the RDA can lead to thyrotoxicosis (enlarged and hyperactive thyroid) in individuals with defective thyroid | |

| | Sources | Functions | Deficiency | Excess | Symptoms of Excess |
|---|---|---|---|---|---|
| Zinc | Liver, seafood, lean meats; lesser amounts in fruits, green leafy vegetables, whole-wheat and rye breads, corn | Essential enzyme constituent; involved in most metabolic processes; important in protein synthesis; helps mobilize vitamin A | Growth failure; small sex glands; loss of sense of taste and smell; loss of appetite; slow wound healing | Twenty to sixty times RDA (excessive intakes may occur when acid foods or drinks are prepared and stored in galvanized containers) | Vomiting, cramps, diarrhea in 3 to 12 hours |
| Fluoride | Seafood; some natural water supplies; fluoridated water supplies | Important in tooth and bone development; important for resistance to tooth decay | Osteoporosis; Paget's disease; dental caries (cavities) | More than 1.5 parts per million in drinking water leads to dental fluorosis; about 20–80 milligrams for several years leads to bone fluorosis | Chronic dental fluorosis (mottled teeth, dull, unglazed, some pitting, dark brown stains); bone fluorosis (symptoms resemble arthritis) |
| Copper | Liver, kidney, shellfish, nuts, dried legumes, raisins, whole-grain cereals | Taste sensitivity; electron transport; bone development; hemoglobin formation; important part of several enzymes | Anemia, skeletal defects, degeneration of nervous system, reproductive failure | Toxic, usually in Wilson's Disease (copper deposits are left in brain, liver) | See column at left. Hepatitis, kidney failure, neurological disorders |
| Cobalt | Milk, muscle meat, organ meats | Integral part of vitamin $B_{12}$ | See $B_{12}$ vitamin deficiency, p. 23 | See $B_{12}$ vitamin, p. 23 | See $B_{12}$ vitamin, p. 23 |

| Mineral | Dietary Sources | Bodily Functions | Deficiency Symptoms | Toxicity Levels | Toxicity Symptoms |
|---|---|---|---|---|---|
| Manga-nese | Nuts, whole grains, some legumes, fruits | Activates important enzymes; important in bone structure, reproduction; normal functioning of central nervous system; constituent of bile; normal lipid metabolism; normal reproduction | Overt manganese deficiency not known in humans | None known | None known |
| Molyb-denum | Beef kidney, some whole-grain cereals, some legumes | Cofactor for several enzymes | Deficiencies produced in animals but unknown in humans | See column at right | Excess results in symptoms of copper deficiency; cattle on high-molybdenum grass get diarrhea, brittle bones, color loss, weight loss |
| Selen-ium | Depends upon soil content of region | Antioxidant; is constituent of important enzymes; enables more efficient use of vitamin E | Possible link to protein-calorie malnutrition; deficiency symptoms in humans unknown. In animals faulty development of vascular system, cataracts, degeneration of pancreas | Excessive amounts toxic in animals and humans | Animals in high-selenium areas get "blind staggers" (stiffness, deformity, blindness, hoof deformity, hair loss, possible death); Oregon schoolchildren in high-selenium area showed increase in dental caries |

| Chromium | All animal protein except fish; whole grains; Brewer's yeast | Vital to normal glucose metabolism | Disturbances in glucose metabolism (even in marginal deficiency states) more likely in old age, pregnancy, and protein-calorie malnutrition | None known | None known |
|---|---|---|---|---|---|
| Nickel, Tin, Vanadium Silicon | Found in many common foods | | Deficiencies of these elements have been produced in laboratory animals, suggesting that they may be essential in the human diet as well. No indications are currently given as to the amounts necessary, but a well-balanced diet should supply adequate amounts. | These may be toxic and should never be taken as supplements | |

loss. Shorter cooking times at lower heat will mean less loss of nutrients. Cooking foods and later reheating them quickly is preferable to keeping them warm over long periods of time.

Some nutrients will dissolve in the water in which they are cooked. In general, one should cook meats or vegetables in as little as water as possible and serve the cooking water with the foods or use it in gravy or soup. If strong-flavored vegetables are cooked in more water, their flavor is somewhat diluted so that the vegetables may be more acceptable to some family members. Though some nutrients will be lost by using extra water, at least the strong-tasting vegetables will be eaten, not avoided.

Contact with oxygen can contribute to nutrient loss. Cooking foods at a hard boil leads to more interaction with oxygen than does cooking at a simmer. Since the temperature is the same whether foods are simmering or are at a rolling boil, no time is saved by rapid boiling, but nutrients could be lost. Cooking food in a tightly covered pot can also help preserve vitamins. Pressure-cooking can be an excellent means of nutrient preservation, as long as minimum cooking times are observed. Careful attention to these cooking suggestions should mean that foods arrive at the table with minimum nutrient loss.

With additional servings of foods from the Minimum Exchanges chart of simple and complex carbohydrates, family members can gain the recommended number of calories as well as protein, vitamins, and minerals. Since a healthy appetite usually serves as a satisfactory calorie counter, there's seldom any reason to turn calorie consumption into a major issue. Enjoyment of a wide variety of foods served in a congenial atmosphere should be the major goal of parents who wish to provide optimum nutrition for their children. The following chapters provide guidelines for the achievement of this basic goal.

# 3
# Infancy—Birth to Three Months

A baby's first three months are among the most critical ones in his entire life. During these early months, his physical growth rate and brain development will be more rapid than ever again. Nutritional inadequacy during this crucial time may mean that physical growth will be retarded or that mental development will be temporarily or permanently slowed. On the other hand, adequate nutrition during this period means a child is not only given every chance for optimum physical and mental development during babyhood, but is also aided in the early formation of sound eating habits, which should enhance his health throughout his life.

There is wide divergence in infant feeding practices, a fact which has led some parents to assume that any method of feeding is satisfactory, as long as a baby grows and doesn't develop serious medical problems. This attitude may be a bit simplistic, for, as Dr. Samuel Fomon, a leading authority on infant feeding practices, noted recently:

*If we detect no differences in health as a result of such divergent feeding practices, it does not necessarily mean that the choice of feeding practice is inconsequential. Rather, the consequences may be too subtle to be detected by casual observation or may be of long-term rather than short-term nature. Little is known about the long-term consequences of infant feeding practices.*

With this quotation in mind, every parent should take seriously the responsibility of meeting an infant's nutritional needs as completely as possible.

Just when an infant is in the greatest need of optimum nutrition, he is unable to digest and fully utilize the wide range of foods which will later give his diet the variety it needs. Instead, the newborn is dependent upon milk, either that of his mother or that prepared from cow's milk or soy milk. If adequate liquid nourishment is not given at this age, evidence of malnutrition will eventually appear, though it may be so slight as to be ignored or attributed to other causes.

## Meeting Nutrient Needs of the Newborn

When setting Recommended Dietary Allowances (RDAs) for infants, scientists have looked to the only substance known to be perfect for the needs of the average newborn—the breast milk of a well-nourished mother with established lactation and an unimpaired let-down reflex.* Despite fairly wide hourly, daily, weekly, and monthly fluctuations in milk protein, fat, and volume, deficiency symptoms are relatively rare in an infant receiving this food for the first four to six months of life.

These daily, weekly, and monthly fluctuations in the nutrient content of breast milk are ideally suited to meet a baby's needs. For example, the gradual increase in fat content during establishment of lactation parallels the maturation of the digestive system of a newborn. Yet such fluctuations make it difficult for researchers to decide just *which* breast milk samples should be used as the standard against which artificially produced formulas will be measured. Currently, RDAs for young infants are based on somewhat out-of-date and incomplete breast-milk analyses. As more precise analysis methods are developed, scientists may alter these RDAs slightly to reflect new findings.

The nutrient content of breast milk serves as the standard RDA for most nutrients, but amounts slightly above the breast-milk level of some nutrients are added to allow for the fact that these nutrients may not be as well utilized when they are provided in manufactured formulas as when they appear in breast milk. For example, bioavailability of zinc is much greater in breast milk than in cow's milk formulas. Ironically, this safety factor has been used by formula manufacturers attempting to prove that formula milk is superior to breast milk. Persuasive sales experts have told doctors and parents, "See, breast milk falls below RDA standards, while our formula exceeds them!" This seems a strong point in favor of formula-feeding, until one remembers that the Recommended Dietary Allowances are deliberately set higher than breast-milk levels as a safety feature.

Though human milk is the ideal food—for reasons which will be discussed later—a bottle-feeding mother who reads the following discussion of Recommended Dietary Allowances for infants should not feel that she has already done grave damage to her child by denying her nature's perfect food. Instead, a bottle-feeding mother should relax and read the RDA in-

---

*The *let-down reflex* is a psychosomatic reflex by which milk is moved from the alveoli to the milk sinuses. The baby's suckling signals the posterior pituitary to release the hormone oxytocin. This hormone causes compression of the milk-producing alveolus and widening of the milk ducts to allow milk to be pushed into the main milk sinuses under the nipple. At the moment let-down occurs milk may even spray from the nipple. The let-down reflex is crucial to successful nursing, since without let-down only the "fore milk" is released and baby is denied the fat-rich "hind milk." Let-down is enhanced by confidence and impaired by anxiety.

formation given here with the firm knowledge that formula-feeding *can* and *does* produce healthy infants. Breast-feeding is no guarantee of an infant's good health, just as bottle-feeding is no guarantee of poor health. By understanding the nutrient needs of an infant, both bottle-feeding and breast-feeding mothers can strive to meet those needs more fully.

## Water

One question asked by almost all new mothers is "How much water does my baby need?" Composed of 10 percent more water by weight than the body of an adult, a baby's body has relatively more surface area from which water may be lost. Thus he must normally replace water amounting to 10 to 15 percent of his body weight per day, while an adult needs only enough daily water intake to replace 2 to 4 percent of his body weight.

An infant's primary source of water should also be his main source of food—human milk or an acceptable, properly concentrated formula substitute. As one pediatrician put it, "Every ounce of water your baby drinks means she will have that much less room to take the breast milk which offers so much more than plain water can." Except in unusual cases, breast milk or formula contains sufficient water to meet a baby's daily needs. Of course, in later months, as milk volume drops and solid-food volume increases, an older infant may want and need additional sips of water.

One recent study of breast-fed infants in Jamaica indicates that breast-fed infants need no additional water for about the first four months of life, even in hot climates. In areas where climate is both extremely hot and extremely *dry*, extra water might be desirable. Giving small amounts of water is certainly acceptable, provided the water is suitable for drinking and the container and feeding bottle are sanitized.

Water from shallow farm wells near barnyards should be analyzed for nitrite content before being given to infants younger than six months of age. High nitrite concentrations can cause methemoglobinemia, an often fatal disease which deprives infants of vital oxygen by robbing them of the oxygen normally carried in the bloodstream. County health departments are usually able to help citizens get their drinking water analyzed.

## Calories

Setting calorie levels according to the amount of milk taken daily by a breast-fed infant poses difficult tasks for researchers, since there is no way to measure the natural flow of milk during breast-feedings. In 1958, researchers Fomon and May attempted to establish the amount taken by feeding babies on demand with measured, pasteurized breast milk. Though this study has long been cited as definitive, the researchers did not take into account the easier flow of milk from a bottle and could not simulate the appetite-controlling effect of the varying fat content of milk during actual breast-feeding. Lowe's 1972 estimate of the ideal volumes of milk for babies is much lower and may be more accurate.

## Recommended Dietary Allowances—Infants

| Age | 0–6 months | 6–12 months |
|---|---|---|
| Energy (cal) | weight in kg x 115 | weight in kg x 105 |
| Protein (g) | weight in kg x 2.2 | weight in kg x 2.0 |
| **Fat-soluble vitamins** | | |
| Vitamin A[a] ($\mu$g* R.E.) | 420 | 400 |
| Vitamin D[b] ($\mu$g) | 10 | 10 |
| Vitamin E[c] (mg $\alpha$T.E.) | 3 | 4 |
| **Water-soluble vitamins** | | |
| Ascorbic acid (C) (mg) | 35.0 | 35.0 |
| Folacin ($\mu$g) | 30.0 | 45.0 |
| Niacin[d] (mg N.E.) | 6.0 | 8.0 |
| Riboflavin (mg) | 0.4 | 0.6 |
| Thiamin (mg) | 0.3 | 0.5 |
| Vitamin B$_6$ (mg) | 0.3 | 0.6 |
| Vitamin B$_{12}$ ($\mu$g) | 0.5 | 1.5 |
| **Minerals** | | |
| Calcium (mg) | 360 | 540 |
| Phosphorus (mg) | 240 | 360 |
| Iodine ($\mu$g) | 40 | 50 |
| Iron (mg) | 10 | 15 |
| Magnesium (mg) | 50 | 70 |
| Zinc (mg) | 3 | 5 |

SOURCE: Adapted from *Recommended Dietary Allowances,* Ninth Edition (1980; in press), with the permission of the National Academy of Sciences, Washington, D.C.

*$\mu$g is the standard abbreviation for microgram, or 1/1000 milligram.

[a]Recommendations for vitamin A are expressed in $\mu$g of R.E. (micrograms of retinol equivalent). One retinol equivalent is equal to 1 $\mu$g of retinol or 6 $\mu$g of carotene.

[b]Vitamin D is expressed as $\mu$g of cholecalciferol, with 10$\mu$g cholecalciferol being equal to 400 IUs of Vitamin D.

[c]Vitamin E is expressed as mg $\alpha$T.E. (milligrams of alpha tocopherol equivalents).

[d]Niacin is expressed as mg N.E. (milligrams of niacin equivalent), with 1 N.E. equalling 1 mg of niacin or 60 mg of dietary tryptophan.

The current (1980) Recommended Dietary Allowance for energy is 115 calories per day for each kilogram of weight from birth to six months. More recent recommendations suggest a range of 80 to 120 calories per kilogram per day during the first year of life, except for premature or ill infants. Using such a range allows more flexibility and enables doctors to take into account differences in activity and growth rate of babies. Ignoring these differences can lead to overfeeding and infant obesity.

With so many factors to be considered, setting a baby's calorie-intake level is obviously a complex task. Fortunately, RDA levels are only intended to serve as *guidelines,* and an infant's own appetite can be trusted to help a parent make the best use of those guidelines. If a mother breast-feeds, chances are good that her baby's developing appetite-control mechanism will do all the work, so that mother need only allow the child to nurse until satisfied. This method works even when there seems to be an insufficient supply of milk, since the constant suckling of a hungry baby will automatically increase a mother's milk supply in twenty-four to forty-eight hours. Having adjusted to this new level, mother and child are again ready to enjoy the benefits of nature's automatic calorie-counting system. Of course, the mother who panics and starts supplementing her baby's diet with formula because she fears he is starving when he demands more frequent nursing removes nature's means of increasing a temporarily inadequate milk supply.

For a bottle-feeding mother, the rule of thumb is to fill the bottle with the recommended amount of formula, then allow the baby to nurse until she is satisfied. Forcing down the last ounce may mean teaching baby to demand more than she actually needs. After all, a hungry infant knows more about how full she feels and how much food she needs than do all the researchers and pediatricians in the world!

The best way to judge whether an infant is eating enough is to have his height and weight checked regularly and compared to a pediatrician's average growth-rate graph. A child whose growth rate approximates the norms on such a chart is probably eating about what he should be eating. Since home measurement of very young infants is often difficult, many parents may prefer to leave such matters to their pediatrician or family physician. The following graph may be useful to those parents who wish to keep their own records of growth. Interpreting the meaning of any serious deviations from the norm is the physician's specialty, but noting those deviations can be a parent's responsibility.

The graphs reproduced in this book feature lines which represent seven different percentiles—from 5th to 95th. If a newborn boy's weight falls into the 50th percentile, this means that 50 of every 100 baby boys weigh less at birth and that 50 of every 100 weigh more. Thus a child in the 50th percentile is at the statistical midpoint when his weight is measured against that of others of his age and sex.

Obviously, a wide range of heights and weights should be considered normal. Since these graphs are for the "average" American child, they may not give an accurate picture of the development of children from certain ethnic groups or from certain areas of the country. For various reasons, some communities seem to have larger or smaller children than the national average. For example, there is some evidence that larger babies are born to women who live in the high-altitude sections of the country. Thus a 7½-pound boy might seem big in Kansas but might be the smallest baby in the nursery in Bozeman, Montana.

If a baby's height (length) and weight fall anywhere between the top and bottom lines of the graph (95th and 5th percentile lines), chances are excellent that that infant's growth is satisfactory. If either height or weight falls outside the given norms, a physician's evaluation of the baby's growth is advisable. In most cases, consistent deviation from the given norms merely means a child is unusually large or unusually small for his or her age. For

## Growth Charts for Infants—Birth to Thirty-Six Months*

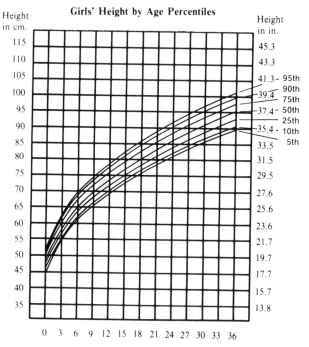

Girls' Height by Age Percentiles

Height in cm.

Height in in.

AGE IN MONTHS

SOURCE: Adapted from Hamill, P. V. V., T. A. Drizd, C. L. Johnson, R. B. Reed, A. F. Roche, *NCHS Growth Curves for Children, Birth—18 years.* National Center for Health Statistics Publications, Series 11, Number 165, November 1977.

*In general, weights and heights that fall within the 5th and 95th percentiles are considered normal. Ideally, height and weight should be within a few percentile points of each other. See pp. 37-41.

example, Don, a full-term baby, was 18 inches (45.7 centimeters) long at birth and weighed 6 pounds, 14 ounces (3.1 kilograms). To his parents, he seemed a big baby—his older sister had weighed only 6 pounds at birth. To the neighbors, he seemed rather tiny—their new daughter, Anne, was 22 ½ inches (57.1 centimers) and 9 pounds, 7 ½ ounces (4.3 kilograms) at birth.

To the pediatrician who cared for both babies, Don and Anne were normal, healthy, well-proportioned infants. Don was in the 5th percentile in height and the 15th in weight, while Anne was above the 95th percentile in both height and weight. In both cases, height and weight percentiles were close enough together that the children were considered neither obese nor underweight.

Even when height and weight both fall within the given norms, there may

# Growth Charts for Infants—Birth to Thirty-Six Months*

## Girls' Weight by Age Percentiles

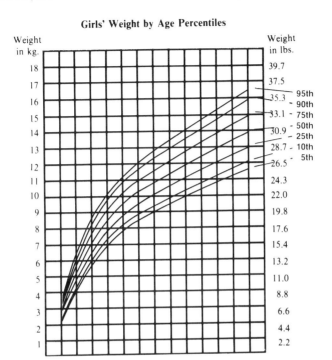

SOURCE: Adapted from Hamill, P. V. V., T. A. Drizd, C. L. Johnson, R. B. Reed, A. F. Roche, *NCHS Growth Curves for Children, Birth—18 years.* National Center for Health Statistics Publications, Series 11, Number 165, November 1977.

*In general, weights and heights that fall within the 5th and 95th percentiles are considered normal. Ideally, height and weight should be within a few percentile points of each other. See pp. 37-41.

still be cause for concern. For example, if a baby's height and weight have consistently been in the 95th percentile and one or both drops sharply and continuously, health problems may be suspected. Furthermore, if a baby's weight is in the 95th percentile, while his height is in the 5th percentile, he is likely to be overweight. Conversely, a baby who is tall for her age (95th percentile) but relatively light in weight (5th percentile), may be underweight enough to need a doctor's care. Thus both height and weight percentiles must be taken into consideration when a parent or physician attempts to evaluate an infant's growth. Any sudden or extreme change in either figure should alert parents to the presence of medical or nutritional problems.

Parents who consult height-weight charts should remind themselves that, contrary to our general twentieth-century American way of thinking, big-

## Growth Charts for Infants—Birth to Thirty-Six Months*

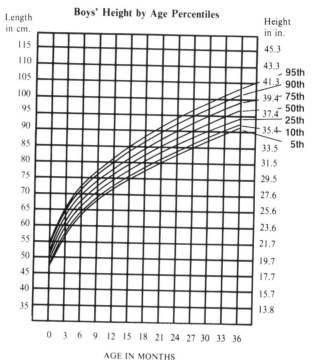

**Boys' Height by Age Percentiles**

Length in cm.

115
110
105
100
95
90
85
80
75
70
65
60
55
50
45
40
35

Height in in.

45.3
43.3
41.3    95th
        90th
39.4    75th
37.4    50th
        25th
35.4    10th
33.5    5th
31.5
29.5
27.6
25.6
23.6
21.7
19.7
17.7
15.7
13.8

0  3  6  9  12  15  18  21  24  27  30  33  36

AGE IN MONTHS

SOURCE: Adapted from Hamill, P. V. V., T. A. Drizd, C. L. Johnson, R. B. Reed, A. F. Roche, *NCHS Growth Curves for Children, Birth—18 years.* National Center for Health Statistics Publications, Series 11, Number 165, November 1977.

*In general, weights and heights that fall within the 5th and 95th percentiles are considered normal. Ideally, height and weight should be within a few percentile points of each other. See pp. 37-41.

gest does not always mean best. Some parents find it hard to accept a son like Don, a boy who falls into the lower percentile rankings while the girl next door is above the 95th percentile. Conversely, some parents find it a real shock to realize that their baby girl is the hospital's record-setter for the year.

Overfeeding a Don to try to change a potential scatback into a tackle will likely damage the boy's self-image and build in a tendency toward overeating and obesity. Starving an Anne to try to make her "petite" can

# Growth Charts for Infants—Birth to Thirty-Six Months*

### Boys' Weight by Age Percentiles

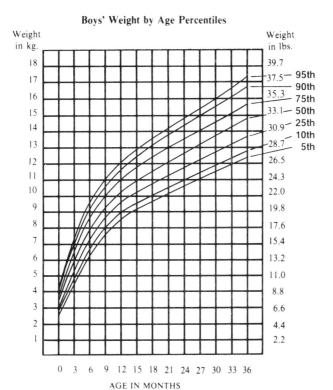

SOURCE: Adapted from Hamill, P. V. V., T. A. Drizd, C. L. Johnson, R. B. Reed, A. F. Roche, *NCHS Growth Curves for Children, Birth—18 years.* National Center for Health Statistics Publications, Series 11, Number 165, November 1977.

*In general, weights and heights that fall within the 5th and 95th percentiles are considered normal. Ideally, height and weight should be within a few percentile points of each other. See pp. 37-41.

only result in clouding her disposition and endangering her health. Whether a baby hovers near the bottom of height-weight charts or soars off the top is determined, in large part, by genetic factors beyond parental control. Once health problems and nutrition imbalances have been ruled out as causes of any unusual growth pattern, an infant's status on height-weight charts should be accepted without further ado. Such an attitude is part of that perfect gift from parent to child—love and acceptance with no strings attached.

## Fat, Carbohydrates, Protein

The calories obtained from cow's milk and human milk are about equal, but the distribution of protein, carbohydrate, and fat calories in the two milks is quite different. The following chart gives the distribution considered ideal by Dr. Samuel Fomon, a noted authority on infant nutrition, plus the distributions found in human milk; milk-based and soy-based formulas; and whole, 2-percent, and skim (less than 1-percent) cow's milk. On the basis of recent research findings, unaltered cow's milk is not currently being recommended for infants under one year of age, and skim milk or skim-milk formulas are not recommended for infants under two years of age. If your pediatrician recommends earlier use of whole or skim milk, question her carefully and refer her to pertinent, up-to-date references before making a final decision.

### Calorie Distributions in Infant Milk

|  | Total Solids (%) | Calories per 100 gm | Percentage of Calories from | | |
|---|---|---|---|---|---|
|  |  |  | Protein | Fat | Carbo-hydrate |
| Human milk | 13% | 75 gm | 6% | 56% | 38% |
| Formulas |  |  |  |  |  |
|   Milk-based | 13 | 67 | 9 | 48 | 43 |
|   Soy-based | 13 | 67 | 16 | 47 | 40 |
| Cow's milk (whole) | 13 | 65 | 22 | 48 | 30 |
|   2% | 13 | 59 | 28 | 31 | 41 |
|   Skim | 10 | 36 | 40 | 3 | 57 |
| Dr. Samuel Fomon's Recommended Calorie Distributions* |  |  | 7–16 | 30–55 | 35–65 |

SOURCE: Adapted from Thomas A. Anderson, "Commercial Infant Foods: Content and Composition," *Pediatric Clinics of North America* 24 (February 1977): 37–47.

*S. J. Fomon, *Infant Nutrition* (Philadelphia: W. B. Saunders, 1974).

Even those formulas which most closely approximate the caloric distribution of breast milk are not nutritionally equivalent to nature's model. For example, fat provides about 50 percent of the calories in breast milk and is the major source of energy for a breast-fed baby. The fat content of cow's milk and human milk is fairly close. However, a newborn may absorb less than 70 percent of the fat in cow's milk, while the average newborn can absorb from 85 to 90 percent of that in human milk. One reason may be that human milk is high in lipase, an enzyme that enhances the availability of essential fatty acids. Furthermore, one fatty acid in human milk (arachidonic) may be better for optimum brain development than the fatty acid (linoleic) found in formula milks.

Human milk contains more cholesterol than does cow's milk. Despite the negative connotations usually associated with cholesterol, this substance is vital to the synthesis of bile acids and of male and female sex hormones. Researchers have theorized that very young infants may need a moderate amount of dietary cholesterol in order to establish mechanisms for the proper metabolism of cholesterol in later life. If this theory is correct, low-cholesterol infant formulas, once thought desirable, may actually be contributing to heart and circulatory problems in later life.

The dominant carbohydrate in human milk is lactose, but other carbohydrates are also important, especially since some of them probably play a vital, though still poorly understood, role in the natural immunities conveyed through breast milk.

Though the protein content of formulas is usually greater than that of human milk, the protein of human milk is easier to digest and thus more efficiently utilized. Human milk is fairly low in relatively hard-to-digest casein, yet high in lactalbumin, long considered the optimum protein for infant growth. The decreased amount of casein in breast milk means that smaller, softer, more easily digested curds form in the infant's stomach. Furthermore, differences in the types and amounts of amino acids of the two foods are quite marked.

## Vitamins and Minerals

In general, fortified commercial formulas meet or exceed Recommended Dietary Allowances for all fat-soluble and water-soluble vitamins and all minerals. Whole or skim cow's milk, soy milk, and cow's-milk and soy-milk formulas which have not been fortified do not usually meet all RDAs. Breast milk meets RDAs, though sometimes (as in the case of vitamin D) the vitamins and minerals may be in a different form or (as in the case of iron) may meet RDAs only because breast milk enhances their absorption.

The following technical overview of the vitamin and mineral content of various milks may be skimmed now and returned to only if the reader wishes to go more deeply into the subject. Certainly, if you wish to know which milks are nutritionally superior and why, this section bears careful reading.

Though many doctors still routinely prescribe *vitamin A* for breast-fed infants, human milk usually provides sufficient quantities of this vitamin, provided the nursing mother's diet is adequate. Generally, since there have been far more cases of vitamin A intoxication in children taking supplements than there have been cases of vitamin A deficiency in children who have good diets and take no supplement, routine prescription of this vitamin seems open to question.

*Vitamin E* stores are very low in premature and low-birth-weight infants, and such babies are susceptible to deficiency symptoms if they are given formulas high in polyunsaturated fatty acids and low in vitamin E. Breast-fed infants receive adequate amounts of vitamin E, and researchers have noted that low at-birth levels of vitamin E rise to normal more rapidly when infants are breast-fed than when they are formula-fed.

*Vitamin K,* synthesized by the intestine after the first week of life, is vital to effective blood clotting in newborns. Since internal hemorrhaging occasionally occurs in newborns during the unprotected first week of life, many pediatricians prefer to increase an infant's clotting ability by routinely administering vitamin K soon after birth. In the absence of vitamin K injections, incidence of bleeding episodes is twice as high in breast-fed infants as in those fed fortified cow's-milk formula. Since breast milk contains less vitamin K than does cow's milk, and since breast-fed babies get little milk during the first two to three days of life, some of these babies may have special need for a doctor-administered supplement. No attempt should be made to give vitamin K at home or without a doctor's supervision, since excessive doses can be toxic to young babies.

Fat-soluble *vitamin D* levels in human milk are known to be relatively low, a fact which has led many pediatricians to the routine prescription of vitamin D supplements for breast-fed infants. Since vitamin D is essential for satisfactory growth and normal bone mineralization, few have been willing to argue with this precautionary dosage, despite the fact that many, many unsupplemented breast-fed infants have shown no signs of vitamin D deficiency. Recent studies have identified a water-soluble form of vitamin D that is as abundant in breast milk as the fat-soluble vitamin D is in fortified formulas; and this discovery has led some doctors to cease routine prescriptions of vitamin D for breast-fed babies. Despite this new finding, many other physicians still feel vitamin D supplements are good insurance and should be given unless there is adequate exposure to sunlight.

Often, vitamin D for breast-fed babies is prescribed in the form of vitamin A and D supplements, presumably because a mother on a vitamin A-deficient diet could produce milk low in this important vitamin. Both A and D are toxic to infants and young children in amounts no greater than those in the most popular dropper-dispensed vitamin bottles. Therefore, such preparations must be stored out of reach of baby and of helpful older children who might decide to give baby as many of the flavorful drops as he will take. In 1976, vitamin and mineral preparations were the third leading cause of childhood poisoning.

*Vitamin C* deficiency in infants has been extremely rare, yet occasional cases of scurvy have been diagnosed in babies fed on unfortified cow's milk which has been boiled, thereby destroying the already-low levels of ascorbic acid found in this milk. Vitamin C levels in breast milk and fortified formulas are normally adequate to meet an infant's needs.

Recently, sporadic cases of scurvy have been seen in infants who were apparently born with a need for abnormally high levels of vitamin C. Such infants, usually born to mothers who have taken megadoses of this vitamin during pregnancy, experience severe hemorrhages and must be gradually weaned from vitamin-C dependency.

Babies fed fortified soy- or cow's-milk-based formulas receive adequate amounts of *thiamin, riboflavin,* and *niacin.* Usually all three of these vitamins are also adequately supplied in human milk, though infantile beriberi has been noted in breast-fed infants when maternal diets were low in thiamin.

*Folic acid* deficiency leading to megaloblastic or macrocytic anemia has been observed in breast-fed babies whose mothers are deficient in this vitamin and in babies receiving unfortified goat's milk or goat's-milk formulas. Since goat's milk is very low in folic acid, supplements should be given to all infants and children who use this milk.

The recommended amount of vitamin $B_6$ *(pyridoxine)* is related to the amount of protein in the diet. Due to the relatively low protein content of breast milk, pyridoxine levels in human milk are sufficient. Vitamin-fortified cow's-milk formulas also provide adequate amounts of $B_6$. Vitamin $B_{12}$ (cyanocobalamin) is often lacking in strict vegetarian (vegan) diets, and breast-feeding vegetarian mothers who do not drink milk, use eggs, or take $B_{12}$ supplements risk passing this serious deficiency on to their infants.

In one case, a six-month-old infant was admitted to a California hospital in a coma. The baby was suffering central nervous system and circulatory system distress due to vitamin $B_{12}$ deficiency. For eight years prior to pregnancy and for the nine months of pregnancy, the baby's mother, a strict vegetarian, had conscientiously excluded all foods containing $B_{12}$ from her diet. While her own $B_{12}$ levels were at the lower end of the normal range, her baby was not so fortunate. After the baby had been treated with $B_{12}$ supplements and had shown improvement, he was discharged to be breast-fed by the mother. Within two months, the child's serum $B_{12}$ had dropped dramatically, and a nine-month checkup showed the baby's development was about that of the average five-month-old. At this point, the mother began taking $B_{12}$ supplements, but the extent of the damage already done to the child may not be known for several years. Fortunately, nonvegetarians, lacto-ovo vegetarians (vegetarians who drink milk and eat eggs), or vegans (vegetarians who avoid all animal products) who use $B_{12}$ supplements can avoid risking deficiency.

The mineral content of human milk differs significantly from that of cow's milk. The higher *calcium*-to-*phosphorus* ratio of breast milk encourages more total absorption of calcium. Convulsions during the first two weeks of life have been traced to low calcium and elevated phosphorus levels in the blood of babies fed a cow's-milk formula. The much higher phosphorus content of cow's milk has been linked to several infant health problems, including defective enamel formation of the teeth.

If a mother uses an *iron* supplement during pregnancy, the iron stores of a full-term, full-weight newborn should be sufficient for the first three to six months of life. On the other hand, if a mother's own reserves were low and she did not use prenatal iron supplements, or if a baby is premature or has low birth weight for gestational age, a breast-fed or formula-fed infant may need iron supplementation almost immediately. Iron supplementation of breast-fed infants has been a point of controversy for some years now. Infant formulas fortified with iron do provide more iron than does breast milk, but since the iron in breast milk is more completely absorbed, supplementation may be unnecessary. (A more complete discussion of this complex subject appears in the next two chapters.)

The sodium content of cow's milk is far greater than that of human milk (25 to 30 milligrams per liter, versus 7 milligrams per liter). Most infant formulas fall somewhere between the two extremes. Since there is evidence that excessive salt intake may lead to high blood pressure at an early adult age in persons predisposed to hypertension, the lower sodium content of breast milk seems highly desirable.

The *zinc*-to-*copper* ratio is much lower in human than in cow's milk. This fact is of interest, since recent research suggests that a proper balance of these minerals may be vital to prevention of heart disease in later life. The zinc requirement during neonatal days is high. The fact that zinc-binding ligand (zbl), not yet developed in the intestines of the newborn, is present in breast milk, has been suggested as a factor in enhanced zinc absorption by breast-fed infants.

*Fluoride* supplements are sometimes recommended from birth unless infants are receiving formulas with at least 1 part per million of this substance. Due to the relatively small amounts of this mineral found in breast-milk, some physicians feel that all totally breast-fed babies should receive fluoride supplements. Other physicians feel that fluoride supplements at this age are not necessary for bottle-fed or breast-fed infants, and some doctors remain frankly undecided on the issue. There is evidence that if a mother drinks fluoridated water, the infant gets enough of this mineral in breast milk to insure good dental health. Since many breast-fed infants also receive some fluoride in water or in baby food during these early months, judging fluoride intake can be extremely difficult. Since excessive fluoride intake can cause mottling of teeth, giving a newborn a fluoride supplement seems unwarranted.

In a 1976 publication by the American Academy of Pedodontics, Dr. Frederick Parkins, professor of pedodontics at the College of Dentistry, University of Iowa, noted that "experts question the value of prescribing fluoride supplements to a child younger than six months of age. Research does not show benefits significant enough to justify [risking] the mottling that may occur when young infants receive [excessive] fluoride supplements."

Many nursing mothers might choose to rely on Dr. Parkin's opinion. Others might prefer to use fluoride supplements recommended by their pediatricians. Until the transfer and utilization of fluoride in breast milk are more completely understood, use of supplements will be a matter of personal choice based on the information available to parents and physicians.

As this overview has shown, an infant's basic nutrition needs may be met by either breast milk or formula, depending upon which method of feeding the mother chooses to use. The following paragraphs will discuss in more detail the advantages and disadvantages of both methods and give advice pertaining to the special problems which may be encountered by mothers using either or both methods.

## Examining Nutritional Options

Through the nine months of pregnancy, a developing infant is totally dependent upon his or her mother's nourishment. What the mother eats and drinks has far-reaching effects upon the child she carries. She is the sole provider of his or her needs. Ideally, she takes this responsibility seriously and seeks and follows the most reliable, up-to-date guidelines for prenatal nutrition.

At birth, the responsibility for baby's nourishment usually remains primarily with the mother. From the earliest days of the human race, the mother has generally met that responsibility by offering the child further sustenance from her own body: breast milk perfectly suited to his needs.

To breast-feed or not to breast-feed is, then, a relatively new dilemma. Prior to this century, choosing *not* to breast-feed was to choose to endanger the life of the child. Sanitation measures were so poor and refrigeration techniques so primitive that pathogens (disease-causing agents such as bacteria) often abounded in cow's milk, making it potentially very harmful for a tiny baby. Nature's way was, then, the only way for a conscientious mother.

Though the first commercial formula was devised in 1919, the great move away from breast-feeding took place only after manufacturers of bottles, canned milk, and infant formula began to realize the financial potential which bottle-feeding offered. Thus, as late as the mid-1940s, 65 percent of infants in the United States were breast-fed as newborns. After World War II, increasing numbers of women were seeking relief from the monotonous routine of round-the-clock motherhood by working outside the home or devoting their energies to charitable activities. Since most occupations and many volunteer activities called for relatively long separation from infants, food processors surmised that these mothers would welcome a nutritional innovation that allowed time to be free from the demands of breast-feeding.

Since bottle-feeding was an extra expense, at first only upper-class women bottle-fed. Gradually, as the practice became more and more of a status symbol, other women made the transition. Often these women lacked proper refrigeration techniques and paid little or no attention to proper sanitation. How many American babies have suffered from intestinal disorders and other illnesses due to the poor handling of bottle-fed milk or formula is not known, but one estimate indicates that diarrhea is more than ten times greater in bottle-fed than in breast-fed babies. Statistics for developing nations indicate that infant-mortality rates for bottle-fed infants are 50 to 75 percent higher than mortality rates for breast-fed babies in these same countries.

Even in the United States, according to a recent survey, less than 1 percent of all infants admitted to a hospital for gastroenteritis were breast-fed. Furthermore, of all bottle-fed infants hospitalized for gastroenteritis, one-third were babies who had been breast-fed at birth and had been switched to a bottle at least one month prior to hospitalization. This recent data would seem to indicate that the difference in bottle-fed versus breast-fed babies in incidence of gastroenteritis is nearly as dramatic in the United States as in the less-affluent populations observed in developing countries, though infant-mortality rates from such illnesses are not as high in the United States.

Statistics such as these lead one to wonder at the ease with which women were led to give up breast-feeding. Of course, such statistics were not available at the time bottle-feeding was becoming the status symbol yearned for by rich and poor mothers alike. Bottle-feeding became so popular that, by 1958, little more than a decade after the end of World War II, only 25 percent of one-week-old American infants were being breast-fed. The decline continued in the 1960s, so that by 1973, only 10 to 15 percent of two-month-olds and 5 percent of six-month-olds were still receiving breast milk from their mothers.

Today a new mother may choose bottle-feeding knowing that formulas are available which closely approximate the composition of human milk and that, with care, she can keep these formulas fresh and uncontaminated. Even so, every woman should be aware that a choice does exist. Although bottle-feeding and breast-feeding are both acceptable ways of nourishing an infant, the decision to choose one method over another should be made only after one has considered all available facts.

If bottle-fed babies can be healthy babies, why is there a gradual return to breast-feeding? Why is this return being led by college-educated, upper-social-class young women, women who could easily afford the cost of high-quality formula and solid food? Why are increasing numbers of physicians urging their patents to breast-feed their babies, at least for the first few months of life?

The answer to these questions lies in a closer look at some persuasive facts about breast-feeding, facts which led the 1969 White House Conference on Food, Nutrition, and Health to conclude that ". . . breast milk is the perfect food for [a baby's] nutritional needs and development; that it is the most natural way to feed babies; and that it provides a protection against infection and allergies that cannot be duplicated."

# Learning Facts and Dispelling Fears
# about Breast-feeding

## Facts about Breast-feeding

The increasing interest in breast-feeding can probably be attributed to the growing realization that breast-feeding has more advantages over bottle-feeding than had heretofore been realized. For both mother and baby, nursing offers unique advantages, most of which cannot be duplicated by even the most advanced formula.

In 1976, the Committee on Nutrition of the American Academy of Pediatrics reported that

*infants grow most rapidly during the first four to six months of life. Nutrient requirements are most critical in this period, during which nutritional deficiencies can have lasting effects on growth and development. . . . Breast milk has not been improved upon as a reference standard.*

Ironically, while breast milk has for some time been used as a "reference standard" against which to measure infant formulas based on cow's milk and soy protein, it has not been seriously reconsidered as the *ideal* formula until recent years. Growing numbers of pediatricians are endorsing breast-feeding, having seen the difference breast-feeding can make in their own patients and having read statistics which indicate the difference it can make in others.

Even so, these physicians may be at some disadvantage since, in 1977, out of the sixteen hundred pages in one major American textbook on pediatrics, only one-and-one-half pages are devoted to breast-feeding, and these pages contained no mention of the "let-down reflex," a crucial term in any discussion of lactation. In the light of relatively little textbook information on the topic, then, what evidence has made pediatricians willing to change their former stance on breast-feeding? What is there about breast-feeding that formula-feeding cannot imitate?

### Nutritional Advantages

Calves grow three times as fast as babies, doubling their birth weight in only forty-seven days, and cow's milk is ideally suited to accomplish this rapid growth. The human child, doubling his birth weight at four to five months of age, has different patterns of development and needs different nutrients to promote optimum growth. Human milk is ideally suited to meet those needs.

The table on page 42 comparing human milk with cow's milk and with cow's-milk-and soy-based formulas shows the extent to which formula makers have attempted to imitate the composition of human milk. As the discussion which follows that chart shows, however, there are many ways in which protein, fat, and carbohydrate found in human milk differ from those found in cow's milk or formulas.

As that same discussion indicates, many doctors now feel that the vitamin and mineral compositions of human milk (including vitamin D and iron) are perfectly suited to an infant's needs for at least the first six months of life. Vitamin and mineral supplements have helped bring breast milk imitations somewhat closer to the original, but, as a careful rereading of the technical discussion of vitamins and minerals in milks should show, significant differences still exist.

### Immunological Advantages

Since technology has finally enabled formula manufacturers to approximate the nutrient composition of human milk more closely, why do leading authorities continue to insist that breast milk must still be considered the ideal food? The World Health Organization, The American Academy of Pediatrics, and the American Public Health Association are a few of the many responsible health-care groups that have agreed that breast-feeding is the best way to nourish young babies. Their conclusion is based on more than a comparison of the nutritional content of breast milk and infant formulas.

Newborns enter life with certain protective antibodies at work which are gained from the mother during the prenatal months. In the most natural birth setting, the mother allows the infant to nurse at her breast within minutes after birth, and colostrum, the yellowish fluid which he receives in this early nursing experience, gives him additional immunity against harmful pathogens.

If a mother has an infection, her colostrum provides her baby with antibodies against that infection. Since a baby is likely to encounter certain harmful bacteria during its trip through the birth canal, such antibodies can prove invaluable in combating those bacteria.

Leukocytes in colostrum may prevent necrotizing enterocolitis, an often deadly intestinal disorder common to bottle-fed newborns who have undergone blood transfusions. High concentrations of certain lymphocytes in breast milk can line part of the baby's intestinal tract and give protection against other pathogens, protection that the baby does not receive in significant degree before birth. Even in high-risk environments, 100 percent breast-fed babies are often able to resist shigella and certain salmonella infections, including typhoid fever.

Lactoferrin, a human milk protein, binds iron. While this iron-binding action does not make a baby iron-deficient, it does create an iron-deficient environment unfriendly to the growth of staphylococci and *E. coli* bacteria (an organism common in the intestinal tract). Human milk also contains a group of complex carbohydrates (starches) that promote the growth of intestinal bacteria which in turn produce an acid environment unfriendly to the growth of disease-causing microorganisms.

One further immunological point should be made: Totally breast-fed infants are less likely to develop cow's-milk allergy—the most common allergy of infancy—when they do begin to drink that substance. It is thought that about 1 percent of all American infants have cow's-milk allergy. Withholding cow's milk for the first three months of life may minimize chances of allergic reaction to it later, since allergy is usually caused by ingesting large doses of allergens at a time when the intestinal walls are relatively open to the absorption of large, foreign, protein particles which would be unable to pass through more mature intestinal walls. Recently, a substance in breast milk has been shown to have an antiabsorptive effect, which seems to prevent development of milk allergy. As a result of this discovery, families with a history of allergies are being strongly encouraged to breast-feed their babies.

Probably because of the combined benefits of fewer troubles with sanitation and milk spoilage, presence of natural immunologic factors in breast milk, and lessened chance for development of milk allergy, significant illness is currently uncommon among breast-fed babies. Of course, the fact that today's American breast-feeding baby often has educationally advanced parents and a mother of relatively advanced maternal age probably also gives these infants a decided health advantage.

One recent study of 164 breast-fed and 162 bottle-fed infants showed that far fewer slight illnesses (22 percent), significant illnesses (9 percent), and hospital admittances (3 percent) occurred among the 50 percent of those infants who were breast-fed. Furthermore, the development of significant childhood illnesses in this group was markedly delayed, with peak incidence occurring during weaning from the breast.

Whatever the multiple, interrelated causes, breast-fed infants are generally healthier than bottle-fed babies, a fact which probably influenced the following comment by Dr. John W. Gerrard in *Pediatrics* (December 1974):

*We now know that breast-feeding insures a smooth transition for the baby from being entirely dependent on his mother for both his nutritional and immunologic requirements to being completely independent. It is this new awareness of the limitations of formula feeding . . . that makes us have second thoughts on breast-feeding.*

### Psychological Advantages

According to a recent work on mother-infant bonding, touch is an important element in establishing a firm bond. Suckling a child is a natural means of enhancing the mother-child relationship.

Both mother and baby can benefit from the close contact essential in breast-feeding. The hormone prolactin is considered a love hormone in birds. There is speculation that the human mother's attachment to her infant may be enhanced by the increased prolactin secretion essential to milk production. This may be nature's way of helping to insure survival of the newborn.

Bonding is further enhanced by the infant's ability to distinguish his or her mother from other mothers by the odor of her milk. A breast-fed baby can make this distinction as early as the fifth day. No such distinction is likely to come this soon to a formula-fed child.

For many mothers, there is a strong sense of pride and well-being associated with being the chief provider of the baby's needs. Almost all nursing mothers enjoy the intimate physical contact which breast-feeding allows, and there is increasingly strong evidence to support the idea that the baby gains a sense of security from this close one-to-one relationship.

### Infant Weight-Control Advantages

One of the most interesting theories being explored by those interested in breast-feeding involves infant appetite control. While an adult's appetite-control mechanism, when properly working, conveys a feeling of fullness after an adequate number of calories has been consumed, the infant's appetite control apparatus apparently responds to volume, not caloric intake.

According to more than one British researcher, breast milk is ideally suited to this method of appetite control because it is not consistently high in calories. At the beginning of a feeding, the milk is thin. It then becomes creamy, moves back to thin, then back to creamy. Thus the baby's thirst can be satisfied by relatively large volumes of breast milk without all milk that is is consumed being high in calories.

Though this theory has not been conclusively tested, it offers one possible reason for the evidence that more bottle-fed than breast-fed infants tend toward obesity during babyhood. In one recent study, one-third as many breast-fed as bottle-fed infants were obese.

Perhaps the simplest explanation for this difference is that the breast-fed infant is seldom urged to eat more than he wants, while the bottle-fed infant may be encouraged to finish every drop of every four-ounce feeding. Since a breast-feeding mother cannot *see* how much milk has been taken, she is forced to rely upon the baby's appetite-control system. When the infant loses interest in the breast, she assumes he has had enough. Since a bottle-feeding mother *can* see that an ounce of formula has not been taken, she may insist on baby's taking that last ounce, though he may not want or need it.

Recent studies of animals have indicated that excessive calorie intake can lead to permanently increased numbers of fat cells. There is evidence that the size of those cells may be decreased by dieting, but the number is *permanently* increased. A significant percentage of obese adults were obese as children, and researchers theorize that the presence of excessive numbers of fat cells gained during infancy and early childhood may increase the chances

of obesity in later life. Though there are problems with this theory
sents one possible answer to the question of why many obese ch
main obese throughout life. No doubt many new theories will be
over the next few decades as scientists try to solve the puzzle of obesity.

As pointed out by British researcher Dr. Barbara Hall, obesity is not a
problem of free-living animals. Perhaps babies fed exclusively on human
milk for the first three to six months of life will also escape the problems of
overweight. Most breast-feeding babies can and do remain relatively slender
during infancy, and Dr. Hall feels that the previously mentioned changing
consistency and flavor of breast milk during the feeding process may be
helping a baby learn appetite control, which will increase the likelihood of
avoiding overeating in later life.

## Other Advantages

The stimulation of the mother's breast during nursing signals the release
of *oxytocin,* a powerful hormone which not only activates the "let-down
reflex" but also causes uterine contractions which help the uterus return to
its prepregnancy size. These contractions may also help prevent postpartum
hemorrhaging.

The *convenience* of breast-feeding is often overlooked by mothers-to-be
who fear being tied down by a nursing baby. After a look at this chapter's
brief directions for formula preparation, a mother-to-be should see at once
the advantages of avoiding all such bother. In contrast, wherever the breast-
feeding mother is, there is also a sterile, nutritious food supply, ready and at
the perfect temperature. Even night feedings are ready in seconds, since
there is no bottle to be heated.

The *economy* of breast-feeding is an increasingly important factor in our
overpopulated world. In some developing countries, bottle-feeding a young
infant may require use of one-quarter to one-half of a family's weekly income. The nursing mother's daily need for additional calories, protein, and
calcium can be met by adding to her normal, well-balanced diet a peanut
butter and jelly sandwich and a glass of milk, at a cost of less than half a
dollar. Extra vitamins and other minerals can be added for very little extra
money. Even if she chooses more elaborate means of meeting her need for
extra nutrients, the formula necessary to feed a child usually costs considerably more and offers considerably less than the breast milk which the
mother can so easily produce. For example, a child nursed through the first
two years of life gets an average of 396 liters (105 quarts) of breast milk. This
is nutritionally equivalent to 437 liters (115 quarts) of cow's milk, at a cost
of approximately $65. Ready-to-use infant formula would cost considerably
more.

Finally, breast-feeding can provide an easy method of *losing a few excess
pounds.* Provided a woman follows dietary recommendations for a lactating
mother and remembers to reduce her own calorie intake as an older baby
nurses less and less frequently, she can meet her own needs and those of her

baby and still whittle away a few pounds. Nursing should never be an excuse for obesity. Instead, it might well open the door to slimness.

In summary, all current medical evidence seems to support breast-feeding as the ideal way to nurture an infant. According to Dr. Jean Mayer, one of America's leading experts in the field of nutrition,

> *natural nursing is a foolproof method which can be duplicated only by intelligent, constantly careful, clinically guided—and costlier—artificial feeding. Under less than ideal conditions, morbidity and mortality are consistently greater in artificially fed infants than in breast-fed.*

Of course, when the art of breast-feeding becomes a fetish or an end in itself, an infant may suffer. For example, infants limited to breast milk alone for periods beyond six to nine months may tend to develop marked deficiency symptoms. The important thing is to seek the best nutritional experience for a newborn, and apparently breast is best, at least for the first three to six months of life.

## Fears about Breast–feeding

If breast-feeding offers so many advantages, why aren't all pregnant women planning to follow nature's way of infant feeding? Unfortunately, many women brought up in homes where bottle-feeding was the norm have very real fears about breast-feeding. By taking a good look at these fears and by trying to deal with them openly and honestly, these women may be able to find the freedom to reconsider breast-feeding in a more objective light.

### Nursing Will Destroy My Sex Life . . .

The breast has been removed from the nursery and placed in the master bedroom, becoming a symbol of sexual gratification instead of a means of infant nutrition. Many young women, viewing the breast as sexual, seem repulsed by the idea of using the breast to meet a baby's needs. Apparently, there need be no either-or decision on this point. Women who nurse their babies report no declining interest in sexual activity. Provided their husbands can be educated as to the advantages of breast-feeding, there seem to be no resentment and no significant modification of lovemaking techniques.

Many fear drastic changes in breast appearance after nursing. While there are no definitive research statistics to disprove this fear, many studies suggest that breast changes are usually the result of pregnancy, not of lactation.

### But I Have to Work . . .

The working mother's hesitation about breast-feeding is legitimate. Obviously, a mother who is able to be at home all day with her baby finds nursing that baby a relatively easy task, while one who works outside the home finds nursing a more complicated art. However, as of March 1973, only 29.4 percent of mothers of children under age three were in the work force. Of that number, an even smaller percentage had babies under six months of age. Based on these figures, over three-quarters of American women could nurse their babies for at least six months without giving up their jobs in order to do so. Though currently more mothers of babies and toddlers are probably in the work force, many of these mothers could find working and breast-feeding compatible.

Even those who must return to work soon after the baby's birth can breast-feed. Some employers offer short nursing breaks in lieu of long lunch hours. Others are even providing day-care facilities, which mean a mother is always fairly close to her child, ready to meet his or her needs. Other mothers leave bottles of formula for a sitter to feed to the baby, and still others hand-express milk or use a pump to fill bottles for their infants. Working and breast-feeding are not mutually exclusive activities. If a mother wants to nurse her child, she can do so, even if she must work outside the home.

### It Might Hurt . . .

When simple prenatal nipple preparation measures can help prevent nipple soreness, "it might hurt" seems a sad reason for giving up the idea of nursing. During the last three months of pregnancy, one can rub the nipples with a Turkish towel, curtail use of soap on the nipple area to allow buildup of protective oils, cut a circle of material from the tips of brassieres to provide nipple exposure to air and tactile stimulation without losing needed support for expanding breasts, and pull out and gently rotate each nipple several times a day.

### But I Wouldn't Know How . . .

Though breast-feeding is a natural act, young women with no nursing mothers or grandmothers to provide examples may indeed *not* know how to nurse. Organizations such as La Leche League International offer technical advice and emotional support to thousands of women each year. Several excellent paperbacks, some of them listed in Appendix D, provide similar advice for women who prefer books to meetings. Many medical personnel are also able to provide assistance.

### I've Heard Nursing Causes Breast Cancer . . .

With breast cancer no longer a hush-hush disease, women are attempting to learn all they can about prevention and early detection of this often-fatal disorder. Many fear that nursing will cause cancer, but current research indicates that, under certain circumstances, mothers who breast-feed their babies for at least nine months may be *less,* not more, susceptible to cancer than nonnursing mothers.

The hormonal changes that are associated with prolonged lactation may offer protection against breast cancer. These hormonal changes, similar to those seen in women who have "stairstep babies," seem to discourage the development of cancer. In short, while there is no evidence to support the rumor that breast-feeding *causes* breast cancer, there is some evidence to suggest that breast-feeding may inhibit the development of breast cancer.

Nursing does not, of course, rule out the possibility of cancer. Even the woman who nurses her children for long periods of time may, under certain circumstances, develop breast cancer. Thus, all women should continue to watch for early signs of this disease.

### I'll Have to Give Up Smoking, Drinking, and Drugs . . .

Since most drugs pass into human milk to some degree, cutting down on both smoking and drinking and avoiding hallucinogens is probably the safest course for both mother and baby. A new mother, having already been through nine months of abstinence or of greatly reduced use of these items, should find continued caution relatively easy. Since prescription drugs can pose mild to severe threats, a lactating woman should always remind her doctor that she is breast-feeding before accepting a prescription. Substitute drugs are usually available.

### But Breast Milk is So High in DDT . . .

Ecological toxicants such as DDT, PCP, and PBB can indeed be present in human milk. Cow's milk is considered safe if DDT levels do not exceed 50 milligrams per liter. Though the ban on DDT has lowered the amount currently found in breast milk, human-milk DDT levels sometimes exceed this arbitrary safety limit. This is probably because ecological toxicants are most concentrated in the highest reaches of the food chain, which are the main components of the human diet. Most experts agree, however, that unless a woman has an unusually high intake of substances such as DDT, the benefits of breast-feeding far outweigh the minimal dangers posed by traces of these chemicals in human milk.

The maximum amount of DDT and its metabolites (Dieldrin, Aldrin, etc.) likely to be ingested by a breast-fed baby is still a thousand times less than the amount known to cause acute intoxication in humans. An infant exposed to insecticides mobilized from maternal tissues prenatally and at birth already has more insecticide stored in her body fat than she is likely to acquire during breast-feeding. Lead, another ecological contaminant causing great concern, probably appears in greater concentrations in evaporated milk and in infant formulas made from evaporated milk than in breast milk.

### What about Contraception While I'm Nursing?

For hundreds of years, breast-feeding provided a fairly reliable means of child spacing, since continuous, unsupplemented breast-feeding stimulates the mother's system to release prolactin, an extremely effective, natural, contraceptive hormone. In cultures where mother's milk is the chief source of calories for baby during the first twelve to eighteen months, average spacing of children is about every two years. Of course, this method is not absolutely reliable, especially in view of the modern trend toward supplementation of baby's diet, with resulting decrease in suckling and in hormone release triggered by suckling. Even so, this natural phenomenon helps increase the likelihood that foams, gels, creams, diaphragms, condoms, or similar mechanical means of birth control will be more successful than under nonnursing circumstances. Of course, as nursing tapers off, ovulation begins, and pregnancy may occur even before the menstrual period returns. Once menstrual periods become regular, a new mother's chances of getting pregnant increase still further.

Most physicians do *not* recommend use of oral contraceptives during the early weeks of nursing, since these drugs interfere with milk production. While some allow use of oral contraceptives after lactation is well established, others warn against regular use of any hormone, since these drugs do pass into breast milk.

Insertion of an intrauterine contraceptive device (IUD) is generally not recommended immediately after delivery. Since uterine tissue is very soft at that time, there is an increased risk that the physician might push the IUD through the uterine wall during insertion. There is greater risk of infection if an IUD is inserted soon after delivery, and there is a greater risk of expelling the device, since the cervical opening remains enlarged for several weeks after birth. For these reasons, most physicians recommend delaying insertion of an IUD until after the six-week checkup. At that time, if the uterus has returned to its prepregnancy condition so that the IUD can be inserted with minimal chances of perforation, expulsion, or infection and if other means of contraception have been used in the weeks since delivery so that there is minimal chance that a new pregnancy has already begun, the doctor may insert the device. As a general rule, IUD insertions are made approximately eight weeks after delivery.

### What If I Don't Have Enough Milk?

Certainly, if a woman chooses breast-feeding, she must do everything possible to insure an adequate milk supply. This means getting enough rest, keeping a positive attitude toward herself and her child, and eating a well-balanced diet, which includes adequate extra calories, protein, vitamins, and minerals to meet the increased demand which lactation places on her body. Since the physiological stresses of breast-feeding are even greater than those of pregnancy, a new mother should not only continue the prenatal diet she has followed for the past nine months, including an extra eight ounces of milk or equivalent high calcium foods, but she should also add to that diet more protein (20 grams over the nonpregnant, nonlactating diet) and more calories (200 over the prenatal diet, 500 over the nonpregnant, nonlactating diet). At one time, authorities felt nursing mothers needed 1000 extra calories, 700 above the recommended prenatal intake, but this figure failed to take into account the presence of postpartum fatty deposits, which contribute needed energy for about three months.

The nursing woman needs a slight increase over prenatal levels in foods rich in vitamin A, vitamin E, vitamin C, thiamin, niacin, riboflavin, iodine, and zinc. Making these additions is quite simple and economical. For example, adding a raw tomato or six ounces of orange juice will give a nursing mother the extra vitamin C she needs, a single plum yields the extra riboflavin recommended, and two-thirds of a cup of green peas and mushrooms can supply the extra niacin. Extra servings of whole grains, leafy vegetables, corn, nuts, and dried split peas can raise vitamin E, pyrodoxine, and folic-acid levels. Since most of these foods are acceptable to vegetarians as well as meat eaters, all nursing mothers should be able to meet the added demands of nursing quite easily.

Since fluid intake/milk-yield studies of dairy cattle have shown that fluid intake increases milk yield, researchers once assumed that increasing fluid intake would increase human milk volume. Experiments with breast-feeding women show, however, that variation of fluid intake has no significant effect on milk supply. Apparently, the body gives very high priority to lactation, since urine and respiratory losses do go down for nursing women on limited fluid intakes. Nutritionists recommend that breast-feeding mothers increase their fluid intake enough to prevent concentration of the urine or constipation due to abnormally dry feces. Water, juices, milk, and moderate amounts of coffee and tea may be taken to maintain fluids at desired levels. There is no indication that forcing oneself to drink more fluids than needed to maintain these bodily functions and sustain normal milk volume will mean a significant increase in milk production.

When a breast-feeding mother gets enough calories, protein, vitamins, minerals, and liquids, her baby usually has sufficient milk of excellent quality. Though there have been reports of an infant's failure to thrive on breast milk, such reports are rare and, with a physician's help, logical reasons for the failure can usually be identified and corrected. Generally, mothers can feel confident that breast-feeding offers optimum nutrition. As noted previously, there is still some debate among nutritionists and pediatricians as to whether breast-feeding babies need any additional vitamins or minerals. This is a matter which can best be determined by the pediatrician's analysis of a particular breast-feeding situation.

Having examined the nutritional options open for her baby, the new mother must decide whether breast-feeding or bottle-feeding seems best suited to her particular situation. No matter how potentially advantageous breast-feeding is for baby, a mother who knows that she cannot feel comfortable in a nursing role should probably not breast-feed. After all, a baby senses adult emotions, and most likely will not receive optimum benefits from a feeding method for which its mother feels strong dislike.

## Learning the Art of Bottle-feeding

The mother who chooses bottle-feeding must decide upon the contents of the bottle, the design of the bottle and nipple, and the method of preparation and sterilization she will use when feeding the baby. Bottle content is, of course, the most crucial of these decisions.

Most physicians now feel that cow's milk alone is not a desirable food for an infant under one year of age. Higher in casein than human milk, cow's milk produces a curd not readily digestible by infants. Use of unaltered cow's milk is thus likely to cause intestinal distress and even internal hemorrhaging severe enough to lead to anemia. Use of undiluted goat's milk is also not recommended, because of the heavy load which undiluted milk puts on the kidneys of the young infant.

In the earliest days of bottle-feeding in the United States, the simplest cow's-milk formulas for newborns usually consisted of 2 tablespoons of corn syrup added to 13 ounces of evaporated milk diluted with 19 to 26 ounces of water. The diluted evaporated milk was easier to digest than regular cow's milk, and the corn syrup raised the percentage of carbohydrates in the final product.

Currently used home-prepared formulas may begin with fresh pasteurized milk, evaporated milk, or even whole dry milk. Raw milk is *not* recommended, due to the danger of infection it poses, especially to young infants. Evaporated milk, which is fortified with 400 International Units (IUs) of vitamin D per 13-ounce can, contains fat in a finely divided form, which produces soft curds. Pasteurized or homogenized fresh milk or whole dry milk may also be used as a formula base, provided the milk is heated or otherwise altered to produce a more easily digested curd. Vitamin C must usually be added, since heating cow's milk destroys most of this vitamin. One Swedish researcher has reported that home-prepared formulas in that country closely approximate available commercial formulas in calorie distribution. However, this would be true only when care is taken to measure all components—including recommended vitamin and mineral supplements —carefully and accurately.

Homemade milk- or soy-based formula should not be prepared without the help of a physician or a nutritionist. Generally, homemade formulas for baby are no longer considered advisable, since the advantages gained by using commercial formulas, with their added nutrients, outweigh their higher cost.

Commercial formulas closely approximate calorie, protein, vitamin, and mineral ratios of human milk. They are easy to use and unlikely to spoil if correctly prepared and stored. They come in various forms, tailored to the economic needs and special circumstances in which they will be used. Ready-to-feed types, the most convenient, are also the most expensive. These mixtures are available in bottles or in cans for quick use. Powdered formulas are less expensive but require mixing with carefully measured amounts of water. The concentrated liquid forms available must also be properly diluted with water before use.

If a mother overdilutes the formula through carelessness or in hopes of saving money, her baby may fail to gain weight satisfactorily. If she uses too little water in order to give baby a "richer" formula, she may overload his kidneys or bring on obesity or other such problems. Especially after a child has been ill, a parent may feel that she needs to use a more concentrated formula. Actually, this is not true, and feeding undiluted, highly concentrated formulas may bring highly undesirable results.

A child suffering from the effects of formula too concentrated for her system may cry. The crying is probably a reaction to the intense thirst brought on by protein overload, yet a mother is more apt to offer still more formula than to offer the water the child desperately needs. Permanent brain damage and severe circulatory problems have been noted in such children. In addition, insufficiently diluted formulas have led to the development of a mass of dense cow's-milk curd that obstructs the intenstine and requires surgical removal. Since most directions for formula diiution have been carefully devised with the health of the infant in mind, mothers should follow these directions with great care.

When infants show symptoms of allergy to cow's milk (as do an average of 0.5 to 1.0 percent of infants in Western countries) or when parents who are vegans (vegetarians who do not consume milk, eggs, or any other animal products) prefer that their children not consume cow's milk, soy-based formulas are an acceptable choice. A number of satisfactorily fortified soy-based formulas are on the market. These formulas provide high-quality protein plus recommended amounts of such key vitamins and minerals as riboflavin, $B_{12}$, calcium, and iron. A word of caution concerning soy formulas and allergies may be in order. A recent Harvard University study indicates that soy-based formulas are at least as antigenic as are cow's milk formulas. Thus, for some children, neither type of formula will necessarily prevent the development of allergies. Breast-milk, again, is the ideal "formula." If breast-feeding is not an option, formulas utilizing predigested cow's milk protein may be recommended for such infants.

Like unfortified cow's milk, *unfortified* soy milk does not contain the vitamins and minerals needed by the newborn and does not closely approximate the protein-fat-carbohydrate ratios of human milk. Almond milk, sesame soy, and soy-tahina mixtures also fall short. Kokoh (sesame seed, brown rice, sweet brown rice, aduki beans, wheat, oats, soy beans, and water) offers excellent protein potential, but in a form so diluted that it can provide only 40 percent of a baby's daily energy need. Since it would be almost impossible for an infant to consume the 60 to 70 ounces of kokoh per day required to meet her energy needs, use of these preparations can retard physical and mental growth and development.

Because infants cannot assimilate enough whole grains, green vegetables, and fruits to offset the possible vitamin-mineral deficiencies of home-prepared formulas, vegetarian mothers should seriously consider using fortified commercial formulas for at least the first six months of life. This excellent nutritional start can help insure a baby's good health until he is old enough to begin a more typical, yet still balanced, vegetarian diet.

The vegetarian or nonvegetarian mother who chooses not to breast-feed or who discontinues breast-feeding after a few weeks or months can be reasonably assured that her child will continue to thrive if she is placed on a reliable soy-based or milk-based formula. Should problems associated with that formula arise, mother and pediatrician can work together to make the necessary changes in formula type, concentrations, or amounts.

## Preparing Formula

When the use of formulas and bottles first became popular, mothers often spent hours sterilizing baby's bottles, then hours more worrying about whether or not they'd done a good job. As mentioned earlier, very young infants are highly susceptible to gastrointestinal infections, and many babies have suffered, and even died, due to unsanitary handling of formula. To be on the safe side, doctors began recommending that mothers use terminal sterilization techniques. By this method, a group of prewashed, glass, formula-filled, nippled, and capped bottles was processed for twenty-five to thirty minutes in a sterilizer. After processing, the bottles were cooled slightly, then refrigerated during the twenty-four-hour period of their expected use.

Though there are some cases in which this method of sterilization may still be warranted, most mothers today use the somewhat simpler "clean" or "aseptic" technique, apparently with no greater incidence of illness. Relaxation of such instructions is always a risky move, since some mothers may feel that being told to give *less* attention to sterilization means they need pay *no* attention to sanitation. At first, doctors recommended that those using the "clean" technique should prepare only one bottle at each feeding time and give that bottle immediately. Today, in homes where general sanitation is not a problem, enough bottles for a twenty-four-hour period may be prepared by this method, then refrigerated at once.

If the baby's doctor feels the "clean" or "aseptic" method is acceptable, every effort should be made to see that the method is, indeed, a *clean* one. Hands should be washed before preparation begins. Then, formula cans, bottles, and nipples should be washed and rinsed, preferably in scalding water. Standard glass or plastic bottles with standard nipples may be chosen (provided nipple openings are not so large that they allow formula to flow too rapidly). Plastic bottles in unusual animal shapes are often very difficult to clean and should therefore be avoided, especially for very young infants likely to be highly susceptible to bacterial infection.

The newer bottles with nipples which simulate the shape of a mother's breast area and presterilized disposable plastic bags which collapse as the formula is sucked out may be preferred by infants who have been breast-fed or by mothers who prefer to clean only nipples, caps, and bag holders. Enough formula for an entire day may be prepared, covered, and refrigerated, provided all bottle parts, plus the metal form over which the plastic bags are stretched, have been properly cleaned before preparation begins. Of course, plastic bags should never be reused.

When a parent chooses ready-to-use formula, the recommended amount of formula is poured into a bottle and any remaining formula in the can is then covered and refrigerated. Unused concentrated formula must also be refrigerated after opening. Although powdered formulas do not require refrigeration before the addition of water, the powder should be stored in a tightly capped container after opening. Preparation of concentrated or powdered formula requires great care, since adding too little or too much water results in a nutritionally unacceptable, possibly dangerous formula.

If refrigeration space is a problem, one might sterilize bottles, nipples, and other equipment and place the appropriate amount of sterile water in each bottle. Then, just before feeding, the recommended amount of powdered or concentrated formula may be added. The bottle may then be capped and shaken to mix. Especially in older houses where pipes may be corroded, it is better to start with *cold* tap water than to risk using hot water, which may contain dissolved lead or other impurities. The cold water may be boiled or not, depending on the purity of the water supply.

Ideally, once the recommended amount of formula has been prepared, heated to room or body temperature, and offered to baby, any formula remaining in the bottle should be discarded since bacterial growth occurs rapidly in warm milk. Saving a few pennies may mean losing them later, when the child develops gastrointestinal illness attributed to spoiled milk. While mothers occasionally refrigerate a partially used bottle and reuse it without any apparent ill effects, one must decide whether the risk of illness is worth the slight saving.

Other mothers, unwilling to risk illness by saving the milk in the refrigerator, attempt to "save" it by force-feeding it to the already satisfied infant. This is an even more serious false economy, in light of what researchers have begun to discover about the relationship between overfeeding and infantile, childhood, and adult obesity.

## Introduction of Solids

The move toward early introduction of solids coincides rather noticeably with the increased production of commercial baby foods. In the 1920s, solids were usually avoided for the entire first year. By the 1930s, about the time of the appearance of the first commercial strained foods, solids were being introduced at four to six months. The age of introduction dropped to two and a half to three months in the 1950s, and by the late 1960s and early 1970s, some doctors were urging use of cereals as early as the first three weeks of life.

The current trend among leading pediatricians with expertise in nutrition is toward postponement of solids. A baby's gastrointestinal tract is highly sensitive to foreign protein and textures for at least the first three months of life. Consequently, babies are more likely to develop food allergies when solids are introduced too early.

One specialist has recommended deferring solids until an infant has head and neck control, can sit with support, and can convey his willingness or unwillingness to accept solids (sixteen to twenty-four weeks). With relatively little saliva excretion and poor ability to push solids back with a tongue accustomed only to sucking, a baby is ill-equipped to handle solids much before that age. Certainly he has little ability to recognize and respond to a spoon. Of course, with modern inventions such as the syringelike infant feeder at her disposal, an enterprising mother can ignore this and push solids down as early as she likes.

Some mothers—and some doctors—insist that children must start solids early in order to learn to eat from a spoon—that they need practice in this important art. While it is true that an infant introduced to solids at three weeks may learn to eat from a spoon at an earlier age than one introduced to solids at six months, the first child may take weeks to learn a skill the second child masters in two feedings.

Some mothers feel that feeding solids early will help a young baby sleep through the night. One leading authority has noted that if solids do help an infant sleep through, this is an indication that the baby has consumed a greater number of calories than he would normally have consumed. This is one form of overfeeding, and such overfeeding will not help an infant establish the habit of eating in moderation. In some cases, early introduction of solids may create digestive disturbances which will disrupt the child's sleep, not help him to sleep for longer periods of time.

Can early feeding of solids be harmful? In many cases, yes. Why force a helpless infant to swallow mouthfuls of strange-textured, strong-tasting vegetables when doing so may cause a long-lasting dislike of these valuable foods? Why risk bringing on food allergies which might be avoided by the delayed introduction of solids? Why risk upsetting a child's developing appetite-control mechanism by overfeeding? Why give solids with the hope of helping baby sleep through the night, only to risk setting off digestive problems that might disrupt sleep patterns for weeks to come? Why risk any of these unpleasant possibilities just to be able to brag about how early a child began eating solid foods?

For the average infant on breast milk or on a properly fortified formula, there is no nutritional reason to introduce foods other than milk before five to six months of age. Especially for the breast-feeding infant, earlier introduction of solids means trading a superior food for an inferior one. Those who do choose to begin solids earlier should at least wait until the baby has the intellectual ability to recognize and respond to a spoon and the physical ability to use the tongue and swallowing mechanisms required for the consumption of nonliquid food (usually three to six months of age).

Since there appears to be no justification for the introduction of strained foods or even juices to infants under three months of age, and since there are indications that the early introduction of solids may lead to overeating and consequent obesity, digestive disturbances, food allergies, or dislike of vegetables, a mother would do well to resist the temptation to rush to solid foods. Her patience will be rewarded if she waits until baby's growing interest in the foods eaten by other family members leads him to accept a spoon and its contents with curiosity and delight, not bewilderment and dislike.

## Psychological Factors in Feeding

As discussed earlier, breast-feeding offers psychological advantages over bottle-feeding because of the completeness of the physical and emotional interaction between nursing mother and suckling child. This does not mean that bottle-fed babies and mothers cannot experience meaningful closeness, merely that such closeness does not come as easily or as automatically for some bottle feeders. What can a mother do to insure that bonding and closeness will be optimum, whether she is breast-feeding or bottle-feeding?

First you can feed the infant as soon as possible after delivery. The breast-feeding mother may give the child little milk in this first meeting of breast and tiny mouth, yet the very act of such intimate, loving contact is one which experts now agree is an excellent beginning for the maternal-infant bonding so essential to the ideal mother-child relationship. Bottle-feeding mothers might ask to hold the child against a bare breast for a few moments on the delivery table, an appropriate beginning for the closeness toward which a mother should work. Later, when water is to be offered, a mother should request the privilege of giving the first feeding.

Second, a new mother can ask to be part of *every* feeding, unless she is physically unable to do so or unless the baby is unable to suckle due to postnatal complications. Closeness comes from familiarity. Baby should *know* to whom he or she belongs as soon as possible. Breast-feeding mothers have more persuasive powers here, for they can request that the baby be brought to them for feedings, even during the night, so that milk will "come in" earlier and baby can receive valuable, protective colostrum at the earliest possible moment. Bottle-feeding moms who want to gain added closeness might also insist upon this privilege.

Third, you can make feeding your baby a special time for mother-child interaction by avoiding the temptation to let all the relatives in on the fun. Here, the breast-feeding mother has a decided advantage, for unless she pumps her breasts or expresses milk by hand, she has the perfect excuse to keep this special time to herself. While there will be times when she would gladly pass this honor on to anyone who offered, she should normally cherish these moments in which she is the sole person responsible for her baby's welfare. Only she can give her or him the maximum pleasure of delicious, warm milk, uninhibited suckling, and delightful skin-to-skin contact. After such pleasure, all the boiled water grandmother offers will hardly be enough to make baby forget who mama is.

The breast-feeding infant is able to distinguish his or her mother's milk from that of any other mother by five days of age. What mother has to give is unique. She is his mother, and he is not likely to forget this fact. Others can show their love in equally important ways, but mother is, and should remain, the focal point of baby's early feeding experience.

The bottle-feeding mother will have a harder time keeping feeding honors to herself. In this day of shared responsibility, there is certainly no reason for father to miss out on the love and joy of infant feeding. Yet, if mother is to be the primary care-giver in the early months, then ideally mother should be the one who feeds baby most often. When this does not happen, as when a premature infant is almost completely isolated from his or her mother for weeks, bonding does not seem to occur as strongly. An estrangement occurs which time does not seem to erase completely. How sad to see the six-month-old who shows no preference for mother or father over baby-sitter, neighbor, or even stranger. Those who exclaim at what a friendly baby he is are probably unaware that a six-month-old infant should definitely know and *care* who his mother and father are. If he does not, bonding has failed to occur or has only partially occurred.

Certainly letting grandparents or a sibling try an occasional feeding will not destroy maternal-infant bonding, but a mother is being wise, not just selfish, to keep most feedings for herself in order to capitalize on these moments when infant and mother are totally absorbed in a mutually satisfying activity.

Fourth, make yourself totally available to your child at feeding time. Though researchers report that most breast-feeding moms maintain excellent, almost continuous eye contact with their feeding infants, breast-feeding does not *guarantee* such intense contact. This does not mean a nursing mother can't manage to read a magazine article as a dozing baby continues to suck at her nearly empty breast, enjoying the closeness and the comfort sucking brings. Indeed, with no bottle to hold, many breast-feeding mothers have found extra reading or television time during nursing periods. Closeness is lost when such outside distractions become the rule, so that baby is offered the breast with a coolness and nonchalance avid supporters of "the womanly art" would prefer to believe belong only to the bottle-feeding mother.

Both breast-feeding and bottle-feeding mothers should realize that feeding time calls for the giving of love and attention as well as nourishment. Unless this opportunity is taken advantage of, a complete stranger might as well be feeding the baby—by breast or by bottle. On the other hand, the mother who talks and smiles to her newborn while offering him his formula is building a strong mother-child bond as surely as is the breast-feeding mother who pays equal attention to the loving and giving aspects of infant feeding.

Fifth, you should be relaxed during feeding time. Tenseness interferes with the let-down reflex crucial to successful breast-feeding. Tenseness is sensed by a child, whether that child is bottle- or breast-fed. At the end of a hectic day, with a two-year-old crying for his supper and the smell of burning pot roast wafting in from the kitchen, relaxing is not likely to be an easy task. Perhaps father can come to the rescue, feed the cranky two-year-old, salvage the pot roast, and bring mom a refreshing glass of lemonade. If baby is a first child and a sibling's demands don't complicate matters, mom can take care of matters herself by tending to the kitchen emergency first, then turning on her favorite music, sitting in a comfortable rocker, and letting herself forget the hassle and concentrate on the tiny miracle in her arms. As mom relaxes, baby probably will, too, and the overall benefit of breast- or bottle-feeding will be increased.

Sixth, a mother should realize that an outpouring of maternal love does not automatically accompany all feedings. For example, if her little blue-eyed miracle has been howling for three solid hours, even the strains of Rachmaninoff's Second Piano Concerto may not dispel feelings of hostility. The bottle-feeding mother can let this be a time for daddy's magic touch, but the breast-feeding mom must either try to relax enough to allow her milk to come or let dad offer water while she takes a warm shower and allows herself a moment of privacy. Usually, after such a break, the milk will flow, baby will eat and sleep, and a night's rest will restore the household's sanity and replenish mother's milk supply, too.

Occasionally, a mother may feel more like "pluck[ing] [her] nipple from his boneless gums, and dash[ing] the brains out" (Lady Macbeth's famous line) than loving and cuddling her baby. Such feelings of hostility are perfectly normal, though extremely frightening when they are first experienced. Acting them out is, of course, not normal. Instead, a mother should be honest with herself—"Yes, this is one of these moments when I wonder why I ever thought motherhood was desirable" or even "Yes, I *do* want to hit him—anything to shut him up," then seek a cooling-off period, a time when she can withdraw and call up her inner reserves. Of course, if such methods don't help to dispel these feelings, professional aid should be sought.

Certainly, baby will pick up even the brief hostile vibrations evident during such a crisis, just as he picks up loving ones at other times. However, unless the hostile moments become increasingly frequent, the positive mother-child relationship already established should be strong enough to withstand relatively infrequent negative moments.

In summary, feeding an infant is a psychological as well as a physical activity. Early moments of love and tenderness can make indelible impressions on an infant's psyche, whether those moments are experienced while breast-feeding or bottle-feeding. In the early months, it is the mother to whom nature has given the responsibility for feeding and it is the feeding, nurturing mother with whom the infant forms her strongest bond.

Of course, a father who has chosen to assume major responsibility for the child while mother works outside the home may be the person with whom baby forms this primary bond. Even a father who does *not* plan to be the primary caretaker can, and should, offer loving handling and cuddling so that the baby becomes attached to him, too. Older children and grandparents may also enjoy such privileges, but mother should usually be the person with whom baby associates the fulfillment of her most pressing need, the need for warm and satisfying milk.

One other point should probably be made concerning the psychological aspects of infant feeding. Though a baby may occasionally wish to nurse at his mother's empty breast for comfort when he is lonely or feeling neglected, neither a breast-feeding nor a bottle-feeding mom should automatically assume that every cry is a hunger cry. To do so may be to set into motion a lifelong cycle of eating out of boredom, frustration, loneliness, and neglect. Food should be used to satisfy hunger, not just to take the place of attention mother isn't willing to give in other ways.

## Common Problems

The common problems associated with infant feeding fall into two broad categories—those which require immediate medical attention and those which may be dealt with by simple, at-home means. Into the first category fall all diseases associated with in-born metabolic problems or other such deficiencies in the way the body breaks down certain essential substances.

Phenylketonuria (PKU), perhaps the best-known of these diseases, is associated with the lack of a specific enzyme necessary for amino-acid metabolism. This easily detected disorder is usually screened for by hospitals at the time of birth; undetected, PKU leads to mental retardation and shortened life span. Over sixty other inborn errors of amino-acid metabolism have been identified, and many of these can cause severe retardation, restricted growth, kidney failure, and other tragic problems if undetected. Fortunately, the most severe of these diseases occur but rarely —less than one in four million live births.

Some infants have an inborn error of metabolism of carbohydrates such as fructose. Given fruit juice, these infants may experience abdominal pain, deformity, and retarded growth. As long as such foods are avoided, an infant with this disorder suffers no mental or physical ill effects. Intolerance to lactose (milk sugar) may also occur. Most instances of lactose intolerance are temporary, coming on suddenly due to an intestinal upset and disappearing after a few days or, at worst, after a few months on a nonmilk formula. Occasionally, infants are born with *true* lactose intolerance stemming from an inborn error of lactose metabolism. In this case, lactose intolerance lasts a lifetime. Though milk allergies of one kind or another occur with some frequency, true lactose intolerance is extremely rare. Fortunately, soy-based formulas can be given to babies who do have this disorder.

In the future, tests may be able to identify parents who are carriers of these disorders, so that their infants may be watched with great care and the diagnosis of in-born errors of metabolism may be made more quickly. Other food allergies need not be discussed here, assuming introduction of solids will not begin until at least three months of age.

In the second category fall those infant feeding problems which beset a child with no known medical disorders and a breast-milk or formula diet. While such problems are not usually life-or-death matters, they are very real concerns for the parents and babies who encounter them.

The following problems can usually be handled by parents and are normally not serious. Of course, if a situation persists, or if baby just doesn't seem himself, a call to the doctor is a good idea.

## Colic

The mother whose hostile feelings toward her screaming infant were described above may have had a "colicky" baby. *Colic* is a vaguely defined disorder which has been attributed to everything from the cabbage a breast-feeding mother ate at lunch to the air a bottle-feeding baby swallowed when grandmother let him suck at any empty bottle. No matter how cloudy the cause, the symptoms are fairly clear. Baby flexes her legs in toward her tummy and screams. Lucky is the mother whose child has only one or two bouts with colic. Some babies go through weeks or even months of discomfort. While mother tries to be a loving, gentle care-giver, baby screams and cries for endless hours. What causes this problem and what can be done to ease the pain for baby and for mother?

Some pediatricians feel that colic may occur because a baby's digestive system is not yet functioning efficiently. Gas becomes trapped and the baby is not able to relax his bowels and expel it. Different methods of burping a child may be experimented with. If on-the-shoulder burping fails, putting baby in a sitting position on one knee, supporting his chin in one hand and patting his back with the other may work. Some mothers find they can "massage" a bubble up by gently rubbing baby's back and sides. Sometimes relief from pain comes by merely holding baby close and allowing skin-to-skin warmth to soothe the distended stomach. At other times, walking the infant about the room, head on shoulder, tummy against breast or chest, seems to help, possibly by distracting him from his pain. Here father can certainly be of aid, bringing welcome relief to a mother who has dealt all day with this distressing disorder.

If none of these methods works, some doctors offer a mild sedative to help baby sleep and pass the gas rectally. If they are not abused, some prescription drugs can give beneficial rest when nothing else seems to work. Parents should *avoid* all self-prescribed cures which involve drugs. Partial knowledge of a "cure" can lead to tragic results. For example, in late 1978 a Florida pediatrician asserted that a colic "cure" mentioned in a popular book on childhood nutrition caused the death of a four-month-old boy. The baby's mother, distraught from the cries of her colicky twin sons, crushed three grams of potassium chloride for each child, then dissolved the mineral in breast milk and attempted to give the twins the concoction. One twin refused the mixture and lived. The other drank the dose, vomited and became listless, then died of cardiac arrest in a hospital intensive-care unit. According to the pediatrician, the dose given was fifteen to twenty times more than a four-month-old infant could safely tolerate, and a check of the baby's blood showed the drug present at a toxic level.

Whether or not the mother managed to read and interpret correctly the cure mentioned is not really the issue at hand. In retrospect, it is easy to say that this parent should not have tried medicating the infant on the basis of experimental results mentioned in a guidebook. Yet the mother probably considered a "natural" mineral such as potassium perfectly safe for baby. Though the courts must decide who was at fault in this case, their decision will not restore the life which was lost.

Other parents can learn a valuable lesson from this tragedy. Vitamins and minerals in supplement (nonfood) form, whether natural or synthetic in name, should be considered as drugs and treated as such. No infant or child should receive vitamins and minerals except under a doctor's supervision and with his or her advice. Very possibly a doctor's more complete knowledge might shed life-saving light on a potentially deadly home remedy.

Even nondrug remedies may be dangerous for babies. For example, one popular home remedy involves dipping a pacifier in honey. Honey has recently been implicated in a number of cases of infant botulism, a disease with symptoms similar to those shown by sudden-infant-death-syndrome (SIDS) infants. (See page 83 for a more detailed discussion of infant botulism.) While there is currently no indication that honey poses health risks for older children or adults, a cautious mother should not use a honey-dipped pacifier to ease a young baby's colic pains.

Since most pediatricians feel that there is no miracle drug or food which can cure colic, they often advise parents to endure the malady gracefully— or, at least, as best they can. This advice, though it is sometimes frustrating, may be the best.

Certainly, many infants never exhibit any symptoms of this exasperating, ill-defined syndrome, but just as certainly, some babies *do* have colic. Mothers who are bottle-feeding must, of course, make certain that a milk allergy or some other formula problem does not exist. This can be extremely frustrating, according to one couple who tried every available formula without success. At three months, their baby suddenly got over gastric distress on his own.

While the breast-feeding mother escapes this problem, since she can be reasonably sure her milk is ideal for the baby, friends, relatives, and even her doctor may try to convince her that baby's distress means that her milk is insufficient for his needs. If she gives in to the pressure and starts to supplement with bottle-feeding, she not only risks causing her milk supply to diminish, she may also cause colic to worsen, due to the shift to unaccustomed formula. Even if she continues to breast-feed, she faces another, almost equally exasperating, dilemma. Could it be that something *she* ate caused baby to have gas pains?

Nursing mothers through the centuries have been warned against eating certain foods that might cause discomfort to the baby. Of course, everyone has a different opinion as to just which offender should be eliminated. Granny insists that a new mother should avoid chocolate. Auntie is just as sure that yesterday's Mexican food caused the problem. In reality, baby may be distressed for reasons totally unrelated to mother's diet.

La Leche International, the largest organization of breast-feeding women, suggests that a nursing mother should not feel that baby's every gas pain is caused by something mama ate. She should try not to feel guilty about eating foods which she has heard might bother her infant, since a nervous, guilt-ridden mother may help bring on a case of colic by transferring to the nursing baby her own anxieties about the foods she has eaten.

A mother who begins a nursing experience with positive attitudes about all foods is more likely to enjoy that experience than a mother who anticipates trouble from the start. The nursing mother should refuse the martyr's role. Instead, she should assume that a normal, well-balanced diet will be satisfactory for mother and baby, omitting certain foods only when she is convinced they are causing trouble.

No scientific method of isolating potential trouble-making foods has yet been devised. Too many variables exist to make a conclusive study of such matters possible. Digestive systems vary from mother to mother and from baby to baby. Highly spiced chili that causes heartburn for one woman may be consumed without ill effects by another. Conversely, the first mother's baby might show no signs of distress after a "second-hand" chili meal, while the second mother's child might scream as if in protest.

How can one be sure the chili caused baby's distress? Only by ruling out every other possible cause (a slight cold, earache, loss of sleep, etc.) *and* by trying two or three more chili meals to see whether similar reactions occur can a mother begin to say with certainty that eating chili bothers baby. Even then, her own fears that colic might occur could be causing more gastric distress to the baby than does the chili.

Actually, a mother who strongly suspects that a chili supper caused pain for baby and a sleepless night for mom and dad is unlikely to want to experiment by eating more chili. Usually, she simply avoids the food and declares, "It gives him colic." This is a perfectly logical path to follow, unless chili happens to be mom's favorite food. In that case, experimentation would be worthwhile, even though baby might react by howling once more. If all is calm after chili supper number two, then mother can usually continue to enjoy the dish.

A verbal survey of any group of nursing mothers usually yields a wide variety of foods avoided for baby's sake. The foods that are named most often may, indeed, *be* colic causers. On the other hand, they may be foods the mothers have been led to *believe* would cause colic. For whatever reasons, some foods do continue to be mentioned more than others.

Gas-causers for mom make up the largest single category. Whether or not some gas-causing element is actually transferred in breast milk, many mothers report problems after eating cabbage (cooked or raw), broccoli, baked beans, onions, fried foods, chocolate, canteloupe, watermelon, and spicy foods.

If a mother is firmly convinced that some food is causing gas for baby, she might choose to eliminate it from her diet. Provided some other equally nutritious food is substituted, this causes no health problems and may give peace of mind to an overanxious nursing mom. On the other hand, some mothers report that eating smaller portions of quality foods such as cantaloupe (high in vitamins C and A) and broccoli (high in fiber and vitamins) causes no distress to baby and allows more variety for mom. Furthermore, some women indicate that many foods which seemed to cause colic to a newborn had no adverse effect after the baby was three to four months old.

Studies concerning the effect of so-called gas-formers on adults have generally shown that gas formation is attributable not so much to individual foods as to the condition of the body that consumes those foods. Since the state of *two* bodies must be considered when evaluating the influence of maternal diet on an infant's digestive system, the probability is great that dietary intolerance for mother and baby is a matter of individual differences.

With this fact in mind, mothers whose systems do not tolerate certain foods will soon learn to avoid those foods, and mothers whose babies have systems which apparently do not tolerate certain "second-hand" foods soon learn to avoid those foods, too. There is no evidence to indicate that *all* nursing mothers should avoid eating certain foods. It's a matter of individual differences.

The most significant recent news concerning colic and breast-feeding babies is a report from Sweden which indicates that breast-feeding babies with intolerance to cow's-milk protein may develop colic if their mothers are drinking cows' milk or eating cow's-milk products. In 13 of 18 cases studied, colic promptly disappeared upon elimination of cow's milk protein from the mother's diet until the baby outgrows this intolerance.

While this treatment of infantile colic in breast-fed infants seems worth trying especially in families prone to allergies, a word of caution is in order. Elimination of all cow's-milk products from the diet of a breast-feeding mother will mean that both mother and child will be deprived of valuable nutrients (especially calcium riboflavin) unless care is taken to add those nutrients to the mother's diet in some other form. Consultation with a physician is advisable in such cases, a small price to pay for conquering that exasperating problem of colic.

For one young mother, finding her previously serene daughter colicky at three weeks was doubly exasperating, for she had long been convinced that colic was a myth, something frustrated mothers made up and mentally imposed on their babies. Furthermore, totally breast-fed babies supposedly didn't get colic. Weeks later, after many sleepless nights, she was no longer a disbeliever. Colic was real, all right, and it was a terror to deal with.

When the heretofore skeptical mother turned to a Korean neighbor for sympathy and advice, she was encouraged to look forward to the infant's

---

Jakobsson, Irene, and Tor Lindberg. "Cows' Milk As a Cause of Infantile Colic in Breast-fed Infants." *Lancet* 2 (August 26, 1978): 437–39.

hundredth day. In Korea, that day often marked the end of colic as well as the end of the critical newborn stage of life. Sure enough, the colic started disappearing shortly before the hundredth day.

Together the two women planned a "Hundred Days Party" for friends who were eager to share in the celebration of an end to the agony caused by the colic which so many people prefer to believe is "all in a mother's mind." Appropriately, a tiny Korean feeding spoon was baby's gift, since in Korea, mothers have traditionally begun to introduce solids to their babies after the third-month birthday.

## Diarrhea

A breast-feeding mom received a frantic midnight phone call from the mother of a breast-feeding friend. "I just *know* this baby's ill," the woman explained. "She's had a bowel movement every time Jan's nursed her and all of them were yellow and ran right out the diaper."

"Relax," came the confident answer, "that's a normal B.M. for a breast-fed baby. Don't worry about it, just learn how to do a *tight* diapering job!" Indeed, many totally breast-fed infants may have five to eight bowel movements a day, all of them the consistency described by the grandmother who'd bottle-fed her own children and therefore thought stools should be firm and brown. Mothers who don't wish to spend hours removing stains soon learn to adjust diapers for a tight fit around the legs and to offer water-proof pads to unsuspecting visitors.

True diarrhea, seen only infrequently in the totally breast-fed infant, is usually dark green in color, foul in odor and extremely watery. Sometimes after gastrointestinal illness accompanied by severe diarrhea, a baby on cow's-milk formula must avoid formula and take only water or a special pediatric electrolyte fluid until his system can again tolerate milk. Diarrhea which is unusually severe, is accompanied by high fever, or lasts beyond a few days should be discussed with a doctor. If it is allowed to continue it may lead to dehydration and even death.

## Constipation

As noted above, the totally breast-fed baby is not likely to be constipated! She may, however, experience changes in her B.M. schedule. After a few weeks, bowel movements may occur only every other day, yet they should still be fairly soft. This reduction in frequency may simply signify that baby is using almost all the nutrients available to her. If the stool is still soft, there is no reason to suspect constipation.

The bottle-fed infant whose formula suits his needs should also have easy bowel movements, though they are usually less frequent and more firm. Should a bottle-fed infant go for more than two or three days without a movement, and should he cry as if in pain, a call to the pediatrician is in order. Occasionally, cow's-milk formulas form hard-to-pass stools and emergency treatment may be necessary. Generally, constipation is not a worry for bottle-fed or breast-fed babies during the first three months.

## Infantile Obesity

When infants are totally breast-fed, infantile obesity is rarely a concern during the early months of life. On the other hand, bottle-fed infants whose formulas are too concentrated or who are being forced to drink more than they really need may be on the road toward obesity.

Studies show that bottle-fed infants gain more rapidly than do breast-fed ones, yet not all bottle-fed infants become obese in later life and not all breast-fed infants remain slender. Bottle-fed infants who are allowed to help regulate their own calorie intakes, who are allowed to say no to the last ounce or two of feeding, and who are *not* given excess calories in the form of solid foods stand an excellent chance of avoiding infantile obesity. This, as a later discussion of obesity will show, is a vital first step in avoiding juvenile, adolescent, and adult obesity.

Biggest is not necessarily best. "Oh, what a fine fat baby" is no longer a compliment to the mother's good care of baby nor a sign of baby's good health.

Food attitudes and habits start at birth. Parents who short-circuit a baby's developing appetite-control mechanism and encourage gluttony may be setting the pattern for a lifetime of overeating. Feed her with love, but don't teach her that the quantity of food given is an indication of the quantity of love extended.

# Practical Meals and Snacks

The newborn makes no distinction between meals and snacks. His hunger pains tell him he needs food, his cry alerts his parents to that fact, and, ideally, his parents satisfy his need for food as soon as possible. Fortunately, few doctors still recommend the rigid scheduling with which our mothers struggled. Generally, doctors recommend feeding a baby when he cries for food, whether or not the "normal" number of hours have yet elapsed.

Recently, the same breast-feeding mother whose baby was thought to have "*terrible* diarrhea" called her friend on another matter. "Ann's had me up all night again. I just can't stand it anymore. The nurse at the hospital said don't feed her more than every four hours, but she starts to cry every three hours and cries for a solid hour every time. What on earth should I do?"

Of course, the more experienced friend suggested that the baby should be fed when she was hungry. Apparently, no one had told little Ann about the four-hour schedule, and she was operating on one of her own. Within a day, mother and daughter were settled into a routine of feeding which sometimes meant four- or even four-and-a-half-hour intervals, but sometimes meant only two-to-three-hour lapses between feedings.

One recent study indicates that breast-feeding mothers who offer feedings at two-hour intervals during the early post-partum period, then allow "on-

demand" feedings thereafter tend to establish lactation sooner and to continue breast-feeding longer than do mothers who attempt to limit the number
of feedings an infant is allowed. That same study recommends continuing
night feedings through the first few months of life, rather than trying to
eliminate them, since the baby's suckling helps establish lactation.

Furthermore, recent studies question the advisability of rushing a child
into a pattern of large, infrequent meals. There is increasing evidence that
large meals at infrequent intervals may promote increased deposit of body
fat, even when calorie intake is less than that of persons eating smaller
amounts of food at more frequent intervals. Increased serum cholesterol
levels and impaired glucose tolerance have been noted in adults who were
fed large meals at wide intervals. Thus, urging an infant to sleep through the
night and to move into a three-meal-a-day routine may not be in that
infant's best interest.

Whether breast- or bottle-fed, babies have different needs at different
times of day. Generally, they seem to nurse longer and go longer between
feedings in the early hours of the day, then demand shorter, more frequent
feedings late in the afternoon and up until midnight. As long as approximately the recommended number of ounces are taken over twenty-four
hours, no one need worry about whether they are taken in *equal*-sized feedings.

Ironically, late afternoons and evenings, hungry times for most babies,
are the very times when a breast-feeding mother is *least* likely to be able to
relax and give the extra love which all those feeding sessions require. When
possible, she should nap or at least rest when baby naps in the early afternoon, thereby giving herself a break before the intense late feedings start.

Babies have low-appetite days and high-appetite days. Brief growth spurts
may cause high intake, while hot weather or too many visitors may cause
low intake. At around three months of age, a pronounced growth spurt
usually occurs. Breast-feeding moms may find baby suddenly wants to nurse
every couple of hours. If he is allowed to do so, the hungry infant stimulates
the breast enough to signal the body to increase milk production. If a
mother's postnatal fatty reserves have been used up by this time, she, too,
may find herself ravenous. As her milk production increases to meet baby's
new demands, she may need to include one or two snacks or extra helpings
to keep her from losing weight too fast and being too tired to meet her needs
and those of her baby. Nursing is a calorie-costly job!

Letting baby suckle more often during his growth spurt or merely letting
him create his own schedule rather than forcing him to comply with the
standard schedule handed out by the prenatal care center or pediatrician's
office may be easier said than done. Friends, parents, or even doctors may
tell a mother, "You're spoiling that baby rotten," the same line which is
often leveled at a mother who rocks a colicky baby and refuses to let him cry
it out.

There is no way to "spoil" a three-month-old baby. At this age, an infant is testing her environment. She has needs—to be fed, changed or just spoken to and cuddled. She has pain—hunger, gas distress, or a sudden feeling of isolation. She reaches out with her cry, calling to the world outside herself.

If her cry brings response in the form of a parent who determines the baby's need and goes about satisfying it as soon as possible, her confidence in her environment is increased. She realizes that she can call again, and she will be responded to. Someone out there *cares* about her needs. If her cries are ignored, if her hunger or her dampness or her pain is not dealt with, she may respond in anger, trying desperately to break down the barrier, to get through to the people "out there." Such a baby suddenly *demands* what she has previously asked for and been refused. Thus, the aggressive, demanding baby is most often the one who has been ignored, not the one whose needs have been met.

Or, the ignored child may stop asking. She may withdraw and begin building a shell which will protect her from the emptiness and lack of response she has felt—and which will also keep her estranged from the parents with whom she should be most intimate.

Meeting a child's needs is *not* spoiling. Loving and cuddling a crying infant or a colicky one is *not* spoiling. Spending longer than absolutely necessary at feeding time is *not* spoiling. Through feeding an infant with love and with an understanding of that tiny person's physical and psychological needs, a parent is conveying, to even the youngest baby, wholesome, healthy attitudes toward food that should form the basis for a lifetime of good eating.

# 4
# Infancy—Three to Six Months

By the age of three months, a baby has usually adjusted well to the breast milk or formula she is receiving and has settled into a comfortable feeding schedule, preferably one of her own making. Her growth rate is still rapid and she is likely to experience rapid growth periods during which she will need more calories. Parents who ignore baby's new needs because they don't fit the feeding schedule the doctor suggested are likely to be in for a few long nights. Those who resist the temptation to force an infant into a set feeding routine and are ready and willing to listen when baby's cries indicate she needs more formula more often will probably be able to satisfy these new demands easily.

## Meeting Nutrient Needs
A review of the RDA chart on page 36 and of Chapter 3's subsequent discussion of nutrient needs should provide excellent background for placing in proper perspective the following information concerning RDAs for three to six month olds. That chapter's discussion of preparation of bottles and of choice and preparation of formula should also be reviewed, especially by mothers who have totally breast-fed their babies for the first three months of life but now wish to begin supplementing breast-milk feedings with formula feedings.

### Calories
From three to six months of age, milk should still be an infant's chief source of energy (calories). While the *protein, fat,* and *carbohydrate* distributions of human milk are ideal, those of formulas can be satisfactory, too. If an infant is weaned from breast to bottle during this time, most doctors now recommend that he be given a formula, not whole or skim pasteurized cow's milk. A baby's intestinal walls, still unready for the complex job of complete digestion of whole milk, may be damaged by an early use of milk, resulting in undetected but potentially significant internal hemorrhaging.

Furthermore, some researchers feel that late-life atherosclerosis may be linked to early feeding of whole cow's milk to infants. Skim milk is not acceptable either, since its fat-protein-carbohydrate proportions are far from those considered ideal for an infant. As Dr. Samuel Fomon has noted, infants fed skim milk may appear to thrive, even though weight gain is less and calorie intake is lower than normal. Nevertheless, Dr. Fomon feels that bodily stores of fat are being used to meet day-to-day energy needs, so that such infants may be at risk in the event of an illness which curtails food intake. Furthermore, the infant who learns to drink large volumes of skim milk to satisfy his hunger may be developing a habit of overeating.

As noted earlier, formulas should be prepared in the recommended concentrations, lest mild obesity or more severe health problems result. If breast-feeding continues to be the chief source of baby's nourishment beyond three months, a mother's fatty reserves will probably be depleted. Usually her own appetite will alert her to the fact that she needs a further increase in calories if she is to produce an adequate supply of milk and maintain her energy at a desirable level. Later, as baby begins to wean herself, a mother should remember that she must wean *herself* as well, gradually cutting down the number of calories she consumes without leaving out the foods essential to her good health and continued milk production.

## Vitamins

A detailed overview of the vitamin content of various milks and formulas was given in the preceding chapter. By referring to that chapter, parents of an older infant can learn the strong and weak points of their chosen milk for baby. In most cases, multivitamin preparations should not be given to an infant who is receiving an approved formula or breast milk unless need has been determined by a physician.

As baby begins to show an interest in solids, strained fruit may provide added vitamins, and, as the chart below indicates, most infants will accept fruits by this age. However, a parent should remember that strained fruits are relatively high in carbohydrates and may raise baby's caloric intake beyond desirable levels unless milk intakes are reduced enough to offset the addition of fruits.

### Acceptance of Various Solids

| Type of Solid | Likely Age of Willing Acceptance |
|---|---|
| Cereals | 2½–3½ months |
| Fruits | 2½–3 months |
| Vegetables | 4–4½ months |
| Meats, meat soups | 5½–6 months |

SOURCE: Adapted from V. A. Beal, "On the Acceptance of Solid Foods and Other Food Patterns of Infants and Children," *Pediatrics* 20 (September 1957): 448–456. Copyright ©American Academy of Pediatrics, 1957.

The totally breast-fed baby receives 35 to 55 percent of his calories in the form of carbohydrates. Early introduction of solids substantially raises the percentage of sucrose and other carbohydrates in the infant's diet and, as the chart below indicates, strained fruits are prime contributors to the carbohydrate load.

## Carbohydrate Percentage of Various Infant Foods

| Food | % of Calories from Carbohydrates |
| --- | --- |
| Breast milk | 37% |
| Cow's milk | 29 |
| Formulas | 42 |
| Meats (strained) | 1 |
| High-meat dinners | 29 |
| Soups and dinners (strained) | 56 |
| Vegetables (strained) | 80 |
| Desserts (strained) | 89 |
| Fruits (strained) | 96 |

SOURCE: Derived from Samuel S. Fomon, *Infant Nutrition,* 2d ed., (Philadelphia: W. B. Saunders, 1974).

Vegetables, though vitamin rich, should probably not be tried this early. Baby's sensitive taste buds may reject their strong flavors now, whereas waiting a few weeks or months might mean a more ready acceptance of these important foods. Furthermore, some vegetables are high in nitrates, which, after preparation and during storage, may be acted upon by bacteria that convert them to nitrites. As mentioned earlier, infants younger than six months of age are susceptible to methemoglobinemia, a potentially fatal disease which interferes with oxygen transport. This disease is caused by excessive nitrites in food or water.

Vitamin-rich beet or spinach purees, carrot soups, and carrot juices may all be quite high in nitrates. Since home-prepared versions of these foods are likely to be processed under less sterile conditions than are commercial baby foods, they usually contain more of the bacteria which are able to convert nitrates to potentially dangerous nitrites. There is no reason to feed these particular vegetables to infants under six months of age, and in view of the potential nitrite problem, parents should save these foods for later introduction. Generally, laboratory tests have shown that commercially prepared, strained versions of these vegetables are not high in nitrites when they are first opened, but allowing jars of these vegetables to stand unrefrigerated for several hours after opening may cause development of nitrites. This is especially true if the container is left open or if bacteria are introduced to the container by use of an inadequately cleaned feeding spoon.

Many meats, such as ham, luncheon meats, bacon, and hot dogs, are high in nitrates (and nitrites) because of the preservatives which have been added to them. These meats should *not* be pureed into homemade baby-food dishes for infants younger than six months.

## Minerals

As the mineral overview in Chapter 3 indicates, fortified formulas and breast milk provide a newborn with adequate amounts of essential minerals. This statement holds true for babies up to six months, with the possible addition of iron. Prenatal iron supplies begin to diminish when an infant is three to six months of age. This fact has caused many doctors to advise bottle-feeding mothers to move to a fortified formula or begin iron-rich solid foods by at least six months of age. Mothers who use iron-fortified formula need not also use iron-fortified cereals.

Until recently, many doctors have recommended that breast-fed babies receive iron supplements or begin to eat iron-rich foods at around three months of age. Though it is true that breast milk has less iron than cow's milk, apparently some factor in breast milk aids in iron absorption. For example, while less than 4 percent of the iron in cow's-milk formulas is absorbed by an infant, around 50 percent of the iron in breast milk is absorbed.

Furthermore, while infants given a 5-milligram dose of iron in cow's milk were able to absorb only 4 percent, iron absorption was increased to 18 percent when that same amount of iron was given with breast milk.

In view of the excellent absorption of the available iron in breast milk, and due to the fact that breast-fed infants generally show no evidence of iron deficiency prior to six months of age, some authorities now feel that there is no need to introduce iron-rich foods or to give iron supplements to full-term babies until after six months of age. The routine prescription of iron to full-term, normal weight, breast-fed infants now seems open to question, especially if iron-rich foods are introduced toward the end of the first six months. There is some evidence that oversaturating the iron-binding lactoferrin in breast milk will inactivate this valuable natural means of warding off gastrointestinal disorders.

Since breast-fed babies do not seem to be iron deficient, and since there is increasing evidence that the relatively low amounts of iron they receive in human milk are extremely well utilized, why risk overloading their systems with iron? In this case, prescribing iron supplements "just to be on the safe side" may actually lower an infant's resistance to disease. Despite this new evidence, some leading authorities in pediatric nutrition still feel strongly that iron supplements should be used routinely for breast-fed babies.

As in most other matters, the needs of a particular baby should be thoroughly assessed by a physician before the question of iron supplementation for that baby is settled. Some premature infants may need iron supplements shortly after birth, but such supplements must be given only under a doctor's supervision. Parent-prescribed iron supplements may interfere with vitamin E utilization, and such interference could be especially dangerous for premature infants.

A mother who is worried about her infant's iron intake might wish to introduce iron-fortified cereals during the three- to six-month period. Since cereals are relatively high in carbohydrates, a parent might wish to consult a pediatrician about making a slight decrease in baby's formula intake at the time cereals are introduced. Unfortunately, very young infants judge satiety by volume and have little or no feel for the number of calories being offered to them. Thus, a baby may take as much high-calorie cereal as he would low-calorie milk, especially if the cereal is diluted with familiar formula and fed in a bottle or syringe. For this reason, spoon-feeding is recommended for even the first introduction of solid foods.

A parent should realize that the calories in solid baby foods are part of the entire day's allotment. While a very active infant who is beginning to roll and pull himself along at four or five months of age might be able to consume the extra calories offered in added cereal feedings plus full milk feedings, an inactive infant might gain excess pounds with the addition of relatively few extra calories per day.

If cereals are to be given chiefly for their iron value, a mother should be sure that the iron is in the form of easily absorbed ferrous sulfate or particle-sized electrolytic iron powder. Cereals specifically intended for infants usually have iron in a readily absorbable form, while those intended for older children and adults may contain iron which is not so readily absorbed. For example, sodium iron pyrophosphate and ferric orthophosphate are poorly absorbed iron sources which should *not* be relied upon. Shaking the cereal box well before each serving is measured may help insure more uniform distribution of iron. Adding milk rather than water means the cereal will provide more satisfactory nutrition, and adding breast milk is even better because of breast milk's ability to enhance iron absorption. Sugar or honey should *never* be added to infant cereals, since nothing is gained thereby except extra calories and adding sugar now may lead baby to develop a preference for sweet foods. Bottled or strained cereals or strained cereals with fruit are usually not a nutritionally or economically wise buy, since they have far less iron than do dry cereals.

## Salt

The sodium content of cow's milk is more than four times that of human milk. Therefore, infants on cow's-milk formula may be receiving more sodium than they really need, especially in view of studies linking high intakes of sodium with hypertension (high blood pressure) in later life. Giving a baby commercial baby food meant, up until recently, adding still more sodium to an infant's diet. Even though the amount of salt in baby foods is not likely to be immediately harmful, there is concern that salt in baby foods may teach a baby that foods must be salty to be flavorful. Strong protests against manufacturers' addition of salt to baby foods led Heinz and Beechnut to discontinue the addition of salt altogether, with Gerber moving toward total elimination of added salt in late 1978.

Home-prepared infant foods can and should be relatively low in sodium content, though some added salt will be present if canned or frozen foods are used. In fact, a recent study showed that the salt content of baby foods prepared at home far exceeded that of commercial baby foods. If family food is prepared from fresh or frozen vegetables and fruits and if baby's portion is removed before the remaining amount is salted, infant salt intakes may be kept to appropriate levels.

## Psychological Factors in Feeding

As a mother continues the communication of love she began during the early breast-feeding or bottle-feeding months, baby's security is further strengthened. Feeding time is still a very personal, very special time for one-to-one contact. It's a time for giving and receiving love and care in ways that will have long-lasting effects on how a child feels about herself and her world.

Parents who know their infant is receiving optimum nourishment should be pleased with that infant's growth and development even if that development does not equal that of a friend's or neighbor's child. Biggest is not always best. For example, the father who is delighted to find his bottle-fed son gaining weight much faster than the breast-fed baby boy across the street may not be so delighted when that "fine fat baby" turns into a butterball at age six or seven and remains soft and pudgy throughout adolescence. Conversely, the mother of a breast-fed child whose weight-gain is not as great as that of the baby down the street should not despair because her little one is "behind." Most bottle-fed babies grow one to three ounces a week faster than do most breast-fed babies for about the first 112 days of life. However, there is no indication that this means growth-stunting for the breast-fed baby or adult obesity for the bottle-fed baby. The rate difference is probably due to a difference in caloric rather than nutrient content of the diet. Breast-feeding mothers don't urge an infant to drink the last ounce, while formula-feeding mothers often do. Since such urging may help develop a habit of overeating, mothers should, within reason, let baby decide when he has had enough to drink.

Provided that a baby's size at birth and rate of gain after birth are within the average range, parents should accept their individual infant's growth and be proud of the child. Avoiding early comments such as "You're a runt, little boy. Eat more and get big enough to play football!" and "My, you're really a *big* girl. Where's that dainty little girl we ordered?" will prevent any chance of these attitudes being conveyed to the child when he or she is old enough to understand them. Acceptance by parents is vital if a child is to learn to feel good about himself. For older children, adverse comments about size or weight during meals can give negative connotations to food in general, sometimes with disastrous results.

As soon as baby is able to sit in a sturdy infant chair or to be secured properly in a high chair, she can become a part of family mealtime. Often a relatively heavy, safety-shell-type car seat provides the perfect resting place, since a young baby can be strapped in and is not likely to tip the heavy seat over. As she watches other people eating, especially siblings, an infant gains interest in trying something new herself. Perhaps she can be allowed to mouth and taste a spoon, giving her growing curiosity room to operate still more fully.

Once the first taste of solids is offered, the family shouldn't be unduly surprised if baby blows out the food or sucks at the spoon, then spits in disgust or annoyance. She has to learn to deal with this strange new method of feeding and should soon settle down to eating, unless family members laugh or otherwise encourage her antics. Parents should approach feeding time with an attitude of confidence and anticipation—"Of course, you're going to enjoy your first taste of applesauce!" Parental attitudes are definitely conveyed to a child, even a very young infant.

Of course, when baby seems to dislike the applesauce and refuses to open her mouth for it after two small bites, staying "positive" seems a bit more difficult! Patience is the key to success. Forcing the food through tightly closed lips will only make mealtime a time of conflict. Waiting until another meal and then trying again is probably the wisest route. After all, since for the average child there is no nutritional reason for beginning any solid food until five to six months of age, there is certainly no need to force a child to take what she does not want.

The same rule holds true for the child who likes and accepts applesauce but indicates that he is satisfied when his dish still has one or two teaspoonfuls left. Usually if mother insists that those last two bites be taken, baby will obey, but to do so may be to introduce the idea that one determines when to stop eating by how much food is left on the dish. This attitude may lead to habitual overeating and subsequent obesity. You can avoid waste by dishing up only small amounts of food, then adding more if baby wants more. In this way, a child's appetite-control mechanism can be allowed to develop naturally, not being short-circuited by well-meant but unwise force-feeding.

Parents who avoid the "eat the last bite" hassle from infancy will go far toward keeping mealtime pleasant for all. The fewer conflicts the better. Adult quarrels should also be avoided at the table. Family arguments destroy the peaceful atmosphere so essential to good digestion and to a good attitude about meals. Not even a six-month-old enjoys hearing two people he loves engaged in a heated argument. Starting early makes setting a pleasant mealtime example easier when children are older and even more likely to be disturbed by mealtime hassles.

# Common Problems

While more and more parents are delaying the introduction of solids until at least six months of age, for others, the introduction of solids is the important nutrition project during baby's fourth, fifth, and sixth months of life. Whenever parents choose to begin solids, they should do so by offering a single food for about a week before moving on to another new food. In this way, they will be able to watch for any signs of food allergy (diarrhea, rash, etc.) and will be more likely to know which food caused the problem. Mixed foods ought to be saved until the period of sensitivity testing is over.

Doctors usually begin by recommending rice cereal, then suggest moving on to other cereals (barley, oatmeal, mixed cereal, and high-protein infant cereals), fruits and vegetables, and then meat. Up until recently, if a mother's main concern was to add an iron-rich food relatively low in carbohydrates, she might have been advised to try the yolk of a boiled egg. Although egg yolk does contain iron, recent evidence suggests that the iron is not easily absorbed by infants. As noted earlier, infant cereal with iron offers an excellent means of increasing baby's intake of this important mineral.

Should baby develop a rash after eating some new food, this does not mean she will remain allergic forever. A young baby's digestive system sometimes just isn't quite mature enough to handle a new food. Thus, another test in a few months may show no adverse reaction to the food.

One important reminder should be added concerning the addition of foods other than formula or human milk to baby's diet. As noted in the previous chapter, recent research has shown that a significant number of California infants fed honey (whether in homemade formulas, as a remedy for colic, for vitamin value, or for supposed allergy control) developed infant botulism. Infant botulism is a disease resulting from the production of botulinal toxin within the intestinal tracts of infants under six to eight months of age. Most adults are familiar with other forms of botulism which occur when food containing botulinal toxin is ingested. In the United States between 1800 and 1977, 2000 cases of food-borne botulism were reported. Before 1949, 60 percent of those cases were fatal. The disease still claims lives, though only 15.7 percent of food-borne botulism cases are currently fatal.

A baby need not ingest botulinal toxin in order to become a victim of infant botulism. Instead, he may ingest *Clostridium botulinum,* an organism common in soil, in the air, and on many foods. If ingested by older children, teens, or adults, *C. botulinum* isn't usually harmful, for the mature human intestinal tract does not provide an environment favorable to germination of the *C. botulinum* spores. In an infant's nonacidic intestinal tract, however, these spores readily germinate, and potentially fatal botulinal toxin is formed. The toxin is carried by the blood to target nerves, and the infant may die before symptoms can be noticed and a diagnosis made.

Indeed, early symptoms of this disease are not so alarming as to cause a parent to rush an infant to a doctor. Constipation, poor feeding, lethargy, weakness, pooled saliva in the mouth, floppiness, loss of head control, weakened crying, and respiratory inefficiency have been observed in infants with this disorder. However, the symptoms are often recalled retrospectively, after the child has suffered fatal respiratory failure due to paralysis of air ways and respiratory organs. In some instances, infant botulism deaths may have first been labeled SIDS (Sudden Infant Death Syndrome). In California, 4.3 of SIDS infants examined harbored *C. Botulinum* spores, while these spores were not found in the intestinal tracts of normal, healthy infants.

Though other foods may cause infant botulism, in thirteen of the forty-three documented cases of this disease reported in California between 1976 and 1978, the infants had histories of honey ingestion before the onset of the constipation that is usually the first symptom of infant botulism. Among ingested foods tested, only honey was found to have *C. botulinum,* and none of the contaminated honey contained preformed botulinal toxin. Because *C. botulinum* spores are heat resistant, even moderately well-cooked foods containing honey may be dangerous to an infant.

Widespread interest in the use of honey versus refined sugar may lead to other such tragedies unless mothers are warned to avoid adding honey to formulas or solid foods or feeding it directly to young infants. When sixty California honey specimens were tested, 13 percent were shown to have *C. botulinum* organisms. Since there is no way for a homemaker to tell whether the honey she is using is contaminated and since honey is not an essential food, the California Department of Health has concurred with the recommendation of the Sioux Honey Association that honey should not be fed to infants under one year of age.

As noted earlier, the environment of the digestive tract of older children and adults apparently does not foster germination of the *C. botulinum* spores and subsequent production of the toxin. Therefore, honey which contains no preformed toxin, yet does contain *C. botulinum* spores, has not been linked to botulism in older children, teens, and adults.

## Dental Problems

A teething baby can often be soothed by allowing her to chew on a cold object such as a frozen popsicle made of unflavored gelatin, well mashed banana, and water. This popsicle won't melt as fast as a conventional one and does not have added sugar. If the popsicle is made in a popular, commercially available plastic holder, the ringed handle can be gripped by an infant as young as five or six months of age. The coolness and firmness of this tasty treat make it a favorite with teething babies.

Early teethers should never be given a bottle in the crib, for the slow action of the oozing milk on the teeth of the sleeping baby may lead to "nursing bottle caries," a serious but avoidable dental problem discussed more fully in the next section. Of course, giving a baby younger than six months of age a bottle in the crib means propping that bottle, as the child is not able to hold it herself. This practice is undesirable for other reasons than tooth decay—it removes the loving parent from the feeding scene; it may mean food is being used to "pacify" baby, not just nourish her; and it may result in accidental strangulation.

Doctor Benjamin Spock has noted that babies allowed to take their bottles to bed by themselves at this age become more attached than ever to the bottle in the last months of their first year, when other infants are becoming less interested in a bottle. This may be because the bottle has become a mother substitute. Mother is no longer holding and cuddling, and the bottle is all the baby has left. Such babies are very hard to wean from their bottles, and, as will be noted later, toddlers who go to sleep with their nighttime bottles are prime candidates for painful "nursing bottle caries."

## Practical Meals and Snacks

As in the case of the very young infant, the three- to six-month-old child learns how to react to life by how life reacts to him. If he cries to be fed and his needs are met, he learns love and trust.

By the age of four or five months, some infants seem ready to drop one of their daytime feedings and move toward three meals a day. Others still seem to need four bottles or feedings. As noted earlier, smaller, more frequent meals may be desirable. An infant should not be rushed into a schedule which conforms to the meal patterns of other family members. Unless solids are a regular part of baby's daily routine, he will probably not be actually eating all meals with the family, though he may be sitting in an infant seat or high chair and observing the family eating habits. Later, when solids are given several times a day, he will begin to feel comfortable with waiting until the others eat. For now, his own personal feeding schedule is the only one of real importance to him. Unless there are pressing reasons not to honor that schedule, life will probably be happier for baby and family if no rigid, adult-imposed schedule is begun. After all, baby's hunger pains are real, and his stomach may be ignoring the clock and setting up rules of its own. In actuality, a four-meal plan is probably easier for mom than a three-meal plan, since baby should be held and cuddled when he is breast- or bottle-fed and this means mama's meals are likely to grow cold before baby has finished nursing.

There is every reason to let an interested baby of five or even four months take a sip or two of formula from a cup during family meals. In this way, he begins to understand that milk comes in a cup, not just from bottle or breast. A breast-fed baby may be given breast milk, water, or (if no allergies are indicated) a bit of formula. This early experience with the cup helps baby feel a part of family meals without giving him food in which he has shown no interest and for which he may not yet be ready. Mealtimes are also good times to offer baby homemade banana-gelatin teething popsicles.

Since baby is becoming more and more interested in her surroundings, she may prefer "people-watching" to feeding. This may pose problems for the breast-feeding mother. Though an efficient baby can get all the breast milk she needs in about five minutes, her reduced suckling time may mean her mother's milk supply will soon diminish. To combat this, she may want to prolong the feeding session by nursing in a quiet room away from the distraction of other people.

Generally, baby profits so much from interaction with others that she should be allowed as much face-to-face contact as possible. Though mealtime with three-year-old brother entertaining four-month-old sister with a constant stream of patter may not be as quiet as mom and dad might like, such meals are the basis for healthy socialization. Relaxed, pleasant mealtimes make children eager to assemble at the table, whereas strict, ritualistic ones may make a small child less and less interested in eating. Even baby's earliest impressions will likely be lasting ones, so smile!

# 5
## Infancy—Six to Eighteen Months

As of 1973, only 5 percent of American infants were breast-fed at the age of six months. Moving from breast to bottle by the age of six months may be necessitated by the mother's health or some other equally pressing circumstance. Unfortunately, such a move usually means a double weaning process—first from breast to bottle, later from bottle to cup. Since nursing after six months takes relatively little time from mother's busy schedule and saves a great deal of time in formula preparation and bottle washing, it seems more logical to let baby drink from a cup at will, yet nurse at the breast to fulfill suckling needs and provide additional milk.

Nursing an older baby has medical advantages as well, since a baby with a gastrointestinal disorder may be unable to digest milk or even formula, but may be able to tolerate breast milk quite well. Since mother's milk is ideally suited to his needs, even a child who has been fed intraveneously and allowed nothing by mouth for forty-eight hours or more will have a head start on recovery if breast milk is his first meal after such an ordeal.

Most pediatricians feel that infants formerly breast-fed and weaned to cup or bottle before twelve months of age should be weaned to formula, not to unaltered cow's milk. In many cases, a baby's intestines are still not mature enough to digest unmodified cow's milk without risk of intestinal bleeding. Though such hemorrhaging may go undetected for months, it may lead to iron-deficiency anemia or other problems. Absorption of fat begins to reach adult levels between the sixth and ninth months of age, and most infants are able to tolerate unaltered, whole cow's milk after one year of age. Once an infant is old enough for whole milk, pasteurized milk is recommended over raw milk. For safety's sake, homemade yogurt should begin with pasteurized, not raw, milk.

If goat's milk is to be used for children of any age, parents should ask their physicians about suitable folic-acid supplements to avoid the risk of megaloblastic anemia. Since high folic acid intake can mask pernicious anemia, supplements should be taken *only* under a doctor's supervision. Skim milk should be avoided before the age of two years, since its low fat content means daily fat intake will be below the desired range of 30 to 55 percent of total calorie intake. Some pediatricians recommend 2-percent milk for infants who are overweight, but others feel that use of 2-percent milk may result in a baby's learning to drink larger amounts of milk than normal, a practice which may lead to the habit of overeating. While some manufacturers offer a special formula for the older than twelve-month baby, most pediatricians agree that whole milk is quite acceptable for the average toddler beyond one year of age.

For the six- to eight-month-old baby, protein, carbohydrate, and fat distributions should be those discussed earlier (see charts on pp. 36 and 109), with energy intake approximately those of RDA but varied to meet individual needs and circumstances. If height and weight gains are within expected ranges, a child's calorie intake is probably satisfactory. Usually, baby's appetite can be trusted to give clues as to how much he needs to eat and drink, though an infant who has become accustomed to adult-instigated overeating may not be able to control his own eating.

Baby's appetite-control mechanism must also begin to cope with solid food at this time. Ideally, *beikost* (from a German word meaning "additional foods") should complement the milk or formula which baby receives and provide vitamins and minerals as well as fat, protein, and carbohydrate.

Many breast-feeding mothers choose to introduce bland foods such as bananas, pureed apples, or pears first, feeling that solids for the breast-fed infant under nine months of age are a taste treat, not a nutritional necessity. On the other hand, some start with pureed meat, giving baby iron and protein, two foods of special importance at this age. Others use iron-enriched cereal. Some introduce the yolk of a boiled egg, assuming this food will provide the baby with iron. Since recent research indicates that the iron in eggs may not be readily absorbed, egg yolk should not be relied upon as an infant's sole source of this valuable mineral. As noted earlier, vegetables have very strong flavors and should probably not be among baby's first solid foods.

Once you choose and offer the first solid food to baby, that same food should be offered periodically during a seven- to ten-day period. During this time, you should watch for any sign of food allergy. If none is evident, another new food may be tried in the same way. This means baby may be receiving only one new food a week for several months, but serving a wide variety of new items at once means there's no opportunity to note allergic reactions and report them to the doctor. Allergy detection is far easier now than it will be later.

Ironically, advertisements are currently suggesting that a new mixed cereal from one of the major baby-food companies should be baby's "first step to solid feeding." Touted as "the complete infant food," this cereal comes in such combinations as rice-banana, wheat-orange, and wheat–

mixed-fruit. Using any of these combinations means complicating the detection of food allergies. Further, an infant who is syringe-fed this superfood will learn nothing about the textures, flavors, odors, and appearances of individual foods. Nor will she have any of the spoon-feeding experience vital to the self-feeding attempts she should be making within a few short months. Since this apparent shortcut to "complete nutrition" may lead to feeding problems later, it is no shortcut at all.

There is no *one* food which can offer optimum nutrient content plus the experience baby should gain by trying individual foods. If a wide variety of fruits, meats, breads, and vegetables is gradually introduced to a six- to nine-month-old, that baby's *vitamin* needs should be easily met. Juices may also be added to baby's diet, especially citrus juices high in vitamin C.

At this point, a mother generally decides whether to use commercial strained baby foods, pureed home-prepared foods, or a combination of the two. Fortunately, recent improvements in commercial baby foods mean that a mother who decides to buy ready-to-use baby food can offer her infant a well-balanced diet, provided she takes the time to read jar labels and choose foods carefully.

Certainly there are many times when the convenience of commercial foods makes them highly desirable. For example, carrying home-prepared foods on a long trip with baby makes refrigeration necessary. For formula-feeding mothers who take along formula in an ice chest, storing baby's solid foods in that same chest is relatively easy. On the other hand, breast-feeding mothers may find that relying upon commerical baby foods is easier than taking along an ice chest just for solids. The same may be true for formula-feeding mothers who use the small, ready-to-feed bottles on trips or for those who carry large containers of water plus sterile bottles with the pre-scribed amount of unmixed, powdered formula in them. Though there's no need to refrigerate jars of commercial baby food before opening, any unused food should be discarded unless it can be refrigerated immediately.

Though commercial baby foods are more convenient, many mothers prefer to prepare baby's food themselves. Some make this decision because they object to the nonessential items added to baby foods. Until 1969, monosodium glutamate was still being added to infant foods. Though this additive has since been eliminated, others that cause concern to parents, pediatricians, and nutritionists are still being used. In general commercial baby foods have fewer additives than many commercial foods consumed by children and adults. For example, most commerical baby foods no longer use sodium nitrate and nitrite as preservatives.

As mentioned earlier, added salt has been a point of controversy for some time. In 1977, the Heinz and Beechnut companies began to produce lines entirely free of added salt, and by late 1978, Gerber was moving toward a salt-free line. If a mother reads labels carefully and buys only those foods without added salt, she need not worry about the sodium content of commercial baby foods.

The question of the safety of certain modified starches added to baby foods has recently been raised. Modified starches help prevent the separation of baby foods that is likely to occur when baby is fed directly from a baby-food jar and the remaining food in that jar is kept for reuse. Amylase, a digestive enzyme in baby's saliva, is transferred to the container by the feeding spoon. This digestive enzyme breaks down unmodified starches in the stored food, causing the food to separate and appear watery. Modified starches aren't easily broken down by amylase; therefore, stored food with modified starch is less likely to become watery. Whether starches such as these are potentially harmful to baby remains a debatable question. Though a 1970 National Research Council Committee did not recommend restrictions on the use of these starches, committees from other organizations (notably the World Health Organization) have since suggested limits on the daily intake of several of these starches.

The latest available word on the subject of modified starches in infant foods comes from the American Academy of Pediatrics. In 1978, the AAP's subcommittee on evaluation of modified starches in infant foods noted that at least two of the chemicals being used to modify starches in infant foods are known to be either carcinogenic or mutagenic, and recommended that food manufacturers not use these chemicals until further studies are done. Since the digestability of modified starches by very young babies remains an unknown factor, some experts question the use of commercial infant foods containing modified starches by infants younger than six months of age.

Under ordinary conditions, infants younger than six months will not be receiving solid foods—whether commercial or home-prepared. Furthermore, modified starches to prevent food separation shouldn't really be needed, for mothers should never feed baby directly from a jar of baby food unless they plan to dispose of any leftover food in the jar. Bacteria, as well as digestive enzymes, can be transferred from mouth to spoon to jar, and some of these bacteria can hasten spoilage of foods, especially if the leftover portion is not promptly refrigerated. Also, if an entire jar of food is heated and baby eats only one-third of that jar, the food may be reheated several times before the food is consumed. With each heating, valuable vitamins are likely to be lost.

By adding relatively inexpensive corn or other such starches to infant foods, a manufacturer saves money by being able to use smaller quantities of fruit, vegetable, or meat. For example, in one baby-food jar labeled Bananas, less than 30 percent of the total solids in the jar was actually bananas. The remaining 70 percent was starch. While added sugar and starch might be expected in baby foods labeled dessert or pudding, most parents are shocked to find that many fruits, creamed vegetables, and high-meat dinners also have added corn starch, milk, and sugar (sucrose).

Sucrose is added to almost all plain vegetables processed by two of the three major companies, and some meats even have added sugar. Many fruits and fruit juices also have added sugar. Though the sugar may be in the form of corn sweetener, it is still sugar and is generally considered an unnecessary, undesirable baby food additive. In the interest of overall good health and of dental health in particular, refined and corn sugars should be kept to a minimum in any diet. Giving baby sweetened vegetables, fruits, and milks may teach him that these items must contain sugar in order to be tasty. Conversely, letting baby enjoy naturally delicious flavors is an excellent way to teach him that added sugar is not a necessity of life.

Commerical high-meat dinners are usually high in starch as well as protein. Though commercial baby-food meats have water added, they still offer an easy-to-use protein source in a form most babies can enjoy. Unfortunately, since at least one manufacturer has recently experimented with doubling and even tripling the amount of *fat* added to the baby-food meats in his line, those meats now offer less protein (and more calories) than most home-prepared meats would offer. Meat sticks, a favorite food of some older infants, are lower in water than the average strained commercial baby-food meats but are relatively higher in fat.

By reading labels carefully, a mother should be able to choose a few fruits and vegetables which do not contain added starches, sugars, or salt. These, plus commercial baby food meats, will enable her to give baby a balanced meal of solids in a convenient, ready-to-use form. Nonetheless, many mothers prefer to prepare baby foods at home.

If a mother decides to use home-prepared foods, she might wish to try some of the basic recipes given in Appendix C of this book or to consult some of the excellent publications available on this topic, some of which are listed in Appendix D.

If quality is a mother's main reason for making baby foods herself, she must give careful attention to the choice, preparation, and storage of those foods. For example, fruits canned in heavy syrup should not be pureed for baby, due to their high sucrose content. Canned vegetables should also be avoided, since most contain added salt. In general, since most frozen vegetables also contain some salt, fresh vegetables are the ideal choice. However, in some areas of the country, fresh vegetables are either unattainable at certain times of the year or arrive at the supermarket in such poor condition that their vitamin content is significantly reduced. In such cases, using frozen vegetables is probably better than using the more expensive, but less satisfactory, fresh ones. A mother tempted to resort to canned vegetables and fruits should be aware that commercial baby foods probably have fewer additives than do standard canned vegetables and fruits. Pureeing canned vegetables and fruits may save a few pennies but offers none of the other advantages of homemade baby foods.

Until a child is able to eat table foods, advance preparation of home-pureed food is necessary to ensure that good food choices are always readily available and to lessen the possibility that baby's needs for well-balanced meals will be ignored. Though well-prepared parent-made baby fruits, vegetables, and meats are generally somewhat higher in vitamins and minerals than are their commercial counterparts, poorly prepared home products may be *lower* in vitamins and minerals. To preserve these nutrients, vegetables should be steamed or pressure-cooked, using minimum water and cooking time. The same vegetables may be enjoyed by baby and family, provided that salt and other seasonings are added after baby's portion has been reserved. For further tips on avoiding vitamin and mineral loss during food preparation, re-read the final pages of Chapter 2.

Vegetables may be pureed in an electric blender, poured into ice-cube trays, cooled slightly, covered with foil or wax paper, then frozen for eight to twelve hours. When the food is well frozen, you can remove the cubes from the tray and bag, label, and store them in the freezer for several weeks. When you want to use them, the cubes may be heated in a microwave oven, a double boiler, a small heat-and-cold resistant custard cup placed in a pan of water, or an electric infant-food warmer. Two or three cubes may be heated in the individual sections of an egg poacher. An even simpler—but somewhat more expensive—method of storing and heating calls for sealing small amounts of food in boil-and-seal bags, then heating them in boiling water at the time of use.

If foods are *not* frozen, refrigerator storage time should be limited, since pureed items are more susceptible to spoilage than most foods. Baby food made from canned or cooked fruit may be refrigerated three to four days; from raw vegetables, two to three days; from raw fruit, one to two days. Soups may be kept for two days and juices for three, but meat and eggs should be used after one day's storage. All refrigerated items should be kept tightly covered.

Since a six-month-old infant may already have a few teeth and be trying chewing motions, her chewing attempts should be encouraged by giving her dry toast or other such items. An adult should stay nearby, since teething toast might crumble and become lodged in baby's throat. Allowing a baby to eat large quantities of toast between meals may mean satisfying her appetite with relatively empty calories so that she is not interested in other foods.

Soon after a baby of this age has begun to accept pureed foods readily, the foods may be blended less completely, giving him the challenge of chewing fine little bits of solid matter. There is some evidence that children kept on strained or pureed foods for too long will not readily move to table food.

One child who was kept on strained commercial food for nearly two years and was never allowed to feed himself or eat table food refused all table food until he reached kindergarten age, preferring to be fed by his mother until he was nearly five. Once he entered public-school kindergarten, peer pressure helped him move to cafeteria foods, and after eating at school, he began to eat table food at home. Though this is an extreme case, it does show that a child's readiness cues should be looked for and respected.

Most babies can eat well-mashed table food before the age of one, though they may be more willing to eat foods run through a small baby-food mill. Such a mill is relatively inexpensive, easily used at home or when dining out, and easily cleaned. Furthermore, unlike a blender, it can be used for very small amounts of food.

Successful transition to table food depends, of course, on those foods being planned to meet a growing baby's needs and prepared with a minimum of excess seasoning. Often baby's portion can be set aside before extra onions or garlic are added. As baby grows older, of course, he will need to be given the opportunity to learn to enjoy the spices which are characteristic of his particular household. For now, heavy spices may make him dislike vegetables and other foods which he might otherwise welcome.

A typical daily food list for a six- to eighteen-month-old baby might include milk (approximately 20 ounces of human or fortified soy or cow's-milk formula given at meals or between), two fruits or juices (including one high in vitamin C and not including those with tiny seeds), two vegetables (green or yellow, plus potatoes several times a week), and high-protein dishes (egg yolk or high-protein cereal with milk for breakfast; meat or cheese for dinner or lunch). According to one leading authority on infant nutrition, an iron-fortified infant cereal should be a part of each day's intake from the sixth through the eighteenth month of life.

The vegetarian infant's protein needs may be met in a variety of ways. Legumes intended for baby should be thoroughly cooked, mashed, and run through a sieve or pureed. Since small bits of legume might choke a baby, careful pureeing is advised. Because excessive use of beans may cause gas, use of beans should be limited to small servings every other day. If nut butter, such as peanut butter, is used, smooth style should be chosen, since whole or chopped nuts may cause a baby to choke, and a small amount of liquid should be added, since unmodified peanut butter tends to stick to the roof of an infant's mouth.

Whole-grain cereals (whole wheat, oatmeal, etc.) should be thoroughly cooked, blended, and sieved to make digestion easier. Since the protein in grains is incomplete, milk or formula to complete the protein should be added to the cereal serving or taken as a drink at the same meal. If cow's milk is not desired, another complementary protein source (see chart on page 17) should be included to offset the missing amino acid(s) in the cereal.

Meat analogs may be mashed or blended with water or formula; some persons object to the color and flavor of additives in these analogs, however. Tofu, the flavorless, custardlike curd of soy beans, can be eaten as is, fried with scrambled eggs, mashed, or cubed and boiled in broth for flavor. Tofu may also be blended with salad dressing and used as sandwich spread or pureed with fruit and eaten as pudding.

Variety is the key to good nutrition, even for the one-year-old. A steady diet of applesauce, given just because baby loves that food, will add too many carbohydrates and too little food value to the diet over a long stretch of time. By starting a few of the foods on this list at the age of six months and gradually adding more as baby learns to enjoy solids, a parent can present a daily menu similar to the one at the end of this chapter by the time the child is eighteen months of age.

Baby should be moving toward a variety of solid foods by that time. Though breast-feeding beyond six months is a marvelous and multi-advantageous way in which baby can obtain her needed milk supply, by nine months a totally breast-fed baby has begun to need more than just milk. Indeed, infants limited to breast milk alone beyond nine months may develop mild deficiency symptoms.

During baby's latter months of infancy, choosing what is *best* for her should still be a parent's primary concern, as it was during the earliest months of this crucial period of growth and development. As her needs change, so should her diet. If solids are added gradually, a well-balanced diet will be eagerly accepted by the average toddler, and she will be learning to enjoy the foods best suited to her individual needs—foods which will enable her to meet or exceed Recommended Dietary Allowances for her age group.

## Psychological Factors in Feeding

Although delaying the introduction of solids until a baby is about six months of age should mean the baby is psychologically ready to eat food from a spoon, the feeding method you use may ultimately mean the difference in acceptance or rejection. Patience and a positive, open attitude are musts during feeding time. A particularly independent six-month-old may occasionally wish to assert her authority by refusing foods she usually takes with enthusiasm. Avoiding a showdown by simply letting the matter pass is better than being caught up in a battle of wills. Slowly, if solid foods are offered routinely and optimistically, baby will learn the fine art of eating with a spoon.

By beginning at six months instead of six weeks, a mother is not force-feeding a helpless infant but is offering food to a small person who is just beginning to realize she can reach for items such as spoons and dishes. At this age, even before efficient self-feeding is likely to occur, a mother can nurture the move toward independence by allowing baby to play with the short-handled, round-bowled spoon which she will eventually use to feed herself. At the same time, she can continue to offer bites of pureed vegetables, fruits, and meat in a long-handled, shallow-bowled spoon made especially for infant feeding.

As baby grows more able to chew soft foods, finger foods such as dry toast, small bits of cheese, diced cooked carrots, green peas, and French-style green beans may be placed on her tray. While she enjoys the diversion of these tidbits, mom or dad can offer spoonfuls of mashed vegetables, fruits, and meats. If patience is exercised, self-feeding and adult feeding should work well together—at least until baby's developing sense of independence causes her to insist on doing it her way entirely!

By that time, the wise parent has learned to protect the carpet or floor by placing baby's chair on a drop cloth of some kind. Old plastic tablecloths, discarded shower curtains, or small plastic drop cloths of the type painters use all make good protective coverings for the floor. This small preventive measure means there is no need to scream at a twelve-month-old who decides to drop her dish just to see it fall. Naturally, such behavior should not be encouraged, but neither should it be the signal for violent reaction from an angry parent.

Milk-spilling, too, is easier on the nerves if the carpet has been covered before calamity strikes. Many parents find it helpful to arrive at an early distinction between baby's mealtime "uh oh!'s" and "on purposes." The former call for a quiet admonition to be more careful, while repeated incidents of the latter type call for firmer disciplinary action. In either case, it is easier to be reasonable and calm when one knows the $17.95-a-yard dining-room carpet has not suffered from the incident.

Milk-spilling and food throwing can be kept to a minimum if baby's eating equipment is wisely chosen. A multisectioned feeding dish is helpful, especially if the dish is relatively heavy or rests on a suction cup. Such a dish is hard for a child to toss—at least until he is old enough to understand that such actions are taboo. The sections are useful, as foods may be kept separate and each food may be pushed against the relatively straight sides of an individual segment, then maneuvered onto the spoon. When individual foods—such as yogurt or ice cream—are served, any dish with fairly deep sides can work well. Often soup can best be managed in a cup, with baby first drinking the broth, then spooning up noodles and vegetables afterward.

A sturdy high chair with a safety strap or harness make the baby feel secure in his new at-the-table world. A *large* bib saves many stained clothes, while a tiny, dainty one usually catches only a fraction of the spills and dribbles.

The short-handled, deep-bowled spoon mentioned earlier seems the most effective style for self-feeding. Some babies enjoy a fork after they are about one year old. Blunt, short tines are ideal, since they are relatively safe. Though some infants prefer sharper, longer tines, parents must realize that sharp forks can damage baby's eyes or cheeks or harm a sibling who ventures too close.

For very young infants, a two-handled, weighted cup is often easier to handle than other drinking utensils. Some older babies refuse such a cup, especially if they see mom and dad drinking from a single-handed cup. Small glasses which can be gripped in one hand are useful as baby's skill improves. Though often warned to "two-hand it," few infants *always* use both hands. Better to use a glass which can be managed in one hand than spend hours wiping up milk spills. Spills will also be less frequent if baby's cup or glass is only partially filled. This means mom or dad may need to refill, but refilling is a far more pleasant task than cleaning up the milk baby has just dumped onto his tray. Besides, letting baby succeed at drinking all his milk is an important way to show him he is capable of eating and drinking as parents and siblings do.

This same principle should be applied to the solid foods you give him. Better to put too few peas on baby's dish and have him finish those and ask for a few more than to load his plate with a mound of food which he cannot possibly finish. The temptation will be to avoid waste by urging the child to finish the last bite, a practice which is likely to lead to negative mealtime attitudes or habitual overeating, which paves the way for obesity.

Better to let baby experience success at eating small portions than to have him faced with constant failure due to overloading his plate. Once parents become aware that babies do not normally consume adult portions, they are usually able to let baby's appetite-control mechanism operate freely. In most cases, unless a child has been patterned into overeating since birth, he will be able to judge for himself how much food he needs and wants. If he is presented with a variety of foods, he soon learns to enjoy most of them, thus assuring a balanced nutrient intake.

Occasionally, a child shows extreme dislike for a certain food. In times past, a mother often ignored baby's dislikes, assuming that small babies have a poor sense of taste. Actually, babies have a very keen sense of taste, apparently from birth. In early childhood, there are taste buds on the insides of the cheeks and in the throat, in addition to those on the tongue. As the child grows older, only those on the tongue remain. Thus, baby should never be considered a tasteless creature!

Fortunately, no one food is absolutely essential to good health. Many substitutes exist, as the six food lists in Appendix A indicate. These exchange lists make it relatively easy for a parent to try several foods with nutrient content similar to that of the refused food. If baby is not force-fed spinach, she may learn to like it later. Better to respect her wishes now than to get into a standoff, "you'll eat this or else" situation, which may make her feel like refusing all foods. In time, she may come to enjoy foods she once seemed to hate. If this doesn't happen, a parent can merely substitute foods she does like that offer the missing nutrients.

Occasionally a child refuses entire categories of foods, such as all vegetables. If this practice persists, of course, a balanced nutrient intake is very unlikely to occur. For a while, careful choices of foods can be made which will cover the vitamins and minerals found in most vegetables. However, if the problem persists, you should probably consult a nutritionist or pediatrician. Since many foods contain valuable trace elements as well as the better-known vitamins and minerals, just giving a multivitamin pill each day is probably not the best answer. This problem may be outgrown if it is handled with patience and understanding.

Sometimes babies who do not like strained vegetables later learn to enjoy vegetables in bite-sized pieces. Often babies who dislike cooked, mashed vegetables learn to enjoy crisp, raw vegetables at a later age. Even at fifteen months, baby has probably learned to distinguish between various textures and colors. If he has been introduced to a variety of foods, he has enjoyed many colors, shapes, sounds, and textures by the time he is eighteen months old.

The very young child learns about food by feeling it as well as tasting it. For example, a six-month-old gave great delight to older children by his examination of a small pancake. First he patted the strange, warm object. Then he tried lifting it as if testing its weight. Finally he brought it to his mouth and tried to chew an edge. To two little girls who were busily eating their own pancakes while watching baby's antics, his actions seemed strange indeed. In actuality, they were perfectly normal reactions to something new and different.

Pancakes later became a favorite food of this particular little boy. In fact, his mother worried about his insisting on this relatively low-protein breakfast food. She soon learned that she could make a protein-rich pancake by using two eggs and adding dried milk solids and wheat germ. Once she had discovered that warm applesauce was as acceptable to baby as pancake syrup, she finally felt relaxed about his several weeks' love affair with pancakes.

Such food jags are not uncommon, and unless they involve high-sugar or otherwise undesirable foods, they are best left to run their course. These favorite items are usually confined to a specific meal, such as pancakes at breakfast, and so they don't often interfere with the eating of other foods at other times of day. Better to let a child enjoy what he likes, as long as that food is relatively nutritious, than to have him grow hostile toward all foods because he's not allowed to let normal food jags run their course.

Avoiding hostile or unpleasant feelings about all aspects of mealtime should be your constant goal. If you keep conversations pleasant, meet accidental spills with matter-of-fact, reasonable actions, and treat likes and dislikes with wisdom and respect, baby's attitude toward mealtime is likely to be positive.

Even after-meal activities such as face washing should be handled smoothly and cheerfully, so that no hint of unpleasantness clouds mealtime. Making a few playful dabs at baby's face with a damp napkin can accomplish the necessary cleanup just as effectively as a rough scrubbing with a cloth. Some parents find that an older baby is quite happy to be held under one arm over the sink while mother washes his hands and splashes his face with water. Such a cleanup involves no painful rubbing at all, yet leaves baby food-free and ready to return to his fun without danger to furniture and walls. From start to finish, every meal should be pleasant and cheerful. Eating together should be a happy, enjoyable family occasion.

# Common Problems

## Food Allergies

Fifteen-month-old Erica, enjoying a meal with her grandparents in the Deep South, was particularly delighted with fresh tomatoes from Papaw's garden. Slice after slice, she eagerly munched the delicious new treat. Suddenly Granny noticed the area around the little girl's mouth was becoming blotchy. Her eyes were red and puffy. She didn't seem distressed, but obviously something was happening to her. She was suffering from tomato allergy.

According to Dr. Jean Mayer, food is the greatest cause of allergy in children under two years of age. Allergies may lead to nausea, vomiting, colic, diarrhea, colitis, spastic constipation, sniffles and dripping nose, red watery eyes, skin disorders, fatigue, irritability, and headaches. In addition, children with milk, egg, or wheat allergies often develop what some doctors call food asthma.

There are two basic types of allergic responses. In the first, signs and symptoms appear within minutes after a food is eaten. Often seafood, berry, and nut allergies display this almost immediate reaction. In the second type, allergic response may be delayed for hours, making diagnosis extremely difficult. Milk, cereal, eggs, chocolate, and pork usually fall into this "delayed reaction" category.

The most common allergy-causing foods in infancy are milk, eggs, cereal grains (particularly wheat), and, occasionally, orange juice. Later, seafood, chocolate, pork, chicken, corn, nuts, and strawberries rank high as causes of allergic reactions. Next in line are oatmeal, rye, oranges, cottonseed, legumes, tomatoes, potatoes, beans, mustard, cucumbers, and garlic. Allergic reactions to rice, lamb, gelatin, peaches, peas, carrots, lettuce, artichokes, sesame oil, and apples are sometimes reported.

Food allergy may be suspected in children who exhibit one or more of the symptoms mentioned, especially if some of the symptoms can be traced to ingestion of a suspect food. If a baby's family has a history of food allergies, the pediatrician should be alerted to this fact early. Even when allergies are suspected, pinpointing them is often extremely difficult. After taking a detailed diet history and having parents keep a diet diary, a physician may use trial diets, elimination diets, provocation diets, and skin tests. Unfortunately, skin tests are only 40 percent effective in showing up food allergies, so they hardly represent a definitive method of detection.

There is growing concern that food allergies may contribute to many physical and emotional problems from infancy through adulthood. As mentioned earlier, in most instances, parents should delay the introduction of solid foods until baby is about three months old, then add solids slowly, one at a time, in order to catch any adverse reaction to a new food. Parents who are able to detect allergies early, while an infant's diet is still fairly simple, may be able to help him avoid years of annoyance or outright suffering due to undetected allergies. Certainly a physician should be notified if you suspect any allergies. Better to eliminate the food you think is causing the problem and substitute another of equal nutrient value than to bring on more adverse reactions. Fortunately, some children seem to outgrow food allergies if they avoid the offending food for a few months or years.

# Diarrhea

Young infants often pick up intestinal disorders which lead to diarrhea. For a child *over twelve months of age,* a strained carrot soup made of equal parts of commercial strained baby-food carrots and water provides a relatively easily digested carbohydrate plus helpful electrolytes. Bouillon (but not bouillon cubes because of their low carbohydrate and high sodium content) or a gelatin-banana mixture may also be used for a child of this age.

In general, an infant suffering from diarrhea should avoid butterfat and eliminate milk formulas, since lactose intolerance is likely to develop during diarrhea attacks. In extreme cases of diarrhea, infants may become lactose intolerant for days or even weeks. In such cases, Lytren and Pedialyte or other special preparations may be prescribed by a doctor. Once the infant begins to recover, he can usually tolerate breast milk. Use of fortified soy-based formula during this time may hasten recovery for the bottle-fed infant. Eventually, the child should be able to resume use of milk products. Diarrhea which lasts longer than a few days, is particularly violent, or is accompanied by high fever or vomiting should be reported to a physician. Dehydration can occur quickly in a young infant when fluid loss and high temperature occur simultaneously.

# Dental Problems

A primary dental problem of the early years is known by a variety of names, including "nursing bottle syndrome," "bottle propping caries," "nursing bottle caries," and "nursing bottle mouth." Lest breast-feeding readers heave a sigh of relief and skip this passage, assuming "This is *one* health problem that doesn't pertain to *my* baby," it should be noted that cases of this disease have been documented in breast-feeding infants and toddlers.

In 1862, Jacobi called attention to the incidence of dental caries (cavities) in children who were offered milk or sugar-water at bedtime. Putting these liquids in bottles, which people began doing in the early years of this century, gives the cariogenic (cavity-causing) agents in these liquids an even better chance to linger on a baby's teeth. While milk drunk from a glass or taken from a bottle at meals or during a regular feeding is not a prime cavity-causing agent, milk taken from a bottle during nap time or throughout the night can and does cause cavities.

When sucking and swallowing action are infrequent, the flow of saliva is minimal; milk remains in the mouth for relatively long periods, and the teeth remain in almost constant contact with stagnant milk. When sweetened milk or highly sugared drinks and juices are used for nap and bedtime bottles, the problem is intensified. Sugared or honey-dipped pacifiers are equally dangerous.

Usually, "nursing bottle caries" is seen in babies or toddlers who have prolonged bottle-feeding beyond twelve months and habitually take the bottle to bed at night and during naps. In classic cases of this disorder, the four upper front teeth (maxillary incisors) are the most affected, while the lower front teeth (mandibular incisors) frequently show no involvement at all. The other primary teeth, usually in the order in which they came in, are occasionally affected, especially if the disease has gone undetected for several months.

Detection is sometimes difficult, since the first sign is an unobtrusive band of dull white along the gum line. This band marks an area from which protective calcium has been removed. Gradually, this decalcified area turns to dark brown or black collars of decay. In very advanced cases, only the root stumps of the upper teeth may remain, while the lower front teeth remain almost perfect. This pattern of decay occurs because the tongue protects the lower teeth during bottle-feeding, while the upper teeth receive a continuous bath of stagnant milk or high-sugar liquid. If the child dozes with the nipple in place, liquid pools against the upper front teeth. Fermentable carbohydrates then act with oral bacteria to form decay-causing acids, which decalcify the teeth and allow proteolytic (protein-decomposing) bacteria to invade the tooth dentine and destroy it.

The pain and discomfort caused by the cavities of "nursing bottle syndrome" may make a child fussy and irritable. Abscessed teeth and inflammation of the facial skin may result. Teeth may be lost because of tongue thrusting, which may lead to poor alignment and improper closure of the permanent teeth. Lisps or other speech impediments may follow loss of incisors, and biting and chewing action are greatly impeded.

Since cavities are caused by a combination of factors, not every child who takes a bottle to bed will develop nursing bottle syndrome. One mother of a two-year-old boy, obviously puzzled by what had happened to her son's teeth, sat in the pedodontist's office waiting for still another expensive treatment. "Dr. Blake has given us a discount, but I still don't see how we'll ever be able to pay for all this. Why, most of my son's upper teeth are gone and even some of his 'jaw' teeth [molars]." When she was questioned, this mother admitted that the child had taken sweetened drinks to bed regularly since he was old enough to hold the bottle by himself, but she hastened to add, "His sister did it too, and *she* never had this happen."

The little girl was lucky. The boy was not. There's just no way to be sure a child's teeth can withstand such abuse until it's too late. Thus, it makes sense to avoid the behavior most likely to cause decay. According to pedodontists, decreased salivary flow during sleep and increased exposure time to milk or sweet beverages are the two prime factors in nursing bottle syndrome. Both factors can be avoided by not allowing baby to take night or nap bottles into the crib or, if baby insists on taking a bottle to bed, by giving only water. This is a small price to pay to avoid this painful, expensive disease of babyhood.

Cleaning teeth with gauze or brushing and flossing them can help lessen the chance that decay will occur. Even among children who pay proper attention to dental hygiene, a few cavities are likely to occur (an average of

1 to 2.5 cavities per child at age three to four), but the ten or more decayed or filled teeth characteristic of the baby with nursing mouth syndrome can and should be prevented.

As we noted earlier, dentists have recently discovered that *breast-fed* babies can also suffer from this disease! Fortunately, this occurs only under special circumstances, but those circumstances should certainly be understood and avoided. While sucrose (refined sugar) is more cariogenic than lactose (milk sugar), lactose can become a cavity causer if it is placed in constant contact with the teeth. Breast milk, the optimum food for babies, is higher in lactose (7.2 percent) than either formula (7 percent) or cow's milk (4.5 percent). Therefore, plain cow's milk, milk formula, human milk, and milk with honey are cavity-causing in the ascending order given.

Obviously, a totally breast-fed baby cannot take a bottle to bed with him —but wait! A mother who nurses her older baby for long hours during the daytime, letting the child doze at the breast with nipple in mouth, sets up a situation very similar to that seen in babies who take a bottle of milk to bed. When long daytime nap nursing is combined with nighttime nursing at will, a mother is often unable to say just how many hours her baby's teeth have been in constant contact with lactose-rich breast milk. If baby has had fruit or sugar prior to nursing and the teeth have not been cleaned, the combination of sucrose and fructose plus lactose makes decay action even more likely.

One dentist reported that decayed upper incisors of breast-feeding babies have a notched effect not usually seen in bottle-fed babies with nursing mouth syndrome. Others have reported no significant difference in decay patterns, but whatever the pattern of a breast-fed baby's nursing mouth caries, the ultimate result is the same—pain, inconvenience, and unneeded expense.

Some breast-feeding mothers have been given so many reasons *not* to breast-feed that they are understandably angered by dentists who inform them that nature's perfect food could cause cavities. This problem must be recognized and discussed among breast-feeding moms, especially those inclined to let their youngsters nurse beyond infancy, an otherwise *helpful* practice. Until mothers have the facts, "at-will" nap and nighttime nursing will no doubt continue to cause occasional cases of nursing bottle syndrome.

Several examples from a group of Colorado dentists make this point well. A twenty-month-old girl who slept with her mother and nursed at will during the night had extensive decalcified areas on her teeth. Yet the mother continued nighttime nursing, dismissing the dentist's comments as still another attack on her right to nurse an older child. The mother of a twenty-three-month-old boy with rampant decay ended prolonged nighttime feeding after her dentist explained the cause of her son's dental problems. Two years after the dentist restored the damaged teeth, the child had no new cavities.

A thirty-one-month-old boy with nine of his seventeen primary teeth decayed and sixteen of the seventeen showing decalcification around the gum area was another victim of prolonged sleeptime-nursing activity. There is cruel irony in seeing breast-feeding mothers, the very mothers who seem most anxious to give their children the best possible nourishment, discover that an otherwise innocent breast-feeding practice has contributed to the development of painful cavities.

Fortunately, as noted earlier, the prevention of nursing bottle caries in breast-fed babies is simple enough. *Do not allow prolonged at-breast feeding while baby is sleeping, at least not after a child's teeth have begun to erupt.* While some dentists go so far as to recommend ceasing nursing as soon as a child can drink from a cup, most agree that the one precaution of avoiding prolonged sleep-nursing can guard against pain and suffering for the infant and high dental bills for his parents. Ignoring the facts and exposing an innocent baby to this known caries-causing condition may mean you are making a costly mistake. As in the case of the bottle-fed baby, not *all* babies fed at will for long hours of napping or sleeping will develop nursing mouth syndrome. Some apparently let the nipple go as they fall asleep. Others may have greater resistance to decay. But why take a chance?

In contrast to reports indicating that breast-fed babies may, in rare cases, develop nursing-mouth syndrome, stands a recent experiment with rats which indicates that most breast-fed babies may have a cavity-prevention edge over their bottle-fed counterparts. In 1979, researchers in the Department of Food Science and Human nutrition at Michigan State University reported that when Lauriciden (monolaurin), a substance found in breast milk, was fed to rats on a high-sugar diet, their cavity incidence was 49% lower than that of a control group whose high-sugar diets did not contain this substance.

While monolaurin may, indeed, give breast-feeding infants added protection against cavities, there is no evidence that its presence in breast milk guarantees total immunity from tooth decay. Since feeding an isolated substance to a laboratory animal can never perfectly simulate natural conditions, mothers should still consider modifying breast-feeding practices which might lead to nursing-mouth syndrome.

Other important items of dental health will be taken up in subsequent chapters. Those parents who can are urged to see a pedodontist early (even as early as nine months), to be sure that no signs of trouble exist and to gain information on ways to prevent tooth decay. In general, parents who avoid conditions conducive to nursing mouth syndrome, brush or gauze a baby's teeth as soon as they come in, and give regular attention to a well-rounded diet that is low in sucrose will probably be giving their infants a fine head start toward a lifetime of good dental health.

## Infantile Obesity

Infantile obesity poses both immediate and long-range problems for a child. During babyhood, there is some evidence that overweight children have a greater frequency of illness in general and a greater frequency of respiratory illness in particular. There is no evidence that they have a higher death rate, despite the higher illness rate.

Though more work must be done before there is sufficient data to show the relationship between infantile, childhood, adolescent, and adult obesity, many studies indicate that juvenile or adolescent obesity began in infancy. For example, an English researcher notes that a high percentage of overweight or obese infants in that country were still overweight at ages six to eight. An American research team compared a group of 158 obese adolescent girls to a group of 158 nonobese girls of approximately the same age and socioeconomic status. No differences were noted in birth weight, height at one year, and age at the start of menstrual period. However, early health records revealed that by one year of age, the group which eventually became obese had gained weight at a significantly more rapid pace and was heavier than the nonobese group at that same age.

The reasons for this apparent relationship between obese infants and obese adolescents are not known, but it seems that overeating does program some infants for later obesity. Of course, it seems equally true that not all overfed babies seem predisposed to be programmed for later-life obesity. Recent reports indicate that once the *number* of fat cells is increased beyond normal, weight reduction can only reduce the size and not the number of fat cells. This could mean that the tendency to fill all available fat cells may be an automatic mechanism which makes weight control extremely difficult in those persons with abnormally high numbers of cells. Other reports question this theory, and there are currently too many unknowns to allow us to draw definitive conclusions.

Even with many questions still unanswered, experts are beginning to agree that parents should probably aim for a rate of weight gain similar to that of a breast-fed baby. Though this goal is most easily attained by breast-feeding, bottle-feeding parents may be able to keep a baby's weight gain to desired limits by (1) avoiding the temptation to force down the last ounce of formula, (2) making sure formulas are in prescribed concentrations, and (3) delaying the introduction of solids until five or six months of age. As in most cases of obesity in later life, the obese infant is one who consistently consumes more calories than he needs for his particular growth, basal metabolism, and activity levels.

Occasionally, early feeding problems seem to cause obesity later. For example, seven of ten obese adolescents in one study had food allergy in infancy. In another group, 28 to 32 percent of ninety-two obese adolescents had a history of feeding problems during the first year of life. These early feeding problems may mean a child is overprotected and perhaps overfed to make up for his earlier trouble. Weight gain becomes a logical goal for a child who has lagged behind due to allergies or other problems, but overcompensation through overfeeding can have long-term, undesirable results.

Other reasons for overfeeding include guilt feelings toward a child of an unwanted pregnancy, insecurity on the part of parents who feel a need to prove their ability to be good parents, and use of food as a reward for good behavior or as the easiest answer to baby's every cry. In the latter case, an overfed baby becomes inactive, passive, and increasingly unable to distinguish hunger from other drives or to tell when his hunger has been satisfied. Such nonnutritive uses of food foster a tendency to rely on food to compensate for emotional and social difficulties throughout life.

Once obesity seems evident in a child younger than eighteen months, a doctor's advice should be obtained. Generally, the goal will be to reduce the rate of gain, not to accomplish weight *loss*. Severe dietary restriction may reduce fat-free body tissues, inhibit growth, and deplete energy reserves that handle stress. The child's diet should be regulated to satisfy normal growth requirements (approximately 90 calories per kilogram per day at six to twelve months), and calories should not be cut beyond that level. If an obese infant's daily volume of milk exceeds 30 ounces, water may be given as needed to satisfy hunger at between-milk feedings. Total calorie intake should remain adequate for normal growth and development. Skim milk is not recommended for infants under twenty-four months of age, though some doctors recommend 2-percent (low-fat) milk for obese toddlers and older children. While 2-percent milk means fewer calories per ounce, allowing an overweight child to drink more of this milk than normal may foster a habit of overeating.

In general, doctors agree that authorities who set energy (calorie) recommendations for infants have paid too little attention to the difference in levels of physical activity among infants. Some babies are not as active as others, even from birth. Less-active infants will be likely to gain weight if they are fed the same number of calories as their more-active peers, yet less-active infants must have enough calories and enough nutrients to meet their growth and basal metabolism needs.

When *actometers* were placed on ankles and wrists to measure infant activity by a mechanism similar to that which powers self-winding watches, no correlation was found between the total calories consumed and the weight of the babies studied. However, a *strong* correlation was found between obesity and activity. The fatter the baby, the less active it was; the thinner the baby, the more active it was. Extremely thin babies moved more and ate more. Extremely fat babies moved less and ate less. The most active baby was twice as active as the least active one.

Differences in activity, not in food intake, seemed the key to infant obesity. Thus, an obese infant may well need all the food she is ingesting—unless, of course, she is being force-fed. Sharply reducing her calories may mean risking disruption of normal physical and mental development. Certainly, leaving her hungry is likely to mean turning her into an unhappy, angry baby.

Infantile obesity is a complex problem involving genetic, environmental, social, and medical factors which influence one another in a wide variety of ways. There are no simple answers to this complex problem. Parents should proceed with caution when attempting to help babies avoid obesity. The primary goal should be slowing weight gain, not causing weight reduction. By encouraging a slow-moving baby to exercise and by *not* encouraging him to drink more formula than he needs, parents can move away from obesity and toward normal gain patterns. By increasing nonnutritive stimulation (visual, vocal, physical), parents can move a baby away from an unnatural dependence on food. Once parents realize that babies fuss for reasons other than hunger, they should be able to satisfy their cries by means other than a warm bottle.

Since even a toddler can sense parental disapproval, mom, dad and others should refrain from cutting remarks about baby's fatness. Especially if a child has been encouraged to overeat and praised for his hearty appetite in the previous weeks or months of his short life, he can become quite confused when he is suddenly berated for these same actions. Any move toward reprogramming baby's eating habits should be made with his emotional as well as his physical health in mind.

## Nutrition Education

Toddlers learn about snacks early, especially if siblings are present. When snacks are nutritious, relatively sugar-free treats right from the first, there is no later tendency to associate snack time with candy, carbonated beverages, or highly sweetened, artificially flavored drinks. A small glass of orange juice and a cube of cheese not only help tide an eighteen-month-old over until lunchtime but also give her vitamin C, calcium, protein, and other valuable nutrients. Bits of peeled, cubed apple provide an equally nutritious afternoon snack which does not interfere with appetite at dinnertime. Now, while baby is too young to look for snacks herself, is the time for programming her snacking habits.

Naturally, parents who munch on chips and candy and drink carbonated beverages should not expect baby to watch and not want to do likewise. Many couples who have long intended to alter their own snacking habits find that baby's "me too" inclinations provide just the push they need to start healthier snacking.

Dessert habits, too, are set at an early age. If baby is urged to have more green beans "so you can have dessert," dessert becomes a more desirable item than beans. If, on the other hand, you offer such items as fresh fruits and banana bread, baby may even be allowed to have these items along with his beans if he so desires. Later, he will probably follow adult example and save dessert until last, but at least he will not have been programmed to feel that dessert is the highlight of every meal.

## Practical Meals and Snacks

A year-old baby can enjoy many of the foods from the basic foods list given in Appendix A. A six-month-old can enjoy many of the same foods in strained form, though calorie needs will be lower. An eighteen-month-old should be able to enjoy a wide variety of foods and will need more calories derived from the same basic foods than will a one-year-old.

Since each baby's "stomach alarm" rings at its own particular time, most parents will find that snacks and meals should be arranged to suit a baby's current inclinations. As these inclinations change, snacks and meals can again be rearranged. *Flexibility* is a must when dealing with feeding patterns of children of any age, and when dealing with infants, flexibility is doubly important.

For an older baby or toddler, a mother should first include foods from all food groups, then add formula, milk, or additional high-quality solid foods in amounts sufficient to provide the recommended number of calories for the baby's age, weight, and activity needs. If these goals are met, the time of day these various foods are taken is of relatively little importance. If a baby prefers peas at breakfast and eggs at dinner, her protein and vitamin needs will be met just as surely as if she takes these foods at more traditional times. If she seems to need snacks, a parent can see that these snacks become an integral part of her overall food plan, not just empty, excess calories. A detailed discussion of snacks, including the views of a heart specialist, pedodontist, and nutritionist, appears in the toddler section. Some of these snack ideas may be applicable to an older infant.

# 6
## Preschool—
## Eighteen Months to Five Years

"Have some of this yummy eggplant casserole," five-year-old Susan urged as she passed little Gary a tin plate containing a mixture of spruce cones and sand.

"No eggplant for me," he replied indignantly, "you know dads don't eat that stuff!"

This scene is amusing enough—as long as it stays in the world of make believe. Unfortunately, the "me too" attitudes of preschoolers usually cross over to the real dinner table as well as the pretend one. Highly impressionable and greatly influenced by all experiences within the family, preschoolers pick up parental food likes and dislikes, snacking habits, and table manners. Since toddlers often pattern their actions after older siblings, the nutrition education the oldest child receives is crucial not only to the development of his own good dietary habits, but also to the development of those of the brothers and sisters who will strive to be like him.

The best way to train a child of this age is by good example. If parents talk about good nutrition but provide twenty-four-hour examples of poor nutrition, the preschoolers' diets are likely to be equally poor. Conversely, if other family members eat well-balanced meals, limit themselves to nutritious snacks, and get plenty of exercise, toddlers and other preschoolers are likely to do the same.

Poor parental eating habits do not have to be passed on to preschoolers. Parents who are sufficiently motivated can change habits which seem especially undesirable. If parents are willing to try such changes, older siblings can even be included in the repatterning process.

Often, a couple does not give serious thought to nutrition until they are faced with the task of feeding a child. Once they see the reasons behind nutrition guidelines and become really interested in following those guidelines, changes can and do take place. Of course, *father* as well as mother must decide to work toward optimum family nutrition. Though the wife has traditionally been the "gatekeeper" who chooses which foods will be made available to the family, her choices are often based on the likes and dislikes of her husband. By the time children are born into the home, family meals may already be severely limited in certain areas.

For example, a 1972 survey of young children revealed that vegetable likes and dislikes in father and children were more similar than in mother and children. Further questioning revealed that 80 percent of the mothers in that survey group rarely served the vegetables they knew father disliked. Consequently, vegetable choices of children in those families were limited by the preferences of the fathers.

Most fathers would probably be quite willing to avoid exerting negative influences upon the eating habits of their children if they realized the long-range effect of those influences. Many studies have noted that food patterns and attitudes established during the preschool years affect food choices and nutrition status throughout life. Furthermore, if parents make diet changes while their children are still young enough to be repatterned with relative ease, they will most likely be rewarded by better nutrition and better health for the entire family, not just for the children.

# Meeting Nutrient Needs

Parents who wish to provide optimum family nutrition should read and understand the reasons behind Recommended Dietary Allowances for pre-schoolers and work toward meeting those allowances. As the chart which follows indicates, nutrient requirements for the preschooler are in most cases slightly higher than for the infant. Still, the same basic foods which give an eighteen-month-old his needed nutrients can provide adequate nutrition for the preschooler. Parents should also remember that children need essential nutrients for which no RDAs have as yet been set. A varied diet that enables a child to meet RDAs will probably also include essential nutrients not listed on the RDA chart.

## Calories

Although the total calorie requirements for preschoolers are higher than for infants, the number of calories required per pound of body weight are *lower* for the preschooler than for the infant (see table on page 109). This drop reflects the fact that the growth rate decreases sharply after the first year of life. The child who showed a weight increase of fifteen pounds in his first twelve months is likely to add only seven pounds during his second year and only five during his third. Unless appetite-control mechanisms have already been confused by force-feeding during infancy, there is a corresponding decrease in appetite between the first and second birthdays. The toddler may begin to look slimmer, since he has begun to use body stores of infant fat as a supplemental energy source.

Deciding how to appease a child's somewhat diminished appetite is important, for high-quality calories and proper calorie distributions are vital to optimum growth and development. An early 1970 study of preschoolers' diets in the northcentral region of the United States showed that protein accounted for approximately 15 to 17 percent, fat 34 to 40 percent, and carbohydrate 43 to 50 percent of the calories consumed each day by the children being observed. Around two-thirds of the children surveyed met the RDA for energy, and nearly all met the protein RDA.

## Recommended Dietary Allowances—Preschoolers

| Age | *1–3 years* | *4–6 years* |
|---|---|---|
| Weight | 13 kg (29 lbs) | 20 kg (44 lbs) |
| Height | 90 cm (35 in) | 112 cm (44 in) |
| Energy (cal) | 1300 (900–1800) | 1700 (1300–2300) |
| Protein (g) | 23 | 30 |
| **Fat-soluble vitamins** | | |
| Vitamin A[a] (*$\mu$g R.E.) | 400 | 500 |
| Vitamin D[b] ($\mu$g) | 10 | 10 |
| Vitamin E[c] (mg $\alpha$ T.E.) | 5 | 6 |
| **Water-soluble vitamins** | | |
| Ascorbic acid (C) (mg) | 45.0 | 45.0 |
| Folacin ($\mu$g) | 100.0 | 200.0 |
| Niacin[d] (mg N.E.) | 9.0 | 11.0 |
| Riboflavin (mg) | 0.8 | 1.0 |
| Thiamin (mg) | 0.7 | 0.9 |
| Vitamin $B_6$ (mg) | 0.9 | 1.3 |
| Vitamin $B_{12}$ ($\mu$g) | 2.0 | 2.5 |
| **Minerals** | | |
| Calcium (mg) | 800 | 800 |
| Phosphorus (mg) | 800 | 800 |
| Iodine ($\mu$g) | 70 | 90 |
| Iron (mg) | 15 | 10 |
| Magnesium (mg) | 150 | 200 |
| Zinc (mg) | 10 | 10 |

SOURCE: Adapted from *Recommended Dietary Allowances,* Ninth Edition (1980, in press), with the permission of the National Academy of Sciences, Washington, D.C.

\* $\mu$g is the standard abbreviation for microgram, or 1/1000 milligram.
[a] Recommendations for vitamin A are expressed in $\mu$g of R.E. (micrograms of retinol equivalent). One retinol equivalent is equal to 1 $\mu$g of retinol or 6 $\mu$g of carotene.
[b] Vitamin D is expressed as $\mu$g of cholecaciferol, with 10 $\mu$g cholecalciferol equalling 400 IUs of Vitamin D.
[c] Vitamin E is expressed as mg $\alpha$ T.E. (milligrams of alpha tocopherol equivalents).
[d] Niacin is expressed as mg N.E. (milligrams of niacin equivalent), with 1 N.E. equalling 1 mg of niacin or 60 mg of dietary tryptophan.

# Growth Charts for Preschoolers—Ages Two to Six*

### Girls' Height by Age Percentiles

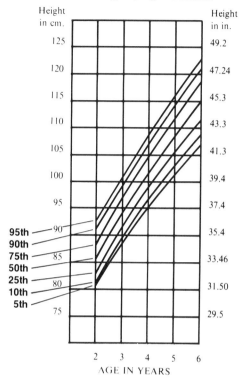

### Girls' Weight by Age Percentiles

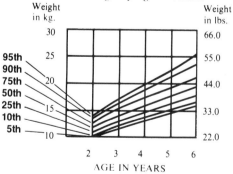

SOURCE: Adapted from Hamill, P. V. V., T. A. Drizd, C. L. Johnson, R. B. Reed, A. F. Roche, *NCHS Growth Curves for Children, Birth—18 years.* National Center for Health Statistics Publications, Series 11, Number 165, November 1977.

*In general, weights and heights that fall within the 5th and 95th percentiles are considered normal. Ideally, height and weight should be within a few percentile points of each other. See pp. 37, 112.

# Growth Charts for Preschoolers—Ages Two to Six*

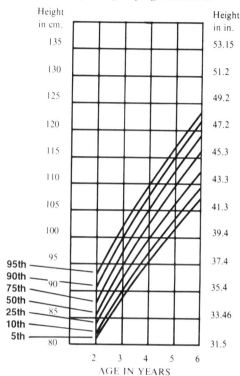

### Boys' Height by Age Percentiles

### Boys' Weight by Age Percentiles

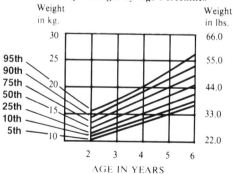

SOURCE: Adapted from Hamill, P. V. V., T. A. Drizd, C. L. Johnson, R. B. Reed, A. F. Roche, *NCHS Growth Curves for Children, Birth—18 years.* National Center for Health Statistics Publications, Series 11, Number 165, November 1977.

*In general, weights and heights that fall within the 5th and 95th percentiles are considered normal Ideally, height and weight should be within a few percentile points of each other. See pp. 37, 112.

Parents may wish to keep watch over a preschooler's growth and development at six- to twelve-month intervals by comparing the child's height and weight to the "norms" given on the NCHS Growth Chart which follows. As noted earlier, these "norms" are not absolutes, and some children who are unusually small or unusually large for their ages may fall outside the 5th or 95th percentile lines.

Don and Anne, the babies whose heights and weights were compared in chapter three, progressed through infancy and into their third years of life with Anne remaining the larger child. Still slightly above the 95th percentile in both height and weight, Anne is a healthy and well-proportioned little girl. Don, finally moving up into the 25th percentile in weight and height is equally well-proportioned.

Parents who use the height-weight charts given below should first look to see that height and weight are in approximately the same percentile. Weight that is 20 percent above height may indicate a tendency toward obesity, and weight that is 15 to 20 percent below height may mean a child is seriously underweight. While skinfold tests and other procedures by a physician may be needed to determine obesity, parents who keep a close watch on height-weight correlations can usually spot a tendency to overweight early, before the child enters upon a lifetime pattern of obesity.

Over the preschool years, any sharp deviation from a child's usual percentile ranking should be discussed with a physician. For example, a physician may decide that a child who consistently hovers around the 5th percentile in both height and weight is perfectly healthy and well nourished, yet a bit small for his age. If no health or nutrition problems are discovered, a child's place on height-weight charts is probably genetically predetermined and parents should love and accept the child as he is, rather than lamenting the fact that he does not fulfill their expectations.

On the other hand, a child who has been in the 50th percentile in both height and weight from birth through three years, then begins to move steadily downward over the next six to twelve months is likely experiencing some health problem. A pediatrician's analysis of the abrupt change is advisable. Whether the problem is a previously undetected illness which requires treatment with drugs or whether it is a problem which can be solved through alteration of the child's diet, a physician's help is needed in order to be sure the child's growth proceeds within normal, accustomed ranges.

## Protein

Though overall growth slows at the end of a baby's first year, brain-cell development is still intense until the end of the second twelve months, and adequate protein intake is essential if optimum brain development is to take place. After one year of age, an infant begins to develop the muscles for standing and walking, and muscle development is also highly dependent upon protein. So rapid is muscle development that half of the weight gained between the ages of one and three is in the form of muscle mass.

As the daily menus at the end of this book show, relatively small portions of milk, meat, eggs, and cheese plus vegetable protein can easily provide the 23 to 30 grams of protein needed by the preschooler. In the north-central region study cited earlier, income status did not seem to have a great bearing on protein consumption. Most children in a nationwide study of preschoolers from low-income families met or exceeded protein RDAs. In fact, some children consume twice the RDA for protein. If these children also consume relatively few carbohydrates and fats, their bodies are forced to rely upon protein for energy, an economically and metabolically unsound practice.

*Vegetarian* diets may also provide completely adequate amounts of protein, though vegans who do not use eggs or dairy products must be especially careful to observe the basics of protein complementarity as given in the chart on page 17.

## Carbohydrates

Many American children derive as much as 20 to 25 percent of their total energy from refined sugar, a simple carbohydrate which provides no nutrients. Their parents may consume 125 pounds of sugar per year or 35 teaspoonsful per day. Most of that 125 pounds is added to foodstuffs, though some of it occurs naturally in various foods.

With the increase in production and consumption of confectionary products such as cookies, candy, and sugar-containing baked goods rising at the rate of 20 percent every four years, intakes of refined sugar continue to spiral upward. Nutritionist Jean Mayer recently told a Senate committee that whereas sugar has been used as an *additive,* it is now consumed in such quantities that it may now be considered a new *food*—one which the human system, at least in many people, is not equipped to cope with.

Despite articles which cite sugar as "fuel for the body's work," other carbohydrates are even more acceptable in this role. Energy needs for a toddler or preschooler can be supplied by other—and better—forms than refined sucrose. Lactose in milk, glucose from starch breakdown, and glucose and fructose from fruit and vegetables can all supply needed energy, as can the sucrose that appears naturally in fresh fruits and vegetables. At fresh weight, peaches, plums, and apricots are 5 to 7 percent sugar, and carrots, peas, and sweet corn are 3 to 5 percent sugar. These foods not only give needed energy but also provide valuable vitamins, minerals, and trace elements.

As we will discuss later, there is mounting evidence that contact of dietary sugar on the teeth is the leading supporting agent that helps bring about tooth decay. Catering to a baby's "sweet tooth" may mean that that tooth, along with many of his other ones, will need to be filled by the end of his preschool years.

As mentioned earlier, parents and siblings in the habit of a diet laden with extra sweets will be likely to influence younger children to imitate their food choices. Using sweets as rewards also reinforces this undesirable habit. If high-calorie, high-sugar foods are eaten in addition to the meals planned for the average preschooler, excess energy intake will likely result in excess pounds.

Complex carbohydrates should also be chosen with care. For example, whole-grain breads and rolls offer vitamins, minerals, and dietary fiber as well as energy. Buying whole grains requires careful label reading. Only those labels that say "whole wheat," "graham," or "entire wheat" signify that no refined flour has been added to the product. Enriched breads such as those labeled "cracked wheat," "wheat," or "rye" are made with white, enriched flour plus lesser amounts of whole grain. "Enriched" flours lose about twenty nutrients during processing. Only four of these are added back in the process of enrichment. Enriched breads *are* nutritious, but they are not as nutritious as whole-grain breads, nor do they add as much roughage to the diet.

## Fats

Dietary fats should also give energy to preschoolers, and the nature of those fats in the diet is important. Some physicians are suggesting that children of this age should be placed on a low-cholesterol, high-polyunsaturated-fat diet in order to guard against late-life atherosclerosis, a disorder which may be associated with high cholesterol intake. Though there is currently no firm evidence that low-cholesterol diets at a young age will have a direct bearing on later cholesterol levels, it seems likely that the children who become accustomed to such diets in their preschool years will have an easier time keeping blood cholesterol low in adulthood.

Because there is reason to believe that relatively high cholesterol intake in infancy helps the body regulate the synthesis of cholesterol in later life and that cholesterol is essential to the synthesis of several bile acids and hormones, most physicians feel that severe restriction of high-cholesterol foods should begin only *after* infancy.

Dr. Samuel Fomon, a leading authority on infant and childhood nutrition, suggests that low-cholesterol diets be begun only after a child's second year. At that point in development, there is no evidence that dietary cholesterol is desirable, though later research might provide such evidence. Still, Dr. Fomon feels the probable benefits of a low-cholesterol diet make this slight risk worthwhile. By using skim or 2-percent milk, lean meat, low- or medium-cholesterol cheeses (those with less than 5 percent butterfat—mozzarella, ricotta, farmer's cheese, Neufchatel) and fewer eggs, a child may lower her cholesterol intake without losing valuable nutrients. Of course, the *calories* lost by using low-fat products will have to be made up in some way. Cholesterol-free margarine and polyunsaturated oils used in baked goods can help fill this gap. Greater use of whole-grain baked items can also supply nutrient-rich, low-cholesterol calories.

Though not all physicians agree with Fomon's opinion of low-cholesterol diets for the average preschooler, most do agree that such diets should definitely be used for preschoolers who have family hypercholesterolemia, an inherited disorder which predisposes an infant to high serum-cholesterol levels, which increase the risk of early onset of heart disease.

Since cases of chronic diarrhea have been reported in children whose fat intakes were cut to 27 percent of total caloric intake, fat-restriction should not be carried to extremes. Fat is an essential part of the human diet, and problems are likely to occur if severe restriction of fat is undertaken. A diet of 30 to 35 percent fat, in which 6 percent of total calories is in the form of saturated fat, should meet the recommendations of the American Heart Association without causing other health problems for the child. However, since the reported cases of chronic diarrhea due to fat-deprivation occurred in children whose diets were 27 percent fat, adjusting a child's fat intake to optimum levels may prove a difficult task. As a general rule, one might reduce animal fats without attempting to bring about drastic reductions in overall fat intake.

## Vitamins and Minerals

Ideally, a preschooler should gain all the necessary vitamins and minerals from the foods she eats. Under ordinary circumstances, and despite persuasive ads for multivitamin compounds, parents should not rely on supplements to do what foods can do better. All too many doctors encourage this practice. At the present, according to Jean Mayer, "Most physicians graduate from medical school with only a cursory understanding of nutrition. Consequently, when the practicing physician is confronted with a nutrition problem, he is forced to rely on pharmaceutical supplements for treatment."

If the family's physician or pediatrician can offer no dietary information and recommends a vitamin supplement, parents can and should consult a nutritionist such as those who work with the U.S. Department of Agriculture's Cooperative Extension Service. For example, their WIC program (Women, Infants, Children) not only offers nutritional counseling but also provides low-income families with adequate food for infants, preschoolers, and pregnant and nursing women. By eating the recommended foods, children not only receive vitamins and minerals but also gain vital calories, protein, carbohydrates, and fats. Consumption of vitamin pills should never be an excuse for poor eating habits.

Vitamin and mineral supplements are *medicine,* especially when they are in megavitamin form. Some of them, notably vitamins A and D and iron, are toxic in even relatively small amounts. While adults might never notice the slight effects of overdoses, children may exhibit a wide variety of symptoms if they are given excessive amounts of these vitamins and minerals. Again, meeting vitamin and mineral RDAs through diet, not through supplements, should be the goal.

Surveys indicate that preschoolers generally get the recommended amounts of most *vitamins.* The most common exceptions are vitamins A and

C. In one recent survey of children aged one through three, only 10 percent of the northern preschoolers and 18 percent of the southern preschoolers ate the dark green and yellow vegetables which offer vitamin A in significant quantities. In a more recent study, 36 percent of the preschoolers had diets judged "below optimal" because they were low in fruits and vegetables known to provide vitamin A. In that same survey, 21 percent of the children studied consumed no fruits during the twenty-four-hour recall period, 13 percent consumed no vegetables, and 4 percent consumed no fruits and no vegetables.

The diets of 55 percent of the preschoolers in the survey were judged "below optimal" because of low vitamin C intake. This figure is hardly surprising, considering the number of children who consumed no fruits and no vegetables in this same study. Vitamin C intakes have been declared low in many surveys of preschool children, with one study of low-income families showing vitamin C intakes which fell below 50 percent of RDA for ages one to three.

Some authorities argue that RDAs for ascorbic acid (vitamin C) are too high, yet the committee charged with setting RDAs for 1980 publication decided to raise ascorbic acid requirements slightly.

Current standards are relatively easy to meet if a child consumes a citrus fruit or juice high in vitamin C each day. Raw citrus fruits offer the surest method of consuming enough ascorbic acid, since there is no vitamin-C loss due to cooking. A glass of orange juice for breakfast is one of the simplest ways of meeting the vitamin C requirement. "Vitamin C added" labels on powdered breakfast drinks and canned orange drinks mean these drinks can provide vitamin C, but beyond this one added vitamin, the drinks offer little more than quick, refined-sugar energy, plus color and flavor additives. For optimum nutrition value, a mother may choose to buy fresh oranges and squeeze them, to buy pasteurized juice from the dairy counter, or to buy frozen orange juice concentrate.

One recent study showed that fresh orange juice has the highest level of active ascorbic acid (vitamin C), with frozen juice a close second and pasteurized juice a far third. At one time, storage of orange juice was thought to lower its ascorbic acid content. According to recent research, total ascorbic acid levels remain constant for about two weeks after frozen orange juice has been blended or stirred with tap water, when stored either at room temperature or in the refrigerator. However, another study cautions that levels of *usable* ascorbic acid may decrease somewhat after only a week of storing. With this in mind, families may wish to mix or squeeze only enough juice for four to five days.

*Mineral* intakes of preschoolers tend to be adequate except for calcium, iron, and zinc. In the north-central region study mentioned earlier, calcium and phosphorus intakes of preschoolers were adequate, but iron intakes were low as judged by 1968 RDA.

*Calcium* remains important in the diet of the preschooler. Although skeletal growth has slowed, there is an increase in the deposit of minerals for strengthening of bones. Adequate calcium is also essential to the development of strong teeth, and a child's permanent teeth are being formed during the preschool years. One recent study found the calcium intakes of *vegetarian* preschoolers ranging from 40 to 48 percent of RDA. Though *lacto-vegetarians* should have adequate calcium intakes, getting enough calcium from nondairy sources is extremely difficult for a vegan preschooler.

When *iron* deficiency is severe enough to cause anemia, such symptoms as fatigue, rapid blood circulation, and irregular, fast heartbeat may be present. Since these symptoms are not likely to be noticed by parents, anemia often goes undetected. To guard against this, the American Academy of Pediatrics recommends that full-term infants be routinely screened for this disorder between nine and twelve months and that preterm infants be screened between six and nine months of age.

Although many pediatricians do this early screening, most do not screen for anemia between the ages of one and two. This is interesting, in view of the fact that most nutrition surveys have found dietary iron intakes particularly low at this age. In fact, one survey of preschoolers from low-income families found that during their second year, some children consume less than half the Recommended Dietary Allowances for iron.

Several studies point to the importance of preventing and correcting anemia. One reported in 1971 that anemic three- to five-year-olds showed decreased attentiveness and narrow attention span, although they did not show lower IQs. Children given iron improved in these traits, while those given no iron did not. In 1973, other researchers reported that children with low hemoglobin levels had low IQ and vocabulary scores, with the younger anemic children showing the greatest deficit.

Though these studies would seem to indicate that anemia causes various types of learning disabilities, anemia *per se* is probably *not* the cause of all the problems described by these researchers, since children with even more severe nonnutritional forms of iron-deficiency anemia do not show these same problems. Still, since such symptoms as reduced work capacity in adults have been traced to iron deficiency, and since the impact of iron deficiency seems greater in children than in adults, avoiding even mild iron deficiencies in preschoolers seems highly desirable.

Currently, some experts feel that recommended allowances for iron are too high, since many persons who do not receive recommended levels of dietary iron do not become anemic. While lowering iron RDAs has been suggested, those who believe that subclinical (difficult to detect) iron deficiency can exist even in those persons who are not classed as anemic on the basis of hemoglobin tests oppose such a move. Even when normal hemoglobin levels are found, other lab tests may reveal subclinical iron deficiencies. Symptoms thought to be associated with those subclinical iron deficiencies include irritability, fatigue, weakness, anxiety, breathlessness and depression. These symptoms respond to iron supplements within a few days, although hemoglobin levels do not show the influence of supplements until much later. If these lab tests are used as criteria, incidence of iron deficiency may be as high as 30 percent in low-income infants and preschoolers.

The 1980 edition of *Recommended Dietary Allowances* discusses the importance of distinguishing between *absorbable* iron and total iron when determining iron intake. Emphasis is placed upon the importance which the nature of an entire meal has upon iron absorption.

Estimates show the average diet for one- to five-year-olds contains five milligrams (mg) of iron for every 1000 calories. This means that a toddler who consumes 1300 calories gains between 5 and 7 milligrams of iron. Since the RDA for ages one to three is set at 15 milligrams, the average toddler is not likely to gain sufficient iron from diet alone. On the other hand, some authorities feel that a diet which supplies the preschooler with 5.5 milligrams of iron per 1000 calories is likely to be quite adequate if that iron is well absorbed. If a preschooler's diet is too high in milk, soft drinks, unfortified baked goods, and other foods relatively high in calories and low in iron, gaining even 5.5 milligrams of iron per 1000 calories will be extremely difficult.

As noted earlier, it is for this reason, some pediatricians have recommended continuing use of iron-fortified infant cereals beyond babyhood. Since cooked infant cereals are not likely to be readily accepted by some toddlers and older children, many mothers prefer to fortify cooked oatmeal, Cream of Wheat, soups, and even baked goods with iron-rich baby cereals.

Iron from unfortified vegetable sources is less well absorbed than that from animal sources. For example, less than 5 percent of the iron in natural cereal products is absorbed, while 23 percent of the heme iron in meat is absorbed. Heme iron, associated with the blood and muscle tissue of animals and fish, is more readily absorbed than is non-heme iron, from eggs, dairy products, and vegetables.

Eating heme iron (meat, fish) and non-heme iron (vegetable products, dairy products, eggs) at the same meal increases absorption of non-heme iron while decreasing the absorption of heme iron. There is some evidence that inclusion of eggs, cheese, and fiber in the diet tends to interfere with iron absorption from other foods eaten at the same time, while *inclusion of vitamin C* in the diet tends to enhance absorption of iron from other foods eaten at the same time. In fact, some authorities feel that fortifying foods with vitamin C may be more effective than fortifying foods with iron to combat iron deficiency in developing countries. The amount of iron present in individual foods is probably less important in determining how well the iron will be absorbed and used than is the influence of all foods taken together at one meal.

In general, iron deficiency is most prevalent in low-income groups that eat few foods high in iron, especially heme iron. However, one study showed that the amount of money a family spends on food exerts more influence on iron intake than either the family's overall income or the mother's level of education. When children from higher income groups are iron deficient, they usually have decreased food intakes due to illness or teething problems or have diets abnormally high in heavily refined, low-iron foods.

Increased use of highly refined foods and decreased use of expensive meat products is also a contributing factor in *zinc* deficiency among preschoolers. In one group of Denver Headstart children chosen from low height percentiles, over two-thirds of the children were lower in both plasma and hair zinc levels than were a control group of children of normal height. From this study, one might assume that low zinc levels may lead to low growth percentiles. Loss of sharpness of the senses of taste and smell is a demonstrated zinc-deficiency symptom, and when these senses are diminished, appetite tends to be low, with resultant low weight gain.

In summary, by eating a well-balanced diet, a preschooler can gain adequate amounts of all the essential nutrients, with the possible exception of iron. Toddlers who show major vitamin or mineral deficiencies are often those who drink too much milk from a bottle, leaving them little appetite for table foods. Older preschoolers who drink too much milk or gain most of their calories from poorly planned meals or improper snacks are also at risk. By making a wide variety of foods available to a preschooler, parents can usually be sure that that child meets or exceeds RDA for all essential nutrients.

## Psychological Aspects

Of course, just buying a wide variety of foods does not make those foods acceptable to a toddler or older preschooler. Children are independent creatures by toddlerhood (if not before!), and they manage to have a great deal to say about which foods they eat and which they reject. To paraphrase, you can lead a child to spinach, but you can't make him eat! That is, not unless you try the force-feeding method adopted by one overanxious mother, who stood by her three-year-old daughter's plate, forked in bits of spinach, and ranted at the girl until every last bite was swallowed.

Whatever good the child might have gained from the spinach was hardly worth the psychological scars such feeding techniques probably left. The unpleasant scene will not likely be forgotten, nor will the fact that the unpleasantness was somehow associated with the eating of spinach. Since appetite for a food is directly connected to pleasant memories of that food, is it likely that this child will ever ask for this vegetable again? Faced with such a situation, a mother might simply acknowledge the child's dislike with "My, you really *don't* like spinach right now, do you? Well, let's just avoid spinach for a while!" By this method, a child's autonomy, his sense of independence, is not sacrificed, and the door is left open for another try at spinach when time and appetite are right.

Studies show that the time is more likely to be right before the child reaches the age of two, at least where new foods are concerned. The following chart, derived from a preschool nutrition survey involving nearly 3500 children, indicates comparative willingness or complete refusal to try new foods.

## Age-related Willingness to Try New Foods

| Age (yrs) | Percent Willing to Try New Foods | Percent Flatly Refusing New Foods |
|-----------|----------------------------------|-----------------------------------|
| 1–2       | 77                               | 6                                 |
| 2–4       | 68                               | 14                                |
| 4–6       | 60                               | 18                                |

SOURCE: Thomas A. Anderson, Stephen H. Y. Wei, and Samuel J. Fomon, "Nutrition Counseling and the Development of Eating Habits," in *The Food That Stays: An Update on Nutrition, Diet, Sugar and Caries,* ed. Edgar A. Sweeney (New York: Medcom, 1977).

When you introduce new foods, you should choose the child's best eating time and serve a favorite food at the same meal. If a child is too hungry, too tired, or too upset to eat even familiar items, she is not likely to welcome a new food. If the new food is a dry one, such as a hamburger patty, it should be served with moist, familiar foods such as creamed corn and green beans. If it is a hot, spicy food such as baked beans, it should be served with a bland food such as potato salad.

Only a small amount of the new food should be placed on the child's plate. Then, if the food is rejected, child and parent aren't faced with a mound of uneaten food, which may seem threatening to the child and wasteful to the parent. Some wasted food may be inevitable for preschoolers. As mentioned in the previous chapter, admonitions to "clean your plate" may lead a child to associate satiety (the comfortable feeling of fullness) with a clean plate rather than with natural cues such as satisfaction of hunger.

A toddler should be offered small portions and allowed the pleasure of being able to finish most of what has been offered and the privilege of indicating when he wants more. He may be praised for eating well, but such praise should not be overdone. By the latter part of his fourth year, a child should be encouraged to select his own portion sizes. At first, parents may need to remind him not to overload his plate, but he will soon learn how much he can eat without waste. Even if he takes too much, he should not be forced to eat it all.

Adults who would never think of forcing a pet to clean his dish often think a child should be forced to do so. A gentle suggestion that a child should eat all she can of what she has taken or an offer to help her get a few stray bites onto her fork might be all she needs to see the project through. If not, the child should be quietly reminded to take less next time, since she can always ask for more.

One overweight young woman remembered being forced as a child to clean her plate and avoid waste because of "all the children in the world who have to go to bed hungry." "By the time I figured out that no matter how much *I* ate, those other children would still be hungry," she explained, "I was already into the habit of overeating. I was determined never to make my boys clean their plates, but my old guilt feelings made me always eat whatever they left. That's disaster for anyone who puts on weight as easily as I do." Her experience should be remembered by those tempted to eat more than they need just to avoid waste. Better to let food go to waste than to waistline. Besides, eating more than one needs is, itself, a highly hazardous form of wasting food for both children and adults.

Children should be encouraged to gauge their appetites and take what they will be able to eat comfortably. This takes practice, and a five-year-old child may frequently overestimate his own capacity, especially until he learns to dish up portions not according to how much he ate last evening but according to how hungry he is this evening. His appetite may vary according to his activity level. When growth spurts occur, the child may become ravenous for days, then dwindle back to a normal appetite.

Except in unusual cases, the hunger drive of a toddler or preschooler is quite strong. He may even have severe hunger pains, and these pains do not always coincide with family mealtimes. Mealtime or not, when a child begins to feel that familiar tension in the stomach, to experience the general weakness and restlessness that follow a drop in blood sugar, he usually calls for food. To meet this emergency, many parents mistakenly rely on cookies, chips, or other empty, high-calorie foods. As noted earlier, building wise snacking habits is a project that pays high dividends, whereas contributing to the formation of poor snacking habits may mean long years of dental bills, obesity, and other problems.

The child who has enjoyed a nutritious snack no closer than forty-five minutes to an hour before mealtime should still have a healthy appetite for lunch or dinner. Even the heartiest appetite, however, may not mean the child will settle down to the business of eating. A preschooler fidgets, squirms, and twists, finding it hard to sit still for long periods of time. Since she may prefer socializing to eating if she begins the meal at the same time as her parents and older siblings, a child of this age may be allowed to start a few minutes early. This head start means a hungry child will be half through before distractions, in the form of those she loves, come in and join her.

If a child dawdles and refuses to finish her food once the family has joined her at the table, she should be told that she may leave the table but there will be no snacks until the next mealtime. A child won't starve because she misses part of a meal, provided the next meal is well balanced.

On the other hand, if a preschooler continues to eat well even in the presence of others, so that she finishes before other family members do, she may begin to rock in her chair or otherwise show that her quiet time is up. At this point, she may be allowed to leave the table and read or play quietly until it is time to rejoin the family for dessert. In this way, her naturally restless spirit need not be forced to conform to a long dinner hour at the cost of her good humor and her parents' nerves. This recognition of a child's limited ability to sit still can save a thousand reprimands over the toddler and preschool years.

Reprimands occur all too often in any family dining situation. When good manners are placed above pleasant atmosphere, tension builds and tempers flare. Eating should be relaxed and natural, with as few artificially imposed injunctions as possible. As one researcher has noted, severe training practices during preschool ages three to five are often associated with severe feeding problems shortly thereafter. Allowed to evolve from the observation of parents and older siblings, acceptable manners do develop, though they may come more slowly than some parents would like. The process may be hastened a bit if parents anticipate and avoid certain problems. For example, by cutting spaghetti into manageable bits, a father is less likely to see a long string dangling a trail of red down his preschooler's chin. Such small bits may be treated as finger foods if appetite outruns dexterity with fork or spoon.

According to child psychologists, a five-year-old who has made progress in eating quietly; is able to use a knife, fork, and spoon habitually and resorts to fingers only rarely; very seldom upsets his milk, uses a napkin properly; and occasionally says please and thank you spontaneously is a five-year-old whose manners should content his parents.

While manners should not be forced on toddlers or very young preschoolers, older preschoolers can be taught that certain behavior is acceptable at mealtime while other behavior is not. Parents who try to explain the *reasons* behind certain rules usually fare better than those who simply lay down ultimatums with a "Because I said so, that's why!" attitude. Better still, a preschooler who has helped set table regulations is more likely to understand and abide by them than is a child who has had no part in determining what constitutes acceptable and nonacceptable behavior during meals.

A child who is regulated without apparent reason is not likely to enjoy meals. Anyone who recalls the countless stories in which small children are required to sit for long periods of time at a formal dining table which looks about as inviting as an iceberg, should be able to feel what a child feels in a situation too formal for his system to handle. Nothing tastes good because nothing, including the food, seems natural. Charles Dickens's orphanage dining room scene in *Oliver Twist,* translated so brilliantly from book to screen in the musical *Oliver!* provides a particularly vivid example of an atmosphere which is *not* conducive to comfortable, spontaneous eating.

In homes where formal dining is preferred, a toddler should probably have her main meal early, so that no one minds if she eats only a few finger foods and then asks to be excused until dessert time. Some families prefer that preschoolers and even young children of school age eat at a small table by themselves. This arrangement may be quite desirable when guests are present. If the guests bring children of their own, host children can help set up a small table away from sensitive adult ears. In this way, the occasion becomes special to both children and adults.

Certainly, if a father can't be home until seven on weeknights, evening meals may be served to the children at five-thirty or six so they can be fed and ready for a story and goodnight kiss when daddy does come in. Starving children until seven can only mean frayed nerves for mom and little ones too. Allowing them an abundance of snacks between the time they get hungry and the seven o'clock dinner hour usually leads to nibbled meals and harsh words from parents. Each family should find the pattern which seems to fit its particular needs, then follow that pattern—whether or not the neighbors approve!

This same rule could be applied to any dining practice: Find out what works well, then use it consistently so that children know what to expect. For example, even when parents provide well-balanced, easily handled glasses and cups, spills do occur and adult reactions to these spills are always important. One parent might slam down his napkin, snatch the startled child from her chair, and send her to her room bewildered and confused. On the other hand, another parent might first ascertain whether the spill was on purpose or accidental, then act in a firm, calm way to set the matter straight.

Usually, children treated with this extra bit of parental understanding feel enough remorse about the accident without being screamed at and humiliated still further. Besides, when dad's own cuff catches on and overturns a water glass, he, too, will appreciate a little understanding from the family.

One notable exception to the general rule about handling spills should be mentioned. A two-year-old is quite likely to grab up his soup dish and call "All gone" as he happily turns the last few spoonfuls of noodles and vegetables onto the kitchen carpet. His antics, though obviously not accidental, must be handled with care, for flying into a rage may be just the act he needs to bring an end to the boredom he's felt all morning. Even a slapped hand may not work, as in the case of one little boy who was promised and given a slap on the hand each time he threw food from his tray. His parents finally admitted they should reconsider this training technique when he began to toss off food with his right hand while holding out his little left hand with a mischievous "Hand, mama, hand!" As mentioned in Chapter 5, a plastic dropcloth can spare nerves and carpet as mom and dad huddle over a new bit of strategy to try on the habitual food tosser or habitual milk spiller. Through all the little traumas of mealtimes, parents need to remind themselves that the formation of wholesome attitudes about food is more important for a preschooler than the acquisition of perfect manners.

Some children develop an unusual fondness for one particular food and demand nothing else. Such food jags are common at various points of development during the preschool years. Fortunately, the favorite food is often requested at only one meal, with other foods being perfectly acceptable at other times of the day. Food jags allowed to play themselves out naturally are likely to be over sooner than those which give rise to great dinner table scenes in which the child and his chosen food item become the focal point of mealtime conversation.

This same generality can be applied to food dislikes. They are usually less likely to persist if treated in a matter-of-fact manner. Usually, the substitution of foods of similar nutritional value is quite simple, especially if a parent works with the Minimum Exchange Chart in Appendix A. On rare occasions, a child dislikes an entire category of food (such as meat). Parents may need to consult a physician or nutritionist if this problem persists beyond a week or two.

In any case, every effort should be made to determine *why* the child refuses a particular food. Has she heard other kindergarteners say that vegetables are yukky? Has she developed a sore throat, which makes citrus juice burn and irritate? Are the meats she's offered moist enough for her to chew and swallow easily? Would she like vegetables if they were raw instead of cooked, cooked for a shorter time, or garnished with a topping of her favorite cheese?

Some children simply don't like some foods. This should not be surprising, for few adults can say with honesty that they like all the foods they've ever tried. If genuine dislike of a food seems evident, you might offer that food periodically, so that the child can observe his parents and siblings eating and enjoying it even when no one offers him a taste. Eventually, he may come around. If not, only parents who have no dislikes themselves should feel the least bit justified in insisting that a child eat something he really doesn't like.

While the introduction of a *new* food is most often successful if the new item is served with an old favorite available for immediate consumption, a food which has been previously tried and rejected may do better served alone. If no other choice exists, the hungry child may try the food again and find he can enjoy it this time. This happens, of course, only if no issue is made over the fact that he has no choice but to eat the previously rejected food or go hungry.

One father of two says that he never learned to eat many vegetables until after he married, because his mother always fixed an alternative to those dishes he claimed to dislike. His wife tended to be tolerant of his dislikes, too, until their first child started to eat table foods. At that point, a truce was drawn, and dad agreed to try a bit of all he was presented with. Today he eats with pleasure a number of those foods he once thought he hated. His children, offered a wide variety of items from an early age and having the benefit of dad's excellent example, are not likely to have to wait so many years before they learn to like the foods they may at first think are not the best.

Unfortunately, in many homes children might have no idea what either parent is eating or even when they themselves are eating, for television has full family attention. In such a situation, family fellowship is completely gone, and whatever food has been prepared cannot be fully appreciated. In fact, if the show is upsetting to the children, they may not even digest their food well.

Families spend all too few hours together in today's hurried society. Mealtimes should be reserved for pleasant interaction, not television viewing. This means, of course, that dad may need to give up a half-hour of World Series game time if he expects the children to stop watching their programs in order to join the family at the dinner table. When children have certain programs which they feel are especially important, a mother may wish to guard against unpleasantness by deliberately avoiding scheduling a meal during the favorite program.

In one family, the preschoolers knew that when "Sesame Street" ended, dinner would be ready. On those occasions when dinner ran a few minutes late, children were told that they could either turn off the TV and read while they were waiting or watch the first few minutes of another program, provided they agreed to leave that program when they were called to eat. This arrangement was adopted after several tearful sessions in which the five-year-old became upset at being asked to leave the second show before it had ended. Once parents and child agree upon the terms outlined above, there were no more tearful outbursts at having to leave the program.

Making the TV off-limits during mealtime serves no useful purpose unless the family makes these mealtimes pleasant. Parents who use lunch as a time to discuss serious problems in an intense manner are likely to find their preschooler doing everything possible to prevent the continuation of this discussion. For a child, acting out is a natural reaction to being excluded. If he can't get attention by eating quietly, he tries a few tactics designed to bring him into the center of things. He may sail a saucer across the room, deliberately spill his milk and then cry about having done so, or even provoke a spanking—anything to avoid being ignored.

Parents who include a child in their conversations and actively seek out his opinion on whatever topics he can handle avoid giving him a reason to act up during the meal. One four-year-old so enjoyed being able to add her opinion and comment to mealtime conversation that she listened intently to adult topics to which she would ordinarily have had no comment to add, then rushed in with "Did you know that Carl [her imaginary playmate] did that just last week? He's such a silly boy!" Often she had no idea of *what* she was saying Carl had done, but being able to add her comments made her feel a part of the curious world grown-ups occupy. Instinctively, she chose to use her imaginary playmate, not a real one, so that both she and her parents would feel no need to question whatever precocious feats Carl might perform.

Imaginary friends are, for many children, a part of being four years old. Four-year-olds often have other rather predictable traits—they talk too much at the table, wiggle constantly, and ask to go to the bathroom during meals. The little girl who related Carl's antics occasionally left the table abruptly with "I've got to go 'poo.' " Letting her know that this was not acceptable table talk without making bathroom business seem taboo became the parents' responsibility. Fortunately, she was so amused by the fact that grown-ups simply say, "Please may I be excused a moment" and slip quietly away that she deliberately and politely asked to be excused at every meal for a week thereafter.

Knowing a few of the likes and dislikes of preschoolers should help a parent plan meals for this age group. Generally, preschoolers are fascinated by differences and by likenesses. They enjoy seeing foods of bright and varied colors served together. They are proud of their newly acquired ability to recognize and name colors, and reciting the colors of various foods makes eating those foods more interesting.

Differences in texture also interest children. Some children do not like foods that stick to their mouths or hands, or fruits with seeds which can be chewed into. Others do not care for rough, dry, or stringy foods. Meals that present several foods with almost identical texture are less enjoyable than those which provide a variety of textures. For young children, each meal might include something soft and easy to chew (such as creamed potatoes), something crisp and fun to listen to (such as carrot sticks), and something chewy enough to require the use of newly learned chewing skills (such as moist hamburger patties).

Chewing skills are developed in different ways by different children. Some children seem to have trouble swallowing and must chew and chew before getting down food which other children swallow with ease. Others tend to hold food in one cheek, chipmunklike, and savor it fully before finally swallowing it. Others are eager eaters who fill their mouths and swallow without chewing well. With maturity, these chewing habits should become less obvious and less offensive to parents. Preschoolers who are constantly berated for chewing too slowly or chewing too fast may deliberately cling to their offensive behavior for effect. Children allowed to outgrow their chewing idiosyncrasies will usually do so on their own.

As mentioned earlier, babies and young children have more taste buds than older children and adults. Perhaps this is why many youngsters seem to prefer bland foods. Others, of course, enjoy highly flavored foods. Pickles, pickled okra, and green chilis may be treats for one five-year old but "yuks" for another.

Extremely tart fruits which are rejected by a child may be mixed with mild ones. For example, apples, bananas, and oranges provide a variety of vitamins in a tasty form enjoyed by most children.

If vegetable flavors seem too strong, you might try cooking the vegetables with more water or without the lid. Unfortunately, such cooking practices diminish vitamins as well as flavor. Perhaps you could add less and less water and allow fewer and fewer minutes of open-kettle cooking as the child's tolerance for strong flavors increases. Cream or cheese sauces can also hide strong vegetable flavors, but such sauces should not completely disguise the flavor of vegetables. Sometimes the strong *smell* of cabbage or Brussels sprouts cooking makes the child unwilling to try these vegetables. For this reason, a kitchen deodorizer might be helpful when strong foods are cooked.

The following tips on vegetable preparation, suggested by Cooperative Extension Service, Oklahoma State University, should help make vegetables more attractive for preschoolers.

## VEGETABLE PREPARATION TIPS

1. Don't overcook.
2. Serve some vegetables raw.
3. Cook vegetables whole for maximum vitamin retention and cut them into bite-size bits when serving so they may be forked easily or eaten as single foods.
4. Note whether a child who will not eat frozen vegetables will eat those same vegetables in canned or fresh form, then use the preferred form as often as possible.
5. Keep servings small, about one level tablespoonful for each year up to age four, so children may enjoy success.
6. Use raw vegetables as a between-meal snack.

Though children's likes and dislikes vary widely, an awareness of common childhood attitudes about various foods may be helpful. The following chart, which represents findings of a 1974 study of food attitudes and snacking patterns of preschool and elementary school children, gives information obtained in interviews with the mothers of the preschoolers in the study.

### Favorite Foods by Categories (Percent)

|                  | Preschool | Elementary |
|------------------|-----------|------------|
| Meats            | 38.8%     | 52.3%      |
| Snack items      | 16.7      | 4.5        |
| Dairy foods      | 11.1      | 4.5        |
| Mixed dishes     | 11.1      | 20.4       |
| Breads, cereals  | 5.5       | 4.5        |
| Desserts         | 5.5       | 9.1        |
| Fruits           | 5.5       | —          |
| Vegetables       | 5.5       | 4.5        |

## Disliked Foods by Categories (Percent)

|                          | Preschool | Elementary |
|--------------------------|-----------|------------|
| Cooked vegetables        | 50.1%     | 47.7%      |
| Mixed dished, casseroles | 14.1      | 10.7       |
| Meat                     | 8.8       | 7.7        |
| Liver                    | 7.0       | 12.4       |
| Raw vegetables           | 5.3       | 6.2        |
| Cottage cheese           | 3.5       | 1.5        |
| Fish                     | 3.5       | 6.2        |
| Fruit                    | 3.5       | 1.5        |
| Eggs                     | 1.7       | 4.6        |
| Milk                     | 1.7       | 1.5        |

SOURCE: Adapted from Nancy R. Beyer and Patricia M. Morris, "Food Attitudes and Snacking Patterns of Young Children," *Journal of Nutrition Education* 6 (1974):131.

As the chart indicates, most children seem to prefer crisp, raw vegetables to cooked ones. The 8.8 percent who disliked meat might have had difficulty chewing and swallowing overcooked, dry meat. Conversely, the 38.8 percent who listed meat as their favorite food might be enjoying small, moist, bite-sized bits.

Children who dislike mixed dishes might simply prefer to distinguish exactly what they are eating, rather than being given a casserole in which no single flavor is evident. Perhaps a child objects to a particular casserole because it runs all over her plate, defying her to eat it with fork, spoon, or fingers. Incidentally, almost as many children listed casseroles and other mixed dishes as their favorite foods as listed such items as disliked foods.

Children who do not care for milk might enjoy it more if they were allowed to pour their own portion from a small, easily-handled pitcher. If this doesn't work, such children can gain the calcium and other valuable nutrients usually supplied by milk from cheese and from powdered or whole milk cooked into puddings, casseroles, and creamed soups.

Some children may prefer their milk at room temperature, since extremely cold foods are often unpleasant to the very young. Most children do manage to eat ice cream before it melts, though some prefer to swirl it into a milky mass before consuming it. Others eat well-frozen ice cream so eagerly that they develop an "ice cream headache." Some children dislike extremely hot foods, though they may be so hungry they dive into a casserole and burn themselves in the process. Dropping a small bit of ice into a soup bowl and allowing the hungry child to stir until the soup cools provides a diversionary activity for the impatient child.

In general, most foods are more acceptable to children if they are served at room temperature. By putting the preschooler's plate on the table before calling him to dinner, a parent gains a few minutes of cooling time for the food on that plate. When he is faced with food that is so hot it cannot be eaten, yet smells and looks so delicious it cannot be resisted, a preschooler is quite likely to express his displeasure in no uncertain terms. Parents who understand his frustration and deal with it matter-of-factly should be able to soothe his nerves and help him relax and eat the food. By that time, it should be cool enough to be safe!

Whatever the mealtime problem, a calm and understanding attitude will usually go far toward solving it, while adult temper flare-ups and overreactions usually make problem situations worse, not better. With a little attention, mealtimes can be pleasant, happy times which give a child a positive, open attitude about eating. As one nutrition team expressed it, "Eating is one of the great pleasures of life and [a parent] should direct . . . efforts toward making it an enjoyable experience. . . ."

# Common Problems

## Dental Caries

Dental caries, the most prevalent disease for all age groups beyond infancy, affects 97 percent of all Americans before they reach adulthood. Over $2 billion a year is spent on repairing teeth in the United States. Dentists estimate that nearly $8 billion would be needed if all the teeth that needed work were treated. If this is true in America, the land of plenty, what must decay be like in less well developed areas of the world?

Ironically, even in areas where malnutrition is common, tooth decay is less common than in the United States. Caucasian citizens of Baltimore, Maryland, have ten times the number of cavities as members of the hill tribes of South Vietnam or the natives of Ethiopia. In general, persons in developed countries such as southern Europe, Canada, and the United States have adequate to good nutrition but a high incidence of caries, while persons in underdeveloped nations have poorer overall nutrition but fewer caries.

A clue to this apparent mystery lies in a brief look at the history of tooth decay. Neolithic and Bronze Age people had relatively few cavities compared to the Romans. As the following chart indicates, Anglo-Saxon and medieval populations had relatively few cavities compared to seventeenth- and nineteenth-century people. If the twentieth century had been added to this chart, even higher percentages of decay would have been evident. Why does tooth decay appear to have risen along with standards of living?

Aristotle pointed toward the answer two thousand years ago when he

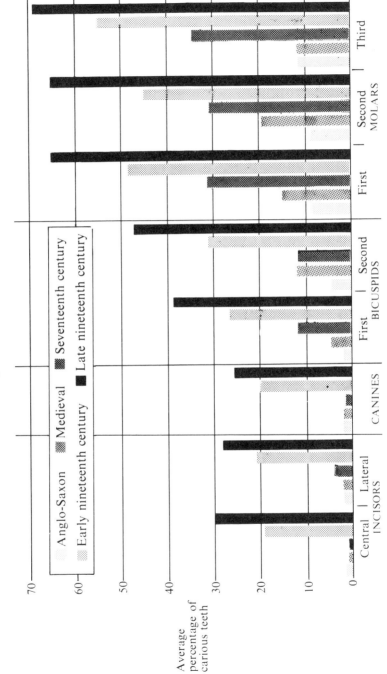

History of Incidence of Dental Caries

Anglo-Saxon   Medieval   Seventeenth century

Early nineteenth century   Late nineteenth century

Average percentage of carious teeth

Central | Lateral    CANINES    First | Second    First | Second    Third
INCISORS                        BICUSPIDS         MOLARS

SOURCE: Edward A. Sweeney ed., *The Food That Stays* (New York: Medcom, 1977).

observed that eating soft, sweet figs resulted in damage of teeth. Even today, tests have shown that increased decay is likely if one eats dried fruits such as figs and raisins, because dried fruits are high in sucrose (sugar) and are likely to stick to the teeth for long periods of time.

Aristotle's population was fortunate—refined sugar had not yet been introduced. After Europe's introduction to loaf sugar during the Middle Ages, more and more sugar was added to food. By the nineteenth century, a new product, white, refined flour, was being turned into cookies, cakes, and other sugar-rich items, and the sugar in these baked goods adhered to the teeth. As the historical chart indicates, caries incidence increased steadily throughout the nineteenth century. The only break in this upward rise in cavities came between the two world wars of the twentieth century, when shipping blockades forced reduction of sugar imports and greater dependence on fresh fruits and vegetables.

Today, about 95 percent of American children are cavity-free at the age of one. However, a marked increase in caries incidence occurs during the preschool years. Five to ten percent of all two-year-olds, forty to fifty-five percent of all three-year-olds, and seventy-five percent of all five-year-olds have some cavities. In fact, the average American five-year-old has 4.6 decayed or filled teeth.

Signs of mild cases of the "nursing bottle syndrome" discussed in the previous chapter are occasionally observed for the first time in a child of five or six. Though enamel damage from ill-advised nursing-bottle use occurred earlier, the affected teeth may be just beginning to show cavity formation. In many cases, vigorous cleaning and topical fluoride applications may stop further destruction and allow remineralization of the enamel to occur.

All too often, parents accept cavities and even teeth completely lost to decay with the attitude, "Well, they were only baby teeth." Premature loss of primary teeth is a common cause of malocclusion (faulty closure) of permanent teeth. When molars are lost, chewing is impaired and the remaining teeth float out of line, so that the permanent teeth come in crooked and out of place. If front teeth are lost, biting becomes difficult and speech problems may occur. Severe abscesses in baby teeth may cause enamel defects in the permanent teeth that will replace them. A young child should be spared the pain and discomfort which accompanies the decay of primary teeth, and should be encouraged to form good dental habits early if she is to be expected to take proper care of her permanent teeth when they come in.

Though many factors contribute to caries development in preschoolers, tooth decay is primarily an infectious bacterial disease. Germ-free animals have no tooth decay, even when they receive a diet which is 65 percent sugar and known to be caries producing under other circumstances.

In 1683, Anton van Leeuwenhoek scraped a sticky, gelatinous substance from human teeth and placed it under his newly invented microscope. With the help of this sensitive optical instrument, he noted the presence of living organisms in this substance. He probably saw *Streptococcus mutans,* the principal microorganism believed to be responsible for tooth decay.

As long as *Streptococcus mutans* bacteria are not attached to tooth enamel, they are constantly being bathed away by saliva and swallowed. However, when *Streptococcus mutans* interact with sucrose (sugar), they form a sticky, gelantinous substance called dental plaque. United in plaque colonies, these decay-producing bacteria are able to stick to the enamel surface of the teeth. Once they are there, the bacteria colonies grow and the dental plaque gets harder and harder to remove.

Refined sugars readily pass through dental plaque, while sugars found in fresh fruits usually do not. As sugar passes through the plaque, it is metabolized by the bacterial enzymes into organic acids. The matrix of plaque protects these acids from the diluting and cleansing action of saliva, thus giving them time to erode tiny pores in the enamel. Proteolytic (protein-decomposing) bacteria then pass through these pores to invade and destroy tooth dentine. Once the dentine is destroyed, the remaining enamel walls collapse and a cavity occurs.

Now that we know the identity of at least one strain of bacteria which produces caries, work is underway to find agents to combat *Streptococcus mutans.* Even if such an agent is found, there are many complex issues to be settled before the public can depend upon an anticavity inoculation with yearly boosters. For now, and probably for many years to come, other means of fighting tooth decay must be employed. According to Dr. Abraham Nizel, use of currently available preventive dentistry measures could reduce caries incidence by 60 to 70 percent.

What are these measures? First, every child should visit a dentist at *least* by age three, for preventive care. Second, children should be taught wise eating habits, including the elimination of sugar-rich snacks. Finally, fluoride dietary supplements should be used unless the water supply has been fluoridated or is naturally high in fluorides.

Since alteration of eating habits is not always carried out, dentists feel that the use of dietary fluoride supplements holds the greatest hope for reduction of tooth decay. The best way to insure proper fluoride use for large populations has been the addition of fluoride to drinking water—the benefits are there every time the tap is opened. When fluoridated water is consumed throughout life, dental caries is reduced by 50 to 60 percent in permanent teeth and slightly less in primary teeth. As of 1972, about 60 percent of the public water supplies in the United States contained fluoride.

Not everyone agrees on the benefits of fluoride. Periodically, articles are written which claim that cancer mortality increased more in cities with fluoridated water supplies than in cities without such supplies. When such claims have been investigated further, additional significant data have usually been discovered. For example, the city with higher cancer mortality rates is found to have had a far larger percentage of residents over age 65 than did the city with the lower cancer mortality rates. Time after time, when such examples have been used to point out the dangers of using fluoridated drinking water, adjustment of the figures to allow for such variables as age, sex and ethnic groups leaves no evidence to support the theory that fluoridated water causes cancer.

In one twenty-year study of 473 American cities, the National Institutes of Health found no consistent relation between fluoridation and observed changes in mortality. Only one city which used fluoride showed an unexplained increase in mortality, while several cities which did *not* fluoridate their drinking water also showed unexplained increases in mortality.

Furthermore, there is no significant difference in microscopic bone structure of persons who have ingested fluoride for a prolonged period of time and those who have not. Even persons living in areas of Texas whose drinking water contains ten times more fluoride than normal do not appear to suffer skeletal abnormalities, though they do tend to have cavity-resistant, though mottled, teeth. Such mottling is common when large amounts of fluoride are ingested prior to tooth formation. In lesser amounts, tooth decay is reduced, but no mottling occurs.

Opponents of fluoridation have pointed out the fact that fluoride gas is poisonous. The same might be said about chloride gas, yet proper chlorination of water supplies does not poison those who use the water. While fluoridated water has been blamed for increase in the incidence of mongoloid (Downs Syndrome) births, cardiovascular disease, and cancer, none of these accusations has held up under investigation.

On the other hand, countless studies have proven that fluoridation of drinking water can and does reduce tooth decay. When fluoride is ingested before tooth eruption, the mineral is incorporated into tooth structure, whereby premature loss of teeth has been reduced by as much as 75 percent. If fluoride is ingested after the teeth have erupted, the mineral washes over the teeth and gets into the crystal spaces, reducing tooth decay by 60 percent or more. This great reduction in cavities means reduction of the number of times a child will need a local anesthetic for dental work. The trauma of visits to the dentist office are lessened, and risk of dangerous abcesses or other serious complications are greatly reduced. The proven benefits clearly outweigh the supposed dangers of fluoride use.

Fluoridated water supplies make a great contribution to dental health and pose no serious threats to overall health of children or adults. Though joining a group opposed to the addition of "chemicals" to a city's water supply might seem to be proof of one's interest in environmental issues, fighting for the right to retain a fluoridated water supply may be more valid proof of one's interest in the health of the city's population. Those communities which have voted to stop using fluoride have returned to the pre-fluoridation status of tooth decay and premature tooth loss within five years of discontinuing fluoridation. When faced with a vote concerning fluoridation, parents who have read all available literature will likely campaign for, not against, fluoridation of drinking water.

Parents of children who do not live in cities with fluoridated water sup-plies should ask their doctor or dentist to prescribe a fluoride supplement for home use. Such supplements must be used with care, since excessive intake of fluoride leads to mottled, grayish enamel. Generally, multivitamin preparations which have fluoride added are less likely to give a child op-timum amounts of fluoride than are separate fluoride supplements, because the composition of such multinutrient tablets cannot take into account the natural fluoride level of the drinking water. Children who also receive topi-cal fluoride application from their dentist at six-month intervals show even greater benefits.

Since children under the age of three probably swallow toothpaste, using fluoride toothpaste several times a day might mean a child could swallow enough fluoride to cause mottling of permanent teeth. If fluoride toothpaste is used with young children, care should be taken to see that the toothpaste is not swallowed. Since preschoolers need help in brushing their teeth, pa-rental supervision is advisable whether or not a toothpaste with fluoride is used.

Regular visits to a dentist and addition of fluoride to the diet are helpful, but attention to overall nutrition, careful management of sugar, and the development of sound snack and treat habits are also necessary for preven-tive dentistry to be effective. Adequate overall nutrition is crucial to the development of sound, cavity-resistant teeth. At ten months, two-and-a-half years, and five years, developing teeth are particularly susceptible to defi-ciencies in the diet. When a child's daily food intake includes an adequate number of calories plus recommended amounts of protein, vitamins C, A, and D, calcium, phosphorus, and fluoride, primary and permanent teeth have an excellent opportunity for optimum development. If any crucial nutrient is lacking at precisely the time of enamel formation in a particular tooth, imperfections in the enamel surfaces of that tooth are likely to occur.

Even if a child gets adequate amounts of all the nutrients essential to the production of strong, healthy teeth, a diet high in sugar, especially refined sugar in the form of candy and other confectionary items, is likely to pro-mote cavities. There is increasing evidence that sugar (especially sucrose) in the diet is *the* leading supporting agent in the promotion of cavities. In order to become a tooth-decay agent, sugar must come in contact with the teeth. Laboratory animals fed through tubes which allow high sugar foods to pass into the stomach without making contact with the teeth do not develop cavities. In lab animals or in humans, foods of high-sugar content must come in contact with the teeth in order for plaque to form and decay to proceed as described above.

Most dentists agree that there are three main factors determining the caries-causing potential of sugar in the diet. First, the *form* of the sugar should be considered. The sugar in a candy bar is solid and readily sticks between and on the teeth. A carbonated soft drink has liquid sugar, which passes quickly and does less damage. One study showed gummy candy such as caramels to be the most retentive form of sugar, with cookies and crackers next in line. Other studies placed baked goods further down the line.

Parents who are tempted to rush to the nearest health food store and buy special snacks for their children should realize that, in terms of potential for causing tooth decay, some health-food snack items may be worse than their grocery store counterparts. For example, in a recent study in Texas, foods were given a ranking of 1 to 10, with 10 indicating the highest cariogenicity (potential for causing tooth decay). An all-natural carob "hi-protein" energy bar received a 10, while a Hershey's milk chocolate bar was farther down the scale. All granola bar items and granola-type cookies ranked 4 to 7, as opposed to bread items like cinnammon rolls and honey buns which rated a 9. Fritos Corn Chips and popcorn received an impressive 0, while cheddar-cheese-flavored club crackers scored 8.

As the above figures indicate, "health-foods" that might, in some ways, be more desirable as snacks for a child than would grocery store snack items might nevertheless in terms of tooth decay be considerably less desirable. Since other researchers have come up with different ways of measuring the sugar-retention potential of snack items, the picture is not yet complete and parents may need to make judgment calls on items which some dentists approve and others disapprove. Nonetheless, parents and children should keep in mind that the *form* of the sugar is a major factor in the cariogenicity of the sugar.

Second, the *time of day* that sugar is consumed makes a difference. Between-meal high-sugar-content snacks not followed immediately by brushing leave sugar on the teeth. Mealtime high-sugar-content foods are usually less harmful because they are eaten with other foods, so that these foods, the saliva produced during chewing, and the liquids drunk with the meal all help remove the sugar from the teeth. Brushing the teeth after every meal also reduces the opportunity for sugar to stay on the teeth long enough to damage them.

Finally, the frequency with which sugar is eaten is important. One candy bar eaten completely means the teeth are subjected to a fifteen- to twenty-minute period of the bacterial acid formation which leads to decay. If that same bar is nibbled every two hours over a six-hour period, there will be three fifteen- to twenty-minute periods of potential decay, three times as much time for tooth destruction. If ten taffy or caramel candies are nibbled at the rate of one every half-hour over an afternoon, every piece of candy provides the teeth with a potentially decay-causing coating of sugar. If all ten candies are eaten at once, the teeth are exposed to only one bath of sugar.

If parents take into consideration the form of the sugar and the time and frequency of its consumption, they need not completely omit sugar from the diet of a preschooler. If they provide sound meals with occasional dessert treats containing sugar, and if high-sugar snacks are avoided between meals, tooth decay from sugar consumption is likely to be minimal. As noted earlier, it's not always easy to determine what constitutes a high-sugar snack. For example, fresh fruits are a better snack than candy, but frequent fruit snacks can also damage the teeth. Raisins are advertised as a snack that's better than candy, but raisins are relatively high in sugar and stick to the teeth. Their nutritive value (especially iron) is higher than that of candy, but their decay-causing potential is as high as that of many candies.

As long as any significant degree of sucrose is in the daily diet (28 grams or 1 ounce per day), any other form of sugar becomes more likely to cause cavities. Indeed, Dr. Richard Parker of the University of Oregon School of Dentistry believes that "the most devastating action occurs when sucrose forms the basic plaque network and glucose-fructose sources hasten its growth." Thus, if a sugar-coated cereal is eaten for breakfast or if sugar is added to cereal which is not presweetened, and a child doesn't clean her teeth well, a colony of sucrose-based plaque is laid down. If the child then eats a banana, that banana becomes three to five times more likely to cause cavities after six hours of interaction with sucrose plaque than it would without interaction with sucrose plaque.

If Parker is correct, following the form-time-frequency plan for eating sugar won't eliminate the possibility of tooth decay. However, following this plan should certainly *reduce* the occurrence of cavities, especially in view of the fact that a large part of the sugar eaten by the average American child is consumed in the form of candy, soft drinks and other high-sugar-content between-meal snacks. Eliminating such snack foods means providing attractive alternatives, such as fresh fruits and vegetables. Accomplishing this goal also means discouraging grandparents and others from attempts to buy affection with candy. Once grandparents see that gifts such as puzzles and books last longer and do less harm, they are usually glad to follow the no-candy policy. Dessert treats with sugar should be kept to a minimum, perhaps by designating one evening per week for the consumption of a special treat such as cake or pie. Other desserts can be fruits or low-sugar treats. But a casual approach should probably be taken, lest children learn to think of cakes and pies as the superstars of the dessert world.

Choosing perfect between-meal snacks means considering *all* aspects of nutrition, not just dental-health aspects. Ideally, a dentist would prefer that a child have no snacks at all, since this would mean sugar and other carbohydrates would be in contact with the teeth only three times each day. On the other hand, some physicians feel that preschool children are not ready for a three-meal, no-snack day. Certainly, many children do get hungry between meals and are irritable and unhappy unless they are fed. Dentists would like to see hard-cooked eggs and cheese as snack items, but those physicians who advocate lowering the cholesterol intake of children feel such snacks are inappropriate. Dentists feel that pretzels are an acceptable snack, but doctors who worry about sodium intakes see salty pretzels as undesirable. Nutritionists feel that peanut butter and crackers make a wholesome snack, but dentists point out that such a snack sticks to the teeth. All of this can be very confusing to parents who wish to choose snack items wisely.

About the only snack items which doctors, dentists, and nutritionists *all* approve are raw vegetables! Dentists like them because they are usually fibrous and require vigorous chewing. Chewing stimulates saliva flow, which washes away decay-causing bacteria, dilutes acids, and provides nutrients which help strengthen enamel. Nutritionists and doctors like the high vitamin and mineral content of fresh vegetables, plus the fact that they are low-cholesterol, low-sodium, low-sugar, and low-calorie items.

While sugarless gum should be acceptable to dentists and doctors alike, *all* sugarless gums are not. Those gums which rely on sorbitol have *not* been proven safe for teeth because *S. mutans,* a major cariogenic microorganism, can use sorbitol much as it uses sucrose. Chewing gums which contain xylitol are preferred by most dentists, since this sugar substitute cannot be metabolized by *S. mutans* bacteria. On the other hand, recent tests show that xylitol may be a cancer-causing chemical for rats. Faced with such choices, parents may have to hope their children dislike chewing gum!

One item *condemned* by all three groups is candy. Cookies remain open to debate. While nutritionists are aware that some cookies, especially those made with raisins and dates, are high in vitamins and iron, dentists see those same cookies as capable of leaving sugar on the teeth. Unless milk or water is taken with the cookies and teeth are rinsed or brushed afterwards, even the most nutritious cookies may contribute to tooth decay.

Parents must view snack choices from all angles, then decide which course they will take in setting snack guidelines for their own families. By using the following list, they can determine which snacks their children can consume regularly. There will always be special occasions when less desirable snacks should be allowed. For example, ice cream cones from a drive-in dairy bar may be the perfect treat for a family returning from a summer boating outing, though ice cream cones would not be a common at-home treat. Parents who make absolutely no exceptions to general snacking rules may find that their children soon rebel against such strictness.

Finding ways in which to make healthful snacks attractive is sometimes a challenge, especially if parents are attempting to retrain older preschoolers who have been accustomed to high-sugar snack treats. Various snack ideas are presented in the menu and snack guides in Appendix B of this book. Other ideas can be obtained from friends, magazine articles, and publications for parents of diabetic children.

Letting a preschooler help pick out supermarket fruits, vegetables, and cheeses means that child will take a greater interest in these items when they are offered as snacks. Even a three-year-old can help wash broccoli and cauliflower and break these vegetables into handy dipping sizes. If you put the washed vegetables in plastic bags or airtight containers, they will be easily available to small hands. Carrots, too, can be prepared ahead of time, and they are less likely to dry out if sliced into handy sticks and placed in a refrigerated glass of water.

## Guidelines for Healthful Snacks

| Food Group | Recommended for Snacks | Recommended for Mealtime Consumption Only (see note below) |
|---|---|---|
| Bread and Cereal | Popcorn; crackers;* pretzels;* chips* | Breads; cereals; cookies; cake |
| Dairy products (filling snacks, so serve well before meals; calcium and phosphorus in these foods may strengthen tooth enamel) | Whole, low-fat, skim milk or buttermilk; plain yogurt; cottage cheese; cream cheese; hard cheese;** low-fat cheese; low-fat spreads and dips | Ice cream; chocolate or other flavored milk; fruited or sweetened yogurt; milkshakes |
| Fruits and vegetables (fibrous fruits and vegetables may help remove other foods from the teeth and do stimulate saliva flow) | All fruit and vegetable juices (though pineapple juice is 8 percent sugar, even when no sugar is added); all fresh fruits (e.g., apples, apricots, watermelon, cantaloupe, cherries, grapefruit, grapes, oranges, peaches, pears, pineapples, tangerines); all raw vegetables (cabbage, cauliflower, carrots, celery, cucumbers, lettuce and other salad greens, radishes, tomatoes, turnips, green peppers) | Sweetened canned fruits; sweetened fruit or vegetable juices; dried fruits such as raisins or dates |
| Meats | Meats;** hard-boiled eggs;*** some bean dips; nuts; peanut butter | Candy-coated nuts; sugar-cured meats (e.g., hams) |
| Other | Olives; coffee and tea (not suggested for preschoolers); dill or sour pickles | Candy; soft drinks; other sweet drinks; sweet pickles; jams, jellies; gelatin made with sugar; sherbets made with sugar; white or brown sugar, honey, or corn syrup |
| Combinations | Carrot pennies for tummy banks (round slices); apple slices with cheddar cheese; cream-cheese balls rolled in chopped nuts; celery stuffed with cottage cheese and chives; baloney slices spread with cream cheese and | |

cut in wedges; shrimp on
toothpicks with cocktail
sauce (no sugar); deviled
eggs;*** pear halves
spread with cream
cheese and sprinkled
with chopped nuts; raw
vegetables with low-
calorie yogurt or cheese
dip; celery stuffed with
peanut butter; peanut
butter and crackers;*
fruit-juice popsicles

---

SOURCE: Adopted from Abraham E. Nizel, *The Science of Nutrition and Its Application in Clinical Dentristry,* 2 ed. (Philadelphia: W. B. Saunders, 1966); and Edward A. Sweeney, *The Food that Stays: An Update on Nutrition, Diet, Sugar, and Caries* (New York: Medcom, 1977).

NOTE: In a letter to the authors, Dr. Nizel cautions that since a major goal of dental nutrition [education] is to *discourage* the 'sweet-tooth' habit . . ." [we] do *not recommend* the use of sweetened foods in general and particularly as desserts. . . ."
NOTE: Asterisks added by the authors.

---

*   Acceptable to some dentists, in moderation.
**  Choose low-cholesterol varieties, if desired.
***Cholesterol level should be considered.

One mother refrigerated tidbits of cheese, celery, and carrots in a clean egg carton. When her son grew hungry, he got out the carton to see what his snack surprises of the morning were. Another parent placed washed apples, nectarines, and other fruits in a small bowl in the vegetable bin of the refrigerator. Her three-year-old daughter took great pride in being able to ask permission for a fruit snack, then getting whatever she wanted from the bowl.

One day the child had just given herself and a friend an apple when the friend's mom came for the little visitor. "I'm so glad to see Melissa eating an apple instead of cookies," she exclaimed. "It seems she only wants sweets at home." This mother was surprised to hear that children who learn that snack time means time for fruits and vegetables enjoy their snacks as much as those who expect and eat sweet snacks. Though her child had been programmed for sweet snacks, the mother decided to try reprogramming. She was successful, even to the point of enlisting the aid of grandparents who had been showering their blond-haired little darling with candies!

## Television Propaganda

"Mama, get up!" came the voice of a five-year-old, "I'm starved from all those 'messages!' "

The "messages" the child referred to were television commercials targeted for children who watch Saturday-morning cartoons and other kiddie programs. In most cases, these commercials cause a child to ask for a bowl of whatever cereal is being advertised at the moment. If there's none of that brand in the house, a temper tantrum in the grocery store that afternoon will make sure there's some there for next Saturday's breakfast.

In a 1972 study, 388 network commercials were monitored during twenty-nine hours of prime time for children's TV shows. Eighty-two percent of those commercials were advertising food, drink, candy, gum, or vitamin pills. If a child began watching programs on CBS at eight o'clock, twenty-seven food and fruit-flavored-vitamin ads would tempt his appetite in the span of an hour.

In 1977, a graduate class at the Minnesota School of Public Health monitored 580 television ads over twenty-seven hours of network shows. Forty-four percent of the commercials they observed were for edible products. The survey revealed that 41 percent of Saturday-morning kiddie-show commercials were for cereals, and that there were five times as many ads for sugar-coated cereals as for those with less sugar.

A sampling of popular ads from three prominent food processors includes Kellogg's Sugar Frosted Flakes (sugar-coated cornflakes), General Mills' Lucky Charms (sugar-coated oat cereal with marshmallow bits), and Post's Super Sugar Crisp (sweetened wheat puffs). These breakfast foods are low in fat and protein, high in calories, and relatively high in carbohydrates, yet they boast that they are "fortified with 8 essential vitamins." They are, of course; but the presence of these vitamins doesn't make up for the absence of other vitamins and minerals or compensate for the undesirably large amounts of sugar. As Gussow observed after her 1972 study, "Cereals in children's television are oversweetened, overpriced, and overpromoted, and, I think, at times overenriched."

Researchers told a 1970–72 Senate Commerce Committee that most ready-to-eat breakfast cereals are not nutritionally valuable and should be labeled "snacks." Certainly they are not the sort of snack dentists would recommend. Nutritionist Jean Mayer's suggestion seems more appropriate: He feels that high-sugar cereals should be relabeled "candy" and placed on the candy counter.

There are those who argue that breakfast cereals *aren't* bad for teeth. These arguments are based on a 1974 study by Glass and Fleisch of fourteen cereals (8 regular and 6 sweetened, 1 or more of them having 45% sugar), which showed that kids who ate larger amounts of these cereals showed no more cavities than those who ate smaller amounts. An examination of the study report shows several important unknown variables—such as whether kids added sugar to less-sweet cereals or whether they ate the cereal at one meal or used it as a snack food several times each day. Furthermore, if a child eats one serving a day of a presweetened cereal with 45 percent sugar content, this adds ½-ounce per day or 3½ ounces per week to his sugar intake. Since the average American eats about 2 pounds of sugar a week, omitting presweetened cereals would cut sugar intake by 1/8! Seen in this light, the sugar content of such cereals can hardly be called negligible. When the child adds varying amounts of sugar to cereals which *aren't* pre-sweetened, sugar levels may be even higher.

# Total Sugar Content (Percent) of Commercial Breakfast Cereals (Includes Both Added and Naturally Present Sugars)

| CEREAL | TOTAL SUGAR (percent) | CEREAL | TOTAL SUGAR (percent) |
|---|---|---|---|
| Puffed Rice (QO) | 0.1 | Raisin Bran (K) | 29.0 |
| Puffed Wheat (QO) | 0.5 | Cracklin' Bran (K) | 29.0 |
| Shredded Wheat (N) | 0.6 | Golden Grahams (GM) | 30.0 |
| Cheerios (GM) | 3.0 | Raisin Bran (GF) | 30.4 |
| Wheat Chex (RP) | 3.5 | Country Morning (K) | 32.0 |
| Corn Chex (RP) | 4.0 | Cap'n Crunch, Peanut Butter (QO) | 32.2 |
| Rice Chex (RP) | 4.4 | Cocoa Puffs (GM) | 33.3 |
| Kix (GM) | 4.8 | Trix (GM) | 35.9 |
| Post Toasties (GF) | 5.0 | Frosted Rice (K) | 37.0 |
| Corn Flakes (K) | 5.3 | Honey Comb (GF) | 37.2 |
| Special K (K) | 5.4 | Alpha Bits (GF) | 38.0 |
| Grape Nuts (GF) | 7.0 | Count Chocula (GM) | 39.5 |
| Rice Krispies (K) | 7.8 | Cap'n Crunch (QO) | 40.0 |
| Wheaties (GM) | 8.2 | Cookie Crisp, Oatmeal (RP) | 40.1 |
| Total (GM) | 8.3 | Crazy Cow, Strawberry (GM) | 40.1 |
| Concentrate (K) | 9.3 | Quisp (QO) | 40.7 |
| Product 19 (K) | 9.9 | Sugar Frosted Flakes of Corn (K) | 41.0 |
| Buck Wheats (GM) | 12.2 | Cookie Crisp, Chocolate (RP) | 41.0 |
| 40% Bran (GF) | 13.3 | | |
| Grape Nuts Flakes (GF) | 13.3 | Lucky Charms (GM) | 42.2 |
| Team (N) | 14.1 | Fruity Pebbles (GF) | 42.5 |
| Life (QO) | 16.0 | Cocoa Pebbles (GF) | 42.6 |
| Fortified Oat Flakes (GF) | 18.5 | Cocoa Krispies (K) | 43.0 |
| All Bran (K) | 19.0 | Cap'n Crunch, Crunchberries (QO) | 43.3 |
| 100% Bran (N) | 21.0 | Cookie Crisp, Vanilla (RP) | 43.5 |
| Life, Cinnamon (QO) | 21.0 | Frankenberry (GM) | 43.7 |
| Country Crisp (GF) | 22.0 | Frosted Rice Krinkles (GF) | 44.0 |
| Quaker 100% Natural, Brown Sugar and Honey (QO) | 22.0 | Corny Snaps (K) | 45.5 |
| Heartland Coconut (P) | 22.0 | Crazy Cow, Chocolate (GM) | 45.6 |
| Familia (BF) | 23.0 | Super Sugar Crisp (GF) | 46.0 |
| Vita Crunch, Regular (OM) | 24.0 | Sugar Corn Pops (K) | 46.0 |
| C. W. Post Plain (GF) | 25.0 | Fruit Loops (K) | 48.0 |
| Quaker 100% Natural, Apple and Cinnamon (QO) | 25.0 | Apple Jacks (K) | 54.6 |
| Nature Valley Granola, Cinnamon and Raisin (GM) | 25.0 | Sugar Smacks (K) | 56.0 |
| Heartland, Raisin (P) | 26.0 | | |
| Frosted Mini Wheats (K) | 26.0 | KEY | |
| Vita Crunch, Raisin (OM) | 27.0 | BF: Bio-Familia | |
| Vita Crunch, Almond (OM) | 28.0 | GF: General Foods | |
| Quaker 100% Natural, Raisin and Dates (QO) | 28.0 | K: Kellogg's | |
| Nature Valley Granola, Fruit and Nut (GM) | 29.0 | N: Nabisco | |
| C. W. Post, Raisin (GF) | 29.0 | OM: Organic Milling | |
| | | P: Pet | |
| | | RP: Ralston-Purina | |

SOURCE: Adapted from Nutrition Composition Laboratory, Nutrition Institute, Human Nutrition Center, Science and Education Administration, Agricultural Research, U.S. Department of Agriculture, Beltsville, Md., 1979.

Highly refined cereals, eaten alone, do not constitute an adequate diet. Even when commercials for cereals carry the added line "part of a balanced breakfast," children are not as likely to develop an appetite for the missing foods being alluded to as they are for the cereal which is being cleverly promoted at that very moment.

Many parents and children are confused by cereal box copy which promises a high-vitamin content but delivers a product high in sugar and low in overall nutritive value. By consulting the accompanying list of the sugar content of popular cereals, a parent can see beyond the information given on the cereal box. As the list indicates, even those cereals which seem desirable because they are high in protein and vitamins have surprisingly high sugar content. Certainly, based on the information here, there's no need to *add* sugar to any cereal—not even Bran Flakes or All Bran. Mom and dad will have to set a good example by removing the sugar bowl from the table during breakfast. If children see sugar being used, they assume that adults like sugar on cereal and that they should like it, too. If the adults don't add extra sugar to cereal, children are not likely to request sugar, either.

Even the subtle aspects of advertisements influence children. In some cases, the only nutrition education a child obtains at home may be from television ads. Such children get an overall impression of what foods they should eat from the composite picture they see. Thus, according to television ads, people drink soft drinks; beer; sugar-based, artificially flavored drinks—but seldom milk. TV shows people eating food *products,* not food. They regularly eat frozen waffles and imitation eggs, but they don't often eat eggs, vegetables, fruits, cheese, and nuts. People in TV ads do drink Florida orange juice, though they are more likely to drink an imitation breakfast juice during prime kiddie viewing time.

When children see these ads and have no knowledge of their purpose nor any way to judge their reliability, they are influenced to want the products which taste "fudgy" and "frosty" or "chocolatey" and which are said to be "fun," "great," and "powerful." When preschoolers go shopping with their mothers, they may ask for, beg for, and even cry for cereals or candies they've seen on TV. According to an unpublished paper from Harvard's Graduate School of Business Administration, mothers of five- to seven-year-olds yield to 88 percent of their snack-food requests, 40 percent of their candy requests, and 38 percent of their soft-drink requests. Mothers of eight- to ten-year-olds yield to cereal requests 91 percent of the time!

These statistics should come as no real surprise. If ads didn't work, would manufacturers be spending over $400 million a year on them? Manufacturers of food products thoroughly research all avenues of advertising before they decide where to invest their money. A 1962 study by the American Newspaper Publishers Association's Bureau of Advertising revealed that breakfast is generally a do-it-yourself meal for American families. In one out of six households, the mother is just getting out of bed when the first person starts eating breakfast, and in one out of four families, a child eats breakfast alone and with no parental supervision.

With such statistics in mind, food manufacturers have moved to capture more of the ready-to-eat cereal market. Children's early-morning television programs were an obvious place for hard-sell tactics, and manufacturers have steadily filled ad spots for these programs with "messages" aimed at hungry youngsters. As the 1977 Senate Report on Dietary Goals for the United States noted, "Persuasive commercial forces work unremittingly to encourage unwise eating habits and to nullify sound [nutrition] education." What can parents do to offset such powerful influences?

They can support the work of interest groups such as Action for Children's Television (ACT), a national nonprofit organization working to eliminate commercial abuses from children's television. As a result of ACT's efforts, advertisement time devoted to children's commercials during weekend programs was reduced by 40 percent, and children's vitamin ads were eliminated from advertisements aimed at children.

A petition concerning the regulation of candy commercials is now pending before The Federal Trade and Communications Commissions (FTC and FCC). Regulations in Holland prohibit the use of a child younger than fourteen in advertisements for candy, soft drinks, and other such items, if those advertisements appear before eight P.M. In addition, candy advertisements must show a toothbrush and toothpaste over 10 percent of the screen. This contrasts sharply with American candy advertisements, which show young children shouting the praises of products which are "chewy" and "made to last," two of the chief reasons sugar in candy form is one of the leading causes of tooth decay.

ACT feels that all ads aimed at children should be banned, because children should be protected from the hard-sell techniques of adults. As ACT President Peggy Charren expressed it, "If adults are encouraged to reach for caramel-coated popcorn, it is unfortunate. But it is totally irresponsible to teach children to prefer food products that will be detrimental to their health. . . ."

Since banning all TV ads aimed at children seems a distant goal, ACT has suggested that the following interim measures be taken: (1) eliminate sticky forms of sugared food (including candy) from ads for children; (2) prohibit use of unfair selling techniques so that the qualities of the food being advertized are shown clearly and simply, not hidden under vague promises of energy power, fun, and friendship or confused by the presence of a familiar face such as that of Donald Duck, by special effects such as twinkling sugar coating, or by prizes in the boxes; (3) encourage greater use of public-service announcements for children that promote good nutrition; (4) encourage food manufacturers to develop products that nutrition-conscious parents will want to buy; (5) encourage more ads by fresh produce and dairy associations; and (6) encourage ads that disclose ingredient information. For further information on ACT's activities, contact: ACT, 46 Austin St., Newtonville, Massachusetts 02160.

Since regulations such as these may not come about until today's preschoolers have children of their own, even though FCC and FTC hearings are under way, parents must find other ways to combat the influence of TV. One very successful tactic is to watch TV with the little ones occasionally and encourage the children to comment on the ads. The typical dialogue we give concerns breakfast cereals, but the same technique can be applied to other food and nonfood ads.

PARENT:  Why do you think this message is on TV?
CHILD:  (*age three*): To tell us about Sugar Flakes.
PARENT:  So we will want some?
CHILD:  And get some!
PARENT:  Do you think they are good for you?
CHILD:  I don't know.
PARENT:  They have lots and lots of sugar.
CHILD:  Then they're yukky. *(Of course, this reaction can be expected only if previous general nutrition dialogues have occurred.)*
PARENT:  Why is sugar yukky?
CHILD:  Bad for your teeth. Makes cavities.
PARENT:  That's right! I'm glad you remembered. We can choose cereals with less sugar, can't we?
CHILD:  Yes. I don't want cavities!

Is this an unrealistic dialogue? Not if nutrition education begins early. In fact, this is very close to an actual conversation between a mother and her three-year-old daughter. By age five, this child enjoyed pointing out fallacies in TV ads on her own, a pastime that educated her little brother to the tricky ways of advertisers through comments such as, "See, those little men didn't *really* come out of that box. It's just a cartoon trick," and "That doll probably works fine on TV, but I'll bet her battery runs down quick once you get her home!"

Consumer education of this sort is an effective weapon against advertisements of any kind. Started as soon as a child can begin to reason out kiddie commercials, it is a process that can lead to a lifetime of wise buying practices. Seen as tools for childhood consumer education, maybe TV ads for kids aren't *all* bad after all!

## Obesity

Long hours of watching television rather than engaging in activities which burn away calories may contribute to obesity in preschoolers. Parents concerned about obesity should be aware of the number of hours a child spends in front of the TV set and encourage him or her to spend more time at activities which require more energy. Lack of exercise causes childhood obesity more often than overeating. Of course, in many cases, overeating is also a prime factor, and both factors are in operation if a child is allowed indiscriminate eating of snack foods during TV-watching hours.

A rereading of the section on obesity (page 73) should be useful at this point, since most of the same suggestions for avoiding or combating obesity in babyhood can be applied to avoiding or combating obesity in the preschooler.

Mothers with an overweight preschooler might observe the child's pace of eating, size and frequency of bites, length of chewing time, and other eating habits. If some of these eating habits seem to contribute to overeating, parent and child could discuss the problem area ("You are taking large bites and eating very fast") and come up with a possible solution ("Let's cut your food into very small bits and try to pause between bites"). Of course, only a child who is old enough to see that such changes may help him or her reach the goal of weight-gain reduction is likely to be motivated enough to try to make the change.

Even a child too young to understand why he is gaining too much weight can be persuaded to get more exercise each day. Few children will refuse a chance for a walk with mom or dad, if only for the delight of having a parent alone for a while. Daily walks of several blocks can be a time for family togetherness, as well as a time for burning up extra calories. The walks can get longer as the child gains stamina. Ideally, parent and child should walk rather than drive wherever they go, whenever possible—whether to preschool classes, a friend's house, or the library.

One overweight five-year-old, conscious of the advantages which walking offered to her chubby little body, deliberately chose to walk an extra block uphill rather than heading home, noting, "I ate an extra cookie at lunch. I want to burn off that cookie calorie!" Though she had no idea of the scientific definition of a calorie, she understood perfectly well that eating too much and exercising too little would keep her chubby.

Helping an obese child become weight conscious without making her feel unwanted or unattractive is a difficult assignment. If a child feels loved and wanted and is made to understand that slimming down will be better for her health, she is likely to accept parental suggestions and work toward slowing her weight gain to normal without feeling depressed or threatened. On the other hand, a child who is constantly ridiculed for obesity and nagged about her laziness and her overeating is likely to feel confused and rejected when weight-control measures are introduced.

Though making needed adaptations may be difficult, the earlier parents face the fact that a child has a weight problem, the better the chances of warding off a long-term problem. Those researchers who agree with the theory that obese children tend to have an excess *number* of fat cells rather than just excess size of fat cells feel that it is crucial to stop the increase in the number of fat cells. If you begin weight-control measures before fat cells reach the number which could normally be present in adulthood, parents and doctor may be able to help the child prevent a further increase in fat-cell number. According to one expert on childhood obesity, ". . . in childhood-onset obesity one should institute dietary regimens prior to age six . . . if a lifelong history of obesity is to be avoided." This researcher suggests that in extreme cases, dietary regimens start before a child's second birthday. Though the fat-cell theory is not definitive, and though doctors disagree about how early weight-control should be begun, most agree that childhood obesity, unchecked, will be detrimental to the future health of the children involved.

As noted earlier, the goal in weight control of obese youngsters is *slowing the rate of gain,* not bringing about weight loss. A doctor's advice is needed before embarking on any childhood weight-control program. For children over two years of age, a pediatrician will probably recommend use of skim milk and avoidance of sweets and empty-calorie snack foods, plus plenty of exercise. He or she should not call for drastic calorie cutbacks which place a child significantly below the recommended number of calories for the age group, though he or she may advocate a slight reduction of calories.

Blond-haired, blue-eyed Joanna, never overweight before, began to take on a pudgy look around the time of her fourth birthday. Her pediatrician was able to convince the child's parents that weight-control measures should start at once in order to prevent the problem from becoming worse. Once they were conscious of the problem, her mom and dad began a one-week food diary to help trace the source of the extra calories. They discovered that Joanna was frequently taking second and third helpings. She was eating no candy or chips, but grandmother prepared home-baked, delicious corn-bread every night, and the little girl customarily enjoyed at least two generously buttered pieces. She sugared her cereal every morning because daddy sugared his, and she often ate two portions of toast and jelly with that cereal.

As the parents looked back, they realized their child's weight increase had begun soon after a second grandmother moved into town to be nearer her little blue-eyed granddaughter. Grandma Sutton baked delicious yeast breads, dinner rolls, and cinnamon rolls and was always bringing by a panful hot from the oven. Cakes were her specialty, too, and she delighted in surprising the family with cakes "just to say I love you." As this pattern became clear to the parents, they realized that they, too, had put on extra pounds over the past year. Admission of this fact suddenly made weight reduction a *family* problem, not a problem limited to Joanna.

At this point, the little girl became particularly enthusiastic about her new program. "Daddy," she announced one morning at breakfast, "you know what Dr. Harris says about sugar! How do you expect to lose those extra pounds if you eat that stuff on your cereal?" Scenes such as this kept parents and child on the route to weight control. The entire family ate well-balanced meals, with minimum amounts of bread and nonsweetened, fresh fruit desserts. Every afternoon mom, dad, and daughter took a long walk. Later, as Joanna learned to ride a two-wheel bike, they biked together.

The parents gradually lost their extra pounds, and their weight steadied. Joanna began to slim down as her height-weight gains began to fall in line with recommended averages. By the time she was in second grade, she could wear normal sizes in most items, though she was still more comfortable in "chubby"-style jeans. Best of all, she had learned eating and exercise patterns which should mean a lifetime free from the obesity toward which she had been headed.

Joanna's parents were interested in the fact that while the tendency toward obesity has not been proven to be *hereditary,* it has been proven to be *familial.* A child born to normal-weight parents has a 7-percent chance of becoming obese. If one parent is obese, the child's chances of being obese are 40 percent, and if both parents are obese, the child's chances are 80 percent. Children of obese parents are likely to fall into the same eating patterns as their parents and to have activity levels which approximate those of their parents.

Even if a potentially obese child does not eat appreciably more than a thin child, he may still eat more than he needs because he has a low activity level. Only when a child gains enough high-quality calories for optimum growth and development and gets enough exercise to burn up any unneeded calories can weight-control measures be said to be working. As Joanna and her parents can testify, a good program of weight control can help the whole family get in shape and stay that way.

## Poor Appetite

While some children eat too much, others seem to eat too little. Often, however, parents only imagine that a child is not eating enough. As we noted earlier, growth rate and calorie requirements per pound of body weight drop drastically after age one. Appetites normally decrease in the toddler and preschool years, increasing during growth spurts and decreasing again once those spurts are done.

Apparently mothers and fathers have long tended to worry about growth. During the 1940s and 1950s, vitamin tonics which claimed to stimulate lagging appetites sold well. Most doctors feel that those supplements were probably useless, but harmless enough. Today, doctors sometimes prescribe a drug which *does* appear to stimulate appetite but may *not* be harmless. Though cyproheptadine (periactin) may merely decrease activity level, so that the child shows a weight gain with relatively little increase in calories, the drug seems to increase appetite as well. If this is so, what if this stimulation cannot be reversed, once the drug is discontinued? Will the child become obese? Most physicians feels that stimulating the appetite by drugs is *not* a wise measure except in extreme cases.

Instead of treating the lagging appetite, mothers should try to discover the reasons behind a child's lack of interest in eating. Some preschoolers have enlarged adenoids, which interfere with their sense of taste and make food less appetizing. A severe cold can have the same effect, and a sore throat can make all spicy foods unattractive. Mild stomach disorders can also cause temporary loss of appetite.

In one case, five-year-old Matt showed a dramatic decrease in appetite one spring. He would appear hungry, take a few bites, then stop eating and idly push the food around on his plate. Even on days when he did manage to finish part of his meals, his mother found chewed bits of meat left on his plate. Eventually, she told the family doctor of the problem. A careful check during the next episode of leftover, chewed meat revealed the problem: Swollen, inflamed tonsils made swallowing extremely painful. Once the tonsils were out, Matt's appetite returned and his weight gain normalized. As Matt's case indicates, if loss of appetite persists or seems related to ill health, a doctor's advice may be needed.

## Childhood Illness

Children who are ill may lose interest in food. If the senses of taste and smell are affected by the illness, as in the case of the common cold, food may not have much appeal. Nonetheless, unless a child has a gastrointestinal disorder or some other illness which requires that he do without food, maintaining a balanced diet is essential to rapid recovery.

If the child has been in bed or has severely decreased his activity level even though he has not been in bed, his calorie needs will be decreased accordingly, and he needs smaller portions than usual. He should not be forced to take food before his appetite begins to return, and once it does return, food should be *offered,* not forced.

Most doctors recommend a bland or soft diet for a child recuperating from illness. Such a diet might include (1) cereals, breads (e.g., gruel, mush, cream-of-wheat, dry toast), (2) chicken or beef broths, (3) plain or creamed soups, (4) simple puddings (rice, custard, tapioca), (5) sherbet or ice cream, (6) strained fruits (if diarrhea is not a problem), (7) poached, scrambled, or boiled eggs, (8) milk, water, or fruit juice, (9) minced or creamed chicken, beef, or lamb, or lean, broiled ground beef. Since some of the above items may be inappropriate, a parent might want to check with his doctor before beginning this recuperative diet.

In general, a sick child responds more favorably to small, frequent meals than to large, infrequent ones. He may not feel like drinking milk, but if milk has been approved by the doctor, a parent can include it in eggnog, custard, creamed soup, ice cream, and cooked cereal. If the child is too weak to sit up and eat alone or to chew very long without tiring, pureed vegetables can be added to beef or chicken broth, and strained fruits may be used instead of fresh ones. As recuperation proceeds and strength returns, a child may enjoy high-energy surprise treats such as sponge cake or angel-food cake. His lagging appetite may be tempted by a tea party with mom or a "let's pretend picnic" served on a tablecloth spread on his bedroom floor.

If antibiotics and antihistamines are being given, extra fluids will be recommended. Letting a child fill her own glass from a new or special pitcher or letting her drink from a straw (especially if it is an unusual, novelty straw) often keeps her interested in drinking more fluids. Fruit juices are ideal, unless the doctor has advised against them. If an ice tray of juice is frozen, the child's glass can be filled with this ice, then with extra juice. Once the liquid juice is gone, the ice cubes themselves can be enjoyed. Children often enjoy vegetable juices after illness. Carbonated drinks, especially sugarless ones, may be used, but colas should be avoided during the hours before bedtime, since their caffeine content may interfere with sleep. If a child has high fever, milk may not be recommended. Water and ice chips may be made available.

## Vegetarian Diets

While serious health problems can and do exist among nonvegetarian children, there is cruel irony in nutrition-related maladies being observed among children whose parents' eating habits are indicative of a life-style that abhors harming or exploiting animals and which is dedicated to the pursuit of physical, emotional, mental, and spiritual well-being. These goals are worthy, yet they must not be pursued at the expense of the health of innocent children. Vegetarians need to realize that severe rickets, advanced pernicious anemia, and irreversible mental and physical retardation have all been observed in young children nurtured on inadequate vegetarian diets. Since vegetarian diets can be among the most healthful for children as well as adults, such problems need not and should not exist.

Extremist diets usually pose the greatest dangers. For example, though Zen-macrobiotic-diet enthusiasts believe that mental and spiritual development should precede physical growth, in actuality, retarded physical development in childhood is usually paralleled by retarded mental growth. Though the "7 percent hungry child" admired by this group may develop the promised "big dream," his physical and mental state may become a real nightmare if he lacks the nutrients necessary for building a strong mind and body. The macrobiotic diet consists of several levels or plateaux, and even the cereal, fruit, and vegetable levels may prove inadequate. When used by children, the brown-rice and limited-liquid level is quite likely to result in severe malnutrition with accompanying long-term mental and physical problems.

Other, less extreme vegetarian diets can be quite satisfactory for a child's growth and development. For example, lacto-ovo vegetarian children who include eggs and dairy products in their diets can easily obtain all the essential nutrients. Such children, who are seldom obese, generally avoid empty-calorie snacks and highly processed foods, have low cholesterol and fat intakes and high fiber and water intakes.

Vegans (strict vegetarians) may have more trouble meeting all their needs. If unfortified soy milk is used by a vegan child, her calcium intake must be carefully monitored, and calcium supplements may be needed. Though other foods contain calcium, the bulkiness of greens and similar high-calcium foods makes getting enough calcium without dairy products or a supplement difficult. Protein complementarity, as demonstrated in the chart in Chapter 2, should be observed so that all essential amino acids are eaten at each meal. Pernicious anemia due to B$_{12}$ deficiency could be a problem unless fortified soy milk is used or B$_{12}$ supplements are taken. High folic acid levels can mask this problem. Since vegetarian diets usually abound in green, leafy vegetables and other foods high in folic acid, pernicious anemia in vegan children may not be detected until irreversible degeneration of the spinal cord or other serious symptoms occurs.

A sample vegetarian menu for the eighteen-month- to three-year-old child appears on page 155. A three- to six-year-old could follow this same menu, adding more whole grains, legumes, yellow and green leafy vegetables, nuts, and nutlike seeds to provide adequate calories for optimum growth and development. If no fish is added, iodized salt should be used. Sea salt, despite its origin, contains no iodine unless it has been added.

There can be many advantages to a lifetime of vegetarian eating, yet these advantages may never be realized unless every effort is made to see that nutrient intakes are adequate for a young child's special needs. Only in this way can a childhood vegetarian diet truly lead to the physical, emotional, mental, and spiritual health and well-being that is its ultimate goal.

## Mealtime Behavior Modification Techniques

Nutritionists who tried to alter children's vegetable eating habits by modifying the method by which those vegetables were prepared found that only 32 percent of the children would even *taste* the vegetable being offered. When nutritionists and psychologists adopted behavior-modification techniques to motivate children to alter their vegetable eating habits, 74 percent of the children *tasted* the vegetables, and greater consumption of vegetables was noted.

To interest the children in trying the vegetables, these researchers offered stickers for each portion the children ate, and these stickers could later be traded for ice cream or pudding at dessert time instead of the customary fruit desserts. This method seems very little different from the "eat your beans or you can't have dessert" method most experts advise parents *not* to use. Perhaps offering *nonfood* incentives would be a better idea, since these researchers were treating ice cream as if it were a more desirable dessert than fruit.

Perhaps children could be given "try-me" stars to put on a small individual vegetable chart. If the children make the charts themselves and discuss the vegetables whose pictures they draw on the chart, they might be quite anxious to add stars showing how many of the new vegetable friends they have tried for themselves. Other studies have shown that children are more likely to be willing to try a new vegetable immediately after seeing a classroom presentation on the vegetable. Home projects could have the same effect, especially if parents and children read stories and poems about a new vegetable, then talk about the vegetable's origins, the vitamins and minerals it contains, and how these nutrients help build strong, healthy bodies. Behavior modification which leads to changed habits for sound reasons seems an ideal goal.

## Preschooler Parties

Since preschoolers have little appetites which are easily distracted by parties and party food, planning a party for mealtime allows children to enjoy fellowship and good food at the same time. In the case of two- and three-year-olds, a noontime party is probably best, since afternoon nap time provides an opportunity for rest after the unaccustomed excitement. Mealtime birthday parties should probably last one to one and a half hours. When toddlers and early preschoolers are involved, a few mothers might be invited to stay to help distribute food items. In general, the younger the child, the fewer the guests is a good rule to follow.

Simplicity is the key to successful preschool parties. Easy, familiar foods may be dressed up for the party, since young children are more comfortable with familiar foods. An older preschooler can help plan the menu. He may even wish to help prepare some of the items. If the party is to serve as a meal, the menu should be as well balanced as possible.

Hot dogs and buns served with a cheese dip for dunking carrot sticks, broccoli spears, and cauliflower bits make easy-to-prepare, usually well-accepted party fare. Fruit juice or milk may be served as a beverage. Older children may enjoy roasting their hot dogs over a small fire, but this is advisable only with adequate adult supervision.

You might provide a snack lunch, in which each child is free to choose his or her own food from items such as hot-dog rounds and cheese cubes alternated on pretzel sticks; thin slices of beef, ham, bologna, or other luncheon meat rolled around a cheese stick; cooked, dried prunes or apricots skewered on a carrot stick; peanut butter spread on a thin apple round with an animal cracker pressed into the peanut butter; peanut butter on a celery stick with raisins on top (ants on a log); raw green-pepper rings topped with cheese-sprinkled meatballs; apple rings topped with Canadian bacon; ground-beef balls and pineapple alternated on a toothpick (not for younger children); or bread cut in animal shapes with a cookie cutter, covered with meat spread, then topped with a cube of cheese and broiled.

Birthday cakes need not be sugary treats. Check the recipe section in Appendix C for carrot cupcakes, green-apple cake, zucchini fruitcake, or pumpkin bread. These are cakes that provide maximum food value with minimum sugar.

### Kids in the Kitchen

"B'ekfast! B'ekfast!" came an impatient voice from the crib. Hungry two-and-a-half-year-old Don Don was ready to eat!

As soon as his dad had sleepily lifted him to the floor, the little boy was toddling downstairs. By the time dad had put on his bathrobe and made it to the kitchen, Don Don was standing by the stove, spatula in hand, saying "Egg! Egg!"

Though he knew he was not allowed to climb up on his stool until grown-ups were present, this little cook was more than ready to scramble his own breakfast egg. Such cooking experiments, when undertaken with great care and maximum attention to safety, can give children renewed interest in food. On a visit to his grandparents' farm, Don had been allowed to gather the eggs, bring them to the kitchen, and scramble them—with grandfather's help, of course. For several weeks after that experiment, cooking his own breakfast became a highlight of his day.

Three-year-old Claire had an equally exciting "food source" experience the day she and her mom gathered fresh salad greens, tomatoes, and carrots from their garden and dug up about a dozen tender russet potatoes. During the digging, Claire proudly produced several worms and begged to go fishing with them. Mother and daughter spent a delightful hour at the creek, returning with two rainbow trout, which they cleaned for dinner. When dad arrived home, he was greeted by an excited child, ready to explain how she and mama "catched our dinner and dug it, too." There was certainly no lag in appetite that evening!

Though such experiences cannot be shared by all children, every child can and should be given an opportunity to learn about the origins of foods. When dinner is only something from a can, it has no interest besides its immediate flavor, smell, or appearance and no value beyond the nutrients it contains. However, if a toddler is asked to go to the cabinet and bring back a can of green peas, the can and its contents take on new meaning. If the child is allowed to pour the peas into the saucepan, add a pat of butter, and place a lid on the pan, he's quite likely to be so proud of what he has cooked that he eats second and even third helpings.

When a five-year-old kneads and shapes whole-wheat bread loaves, helps add mushrooms, sausage, green peppers, and cheese to a pizza, or washes and separates broccoli for an afternoon snack, she has an interest in these foods which can be gained only through personal involvement in their preparation. Starting this involvement during the preschool years is an excellent way to increase a child's awareness of the hows and whys of good nutrition. It is also an excellent way for parents and children to spend happy, productive hours together.

## Nutrition Education

The best nutrition education which can be given to a child before the early school years is an opportunity to develop desirable attitudes about food. While this general concept has been stressed in both this chapter and the preceding one, the following box gives a few special suggestions for fun activities which teach food concepts and other things as well.

At first glance, the nutrition-education approach given here may seem idealistic. True, no parent is likely to try all of these ideas. Still, these and many other activities can teach food facts, plus math and reading-readiness concepts in a natural and enjoyable way.

As parents watch a child move from food-tossing babyhood to a state of four-year-old maturity which warrants inviting him to join them in an occa-

# A Sensory Approach to Learning about Foods

| | |
|---|---|
| **Touch and Sight** | What do you have on your plate that's crunchy and orange? Long and green? Slippery and red? *(Later)* What protein do you have on your plate? Carbohydrate? Vitamin C? *(For fun)* Make a "feel box" in which food items of various shapes are placed. Cut a circle in a shoe-box lid, making it just large enough for a small hand. Place several objects in the box, then let the child feel inside and try to guess what's there (orange, banana, carrot, tomato, etc.). This teaches *observation skills* as well as food identification. |
| **Taste** | Compare lemons, limes, oranges, and bananas as to taste. Ask which one of these things doesn't belong, then explain the citrus family and its value. Discuss sections, skin feel, shape, color, etc. Compare potatoes—baked, mashed, fried, and as chips—and discuss their food value. Compare eggs—scrambled, hard-cooked, and in custard—and discuss their food value. Compare greens (lettuce, cabbage, spinach) and discuss their value and preparation. Compare beans (green, dried, cooked) and their food value. |
| **Smell** | Place a little extract (vanilla, peppermint, lemon, almond) in baby-food jars and have child sniff and identify smell or food he associates with smell. |
| **Sight** | Open various fruits and see what's inside. Exotic fruits such as papaya, mango, avocado are especially exciting because their seeds are so different from those of common fruits. |
| **Changes** | Demonstrate and discuss how foods change. Popcorn when popped, egg when put into a cake or as meringue on pie, water when frozen, dried pinto beans when soaked and cooked. |
| **Sources** | Pick apples; make pies, tarts, and applesauce. Discuss seeds and read *Johnny Appleseed* as pie is cooking! |

SOURCE: Adapted from the Food and Nutrition Committee of the Missouri Home Economics Association, *Teaching the Young Child Good Eating Habits for Life,* 2d ed., Jefferson City, Mo., Missouri Division of Health, 1971.

sional candlelight dinner featuring the best china and silver and a Brahms violin concerto as background music, they can feel that years of attitude training have paid off. Food and family fellowship have special, positive meanings to such a child, meanings that are likely to remain as firm foundations for a lifetime of optimum nutrition.

## Practical Meals and Snacks

Three-year-old Mary Elizabeth, perched on the kiddie seat in her mother's grocery cart, grew more and more fretful as the cart was pushed from aisle to aisle. Finally, in the produce section, she demanded to eat a banana—at once. When her mother denied her request because she hadn't yet paid for the fruit, the normally reasonable child burst into tears and kicked at the cart. Furious, her mother threatened, spanked, then somehow managed to get the sobbing child through the checkout stand and to the car.

At home, the little girl was too upset for lunch and went to sleep instead. Exhausted, her mother sank into a chair to ponder what went wrong. Suddenly the clock in the living room sounded. One-thirty! Two hours past Mary Elizabeth's usual lunchtime. No wonder she had been so cranky!

Young children are comfortable with schedules. They may need to deviate from them to ask for an unaccustomed snack after unusually hard play or during a growth spurt, yet they don't react very pleasantly to having grown-up activities *force* postponement of a scheduled meal. Though the average preschooler can't usually tell time by a watch, she *does* have an extremely accurate stomach clock! Unless her appetite is tricked by an extra snack or a late, late breakfast, that little stomach clock usually lets her know when lunch should be ready.

Ideally, a preschooler's daily meal and snack schedule should be arranged to meet her needs and those of other family members. However, *when* a child receives the items from the basic food lists is less important than the fact that she *does* receive most of them within a twenty-four-hour period.

One simple way to check the quality of a preschooler's diet is to make a twenty-four-hour recall of her food intake. You can then place each food on your list under one of the headings of the six exchange lists: milk, vegetable, fruit, bread and cereal, meat and other protein dishes, and fat. Refer to the Family Guide to Minimum Exchanges on page 254 to see whether your preschooler received the recommended number of servings of foods from each group.

If your child consumes the recommended number of servings and enjoys height-weight gains in the normal range, he is probably well-nourished. If he falls short in any of these areas, adding additional foods from the first five exchange lists in Appendix A should help bring his diet up to desired levels. The menus shown in Appendix B, featuring exchange-keyed recipes which appear in the recipe section of the book, can be enjoyed by the entire family. Only portion sizes of key items need be changed to meet the energy needs and the specific nutrient needs of children and adults of all ages. As mentioned earlier, a portion of fruits, vegetables, or cereal for a preschooler is approximately one tablespoon for each year of age to age three. Once a homemaker grows familiar with the principles of the exchange system, she should be able to follow it with ease.

Vegetarians may need to adapt the food lists given in Appendix A by adding special foods not enjoyed by nonvegetarians. Since deciding which food list to place a favorite food on calls for greater knowledge than most laypersons possess, consultation with a nutrition specialist is probably advisable. The following vegetarian menu is typical of that enjoyed by many toddlers and young preschoolers.

## Typical Vegetarian Menu for Ages Eighteen to Thirty-Six Months

**Breakfast:** Egg (optional)
1/3–1/2 cup cereal (high protein with milk, or cooked whole-grain cereal)
3/4 ounces citrus juice
1/2–1 slice whole-wheat bread with margarine
Milk*

**Lunch:** 1/2 cup vegetable soup (with legumes)
1/2 to 1 peanut butter sandwich (whole-wheat bread, optional alfalfa sprouts)
Fruit**
Milk*

**Dinner:** 1/3–1/2 cup legume or legume-mushroom-grains dish
Potato (1/4–1/2 medium-sized)
1/3–1/2 cup yellow vegetable
1/4–1/2 cup tomato-lettuce salad
1/4–1/2 slice bread or whole-wheat roll with margarine
Fruit**
Milk*

*Six ounces whole cow's or fortified soy
**May be taken as snack

# 7
# Elementary-school Years—
# Six to Ten

Once a child enters school, he or she leaves behind the protection and guidance of mother and father and faces alone many decisions about what to eat. Whether the child refuses or accepts candy from a friend at recess, eats his green beans in the cafeteria at noon, or chews bubblegum on his way home from school will be his own decision. Hopefully, he will retain the nutritional values he has learned from birth, despite negative peer pressure. Though there will certainly be days when doing what everyone else is doing seems more attractive than doing what his training has taught him is better for his health, there will also be days when his firm foundation in sound eating habits enables him to make wise food choices.

This move from a total dependence upon parental standards to partial reliance upon the standards of peers is a tentative step toward maturity. Though it is sometimes difficult for a parent to accept, such assertions of independence are a necessary part of growing up. The child who continues to look to mama and daddy for every decision is not readying herself for the years ahead. During the elementary school years, parental values may be tested, temporarily rejected, then accepted as the child's own. It is toward this end that all preschool training has moved, not toward perpetual parental dominance of the child's life.

## Meeting Nutrient Needs

Meeting nutrient needs of the six- to ten-year-old basically means eating more of the same foods which met his needs during the preschool years. Since there is no drastic increase in the need for any one nutrient, increasing the amounts of fruits, vegetables, breads, cereals, meats, and dairy products in a child's diet means gaining adequate nutrients and an adequate number of calories. Of course, children who satisfy their appetites on candy and other empty, high-calorie treats are not likely to eat the recommended amounts of other, more nutritious foods. These children may fall below the RDAs in several areas, and their diets may be low in essential nutrients for which no RDAs have, as yet, been assigned. To insure optimum nutrition, parents should introduce children to a wide variety of good foods.

## Calories

The slowed growth rate between the ages of six and ten means a decline in food requirement per unit of body weight (calories per kilogram). From age one to age six, the average child adds 16 to 17 inches of height, at a rate

### Recommended Dietary Allowances—Elementary-school Years

| Age | 4–6 years | 7–10 years |
|---|---|---|
| Weight | 20 kg (44 lbs) | 28 kg (62 lbs) |
| Height | 112 cm (44 in) | 132 cm (52 in) |
| Energy (cal) | 1700 (1300–2300) | 2400 (1650–3300) |
| Protein (g) | 30 | 34 |
| **Fat-soluble vitamins** | | |
| Vitamin A[a] (*$\mu$g R.E.) | 500 | 700 |
| Vitamin D[b] ($\mu$g) | 10 | 10 |
| Vitamin E[c] mg $\alpha$T.E.) | 6 | 7 |
| **Water-soluble vitamins** | | |
| Ascorbic acid (C) (mg) | 45.0 | 45.0 |
| Folacin ($\mu$g) | 200.0 | 300.0 |
| Niacin[d] (mg N.E.) | 11.0 | 16.0 |
| Riboflavin (mg) | 1.0 | 1.4 |
| Thiamin (mg) | 0.9 | 1.2 |
| Vitamin $B_6$ (mg) | 1.3 | 1.6 |
| Vitamin $B_{12}$ ($\mu$g) | 2.5 | 3.0 |
| **Minerals** | | |
| Calcium (mg) | 800 | 800 |
| Phosphorus (mg) | 800 | 800 |
| Iodine ($\mu$g) | 90 | 120 |
| Iron (mg) | 10 | 10 |
| Magnesium (mg) | 200 | 250 |
| Zinc (mg) | 10 | 10 |

SOURCE: Adapted from *Recommended Dietary Allowances,* Ninth Edition (1979, in press), with the permission of the National Academy of Sciences, Washington, D.C.

*$\mu$g is the standard abbreviation for microgram, or 1/1000 milligram.

[a]Recommendations for vitamin A are expressed in $\mu$g of R.E. (micrograms of retinol equivalent). One retinol equivalent is equal to 1$\mu$g of retinol or 6$\mu$g of carotene.
[b]Vitamin D is expressed as $\mu$g of cholecalciferol, with 10$\mu$g cholecalciferol equalling 400 IUs of Vitamin D.
[c]Vitamin E is expressed as mg $\alpha$T.E. (milligrams of alpha tocopherol equivalents).
[d]Niacin is expressed as mg N.E. (milligrams of niacin equivalent), with 1 N.E. equalling 1 mg of niacin or 60 mg of dietary tryptophan.

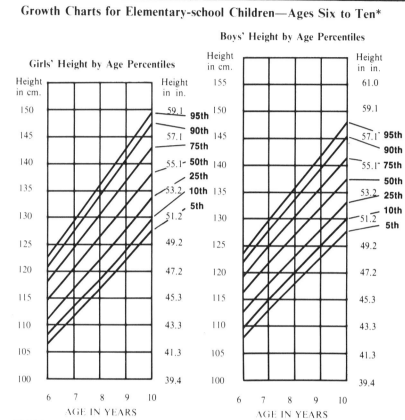

## Growth Charts for Elementary-school Children—Ages Six to Ten*

SOURCE: Adapted from Hamill, P. V. V., T. A. Drizd, C. L. Johnson, R. B. Reed, A. F. Roche, *NCHS Growth Curves for Children, Birth—18 years.* National Center for Health Statistics Publications, Series 11, Number 165, November 1977.

*In general, weights and heights that fall within the 5th and 95th percentiles are considered normal. Ideally, height and weight should be within a few percentile points of each other. See pp. 157, 160.

# Growth Charts for Elementary-school Children—Ages Six to Ten*

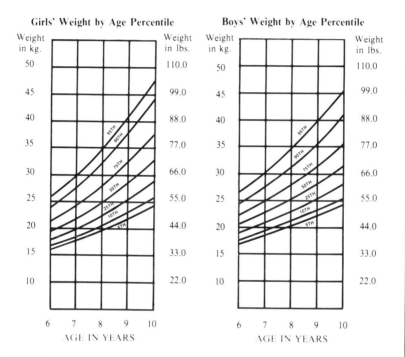

### Girls' Weight by Age Percentile

### Boys' Weight by Age Percentile

SOURCE: Adapted from Hamill, P. V. V., T. A. Drizd, C. L. Johnson, R. B. Reed, A. F. Roche, *NCHS Growth Curves for Children, Birth—18 years.* National Center for Health Statistics Publications, Series 11, Number 165, November 1977.

*In general, weights and heights that fall within the 5th and 95th percentiles are considered normal. Ideally, height and weight should be within a few percentile points of each other. See pp. 157, 160.

of 3 to 4 inches per year, but from age six to age ten, average height increase is only 8 to 10 inches, at a rate of 2 to 2 ½ inches per year. Though growth is slower than during preschool years, adequate calories are still needed if the growth rate is to be satisfactory. A deficit of only 10 calories per kilogram of body weight (1 kilogram equals 2.2 pounds) can result in failure to grow at expected rates.

Parents who wish to chart childhood growth rates may use the preceding graphs. As discussed in earlier chapters, height and weight below the 5th percentile or above the 95th percentile may still be considered "normal," provided both height and weight are close to the same percentile. For example, six-year-old Anne, just outside the 95th percentile in both height and weight, is a well-proportioned first-grader. Her friend Don, a 25th percentiler in both height and weight, is equally well-proportioned. The two have maintained their places on the growth curves from birth to six years of age, and their physician has observed their growth patterns and seen them as normal.

Conversely, six-year-old Rodney, a child who has never been under the care of a physician except for pneumonia at age three, seemed normal in his growth until first grade. At the end of the year, his teacher recommended that Rodney be taken to a pediatrician, since he started the year in the 16th percentile in both height and weight but, by late May, had dropped below the 5th percentile. A medical examination and laboratory tests revealed a serious kidney disorder which had hampered his growth but had produced no other easily observable symptoms. While this medical problem was not related to Rodney's diet, had his parents been watching his height-weight patterns as indications of his nutritional status, they might have found the problem earlier.

Parents of elementary-school-aged children should watch for any sharp deviation from well-established height-weight growth patterns. They should also be on the alert for any pronounced increase or decrease in weight which might indicate a move toward obesity or toward an underweight state. If no health or nutrition problems are observed and a child remains unusually small or large for his or her age, parents should offer love and acceptance of the child as he is, rather than lamenting the fact that his size does not meet their earlier expectations. In this way, the child learns to accept and love himself, a vital prerequisite for his present and future happiness.

Until age eleven or twelve, boys are usually heavier and taller than girls. For both sexes, weight gains are generally more rapid in fall and winter than in summer and spring. Between the ages of ten and twelve, an increase in energy (calories) will be required as preadolescents lay down reserves for the demanding growth spurt of adolescence. Any serious deviation from the heights and weights given in the chart below should be discussed with a physician. Children who maintain growth rates within the expected margins may be assumed to be consuming approximately the right number of calories. Generally, healthy appetites are accurate calorie guides.

A major problem faced by *vegetarian* parents is getting children to eat enough of the relatively low-calorie vegetable foods to gain sufficient calories for optimum growth and development. Unrefined grains and leafy vegetables are high in bulk but relatively low in calories. If a child does not eat sufficient cereals and breads, valuable protein will be used as a source of energy, at the expense of growth. Though vegetarian children need to be sure they receive an adequate number of calories, they cannot afford to fill up on highly refined junk foods or other high-calorie, low-nutrient items. They should use high-quality calories such as whole-grain cereals and breads, thereby gaining protein, iron, and B vitamins as well as energy.

## Protein

One researcher who feels that American youngsters should reduce their cholesterol intake in the hope of avoiding atherosclerosis problems in later life has suggested that this goal may be reached by lowering the amount of protein from animal sources to RDA levels. Since many American children eat more than double the recommended amount of protein, this suggestion may be valid for some families. If you follow the suggestion of cutting the amount of animal foods, however, you should take care to include enough dairy products to meet calcium RDAs and enough meats to allow for optimum intake of trace elements.

Animal and nonanimal protein intake should remain at 12 to 15 percent of total calories consumed each day. Since consuming more protein than necessary is ecologically wasteful and economically expensive, many parents may find it makes sense to lower animal protein intake, which automatically lowers cholesterol intake as well. Because some children with unusually low serum cholesterol levels might be unable to adapt to a low-cholesterol diet, consultation with a physician before beginning such a program is wise.

## Carbohydrates, Fats

Carbohydrates and fats should supply a major portion of needed energy, and the use of polyunsaturated fats may help keep cholesterol levels desirably low. As noted earlier, families who wish to lower fats in the diet should not lower fat intakes too drastically. The American Heart Association has recommended that fat intakes not exceed 30 to 35 percent of total caloric intakes, yet cases of chronic diarrhea have been reported in children whose diets were restricted to 27-percent fat intakes. Since a 3-percent difference does not allow much margin for error, parents should be aware of problems which might arise due to fat deprivation and should be prepared to increase fat intakes, should such problems arise. Carbohydrates high in fiber can add bulk to the diet, thereby helping a child have easy-to-pass bowel movements. By concentrating on complex carbohydrates, a child can gain many valuable nutrients, not just energy.

Just at the time a child moves away from constant parental supervision, she is often offered high-sugar treats in school candy and gum machines.

These machines, ostensibly operated to raise money for school projects, cost parents and children far more than the nickels, dimes, and quarters spent in them each day. By supplying exactly the kinds of sugar most likely to cause tooth decay, these machines lead to high dental bills for parents and tooth-decay pain for youngsters.

Even children who have been used to nutritious snacks may be tempted to buy candy if candy is the only snack available. Parents who are concerned should request that candy and soft-drink machines not be available at school, or that vending machines be stocked with fresh fruit, nuts, cheese, milk, and other more desirable snacks. Though vending machines for these products cost more initially, they can be money-makers for school groups if they are well handled. Even if operating these vending machines is only a break-even proposition, parent groups should consider provision of high-quality school snacks a worthwhile group project.

Deciding which foods should be allowed in vending machines has posed problems for many groups. According to Carol Tucker Foreman, Assistant Secretary of Agriculture for Food and Consumer Services, the United States Department of Agriculture (USDA) has been asked to determine which vending machine foods should be considered "junk foods" and which should be considered nutritious foods. At present, USDA recommends that foods which do not supply at least five percent of one or more of eight common nutrients should not be sold on school property until after lunch period each day.

Many parents protest that this standard is too lax, since manufacturers will be tempted to fortify candy bars with vitamins in order to have their products accepted for use in school vending machines. While this standard does leave room for improvement, it at least represents a move in the right direction. Ideally, parents within a school system should work to establish their own standards for vending machine items, rather than leaving the problem up to government officials.

## Vitamins, Minerals

A school-aged child's increased need for vitamins and minerals can easily be met if the child chooses to gain the extra calories he needs by eating quality foods such as fruits, vegetables, breads, meats, and dairy products. Despite many advertisements which urge routine use of multivitamins, children with a well-balanced diet should not need supplements. While there is some evidence that use of a multi-vitamin/mineral supplement can help some children meet RDAs, dependence upon such supplements may cause parents to be less inclined to work toward providing the child with a well-balanced diet. Such laxity may mean the family will be deficient in trace elements and other items not found in commercial vitamin supplements.

Advertisements and health-magazine articles also urge parents to give their children megadoses of certain vitamins. Seeing their children plagued by winter colds, many parents are intrigued by the claims of Linus Pauling and others that large doses (from 0.5 to 10 grams per day) of vitamin C may reduce the frequency and severity of the common cold. Typical of such reports are two by Coulehan and colleagues concerning the administration of one gram per day of ascorbic acid (vitamin C) to Navajo children in a boarding school. In 1976, Coulehan reported that there was no difference in the incidence of illness episodes of children receiving vitamin C and those not receiving the vitamin, but noted that colds seemed less long-lasting in those children taking vitamin C. Earlier, Coulehan had reported that although children taking vitamin C had fewer positive throat cultures than those not receiving the vitamin, he still felt widespread usefulness of vitamin C as a cold remedy was not justified. Another researcher favored the use of vitamin C, noting that subjects given vitamin C dosages of 3 to 6 grams per day immediately after a cold began seemed to get over their colds faster than those who took only the placebos (sugar pills).

Conversely, in 1977, a five-month study of identical twins showed that genetic, environmental, or subjective factors probably exert a greater influence on frequency and duration of colds than do vitamin C intakes. This study concluded that the effectiveness of vitamin C therapy varies with the age, sex, and possibly genetic constitution of the subject, and that younger children seem more receptive to the cold-prevention benefits of high intakes of vitamin C than do older children.

Although the latter study reported no measurable ill effects from the high dosages of vitamin C taken by the children in the study, a 1978 report indicates that in some cases, megadoses of this vitamin may lead to blood-sugar problems and kidney stones. As early as 1975, researchers warned that extremely high intakes of vitamin C may tend to interfere with tests for diabetes, bring on diarrhea, and increase urinary excretion of oxalic acid.

The iron needs of elementary-school-aged children, which are somewhat lower than they were for the preschool years, should be met if a well-balanced diet is consumed. Since calcium need remains set at 800 milligrams per day until preadolescence, there are those who feel that too much emphasis is placed on milk drinking by elementary-school children. Generally, physicians agree that after the age of eighteen months, milk intake should not exceed one-third the total number of calories taken per day. Two to three glasses (16 to 24 ounces) of whole milk would, by this standard, be adequate. Falling below the recommended 800 milligrams of calcium is not recommended, especially for the older elementary child, who will soon need to call on calcium stores during the rapid-growth years of adolescence. Since all nonmilk foods in the diet of the average elementary-school child can yield but 300 milligrams of calcium and since the RDA is 800 milligrams, gaining enough calcium is extremely difficult when one totally excludes dairy products from the diet.

When an antimilk movement began to cause alarm in the early 1970s, an American Academy of Pediatrics (AAP) committee was called upon to study the problem. Having explored the three main areas of concern raised by the antimilk spokespeople, this committee issued a statement on the topic reflecting the following findings. While it is true that some children do show an enzyme deficiency which makes them unable to tolerate milk, most children do not have severe enough enzyme-deficiency problems to cause adverse effects from drinking milk, unless milk is taken in excessive quantities. In view of the fact that the protein and calcium content of milk is too important to be lost, the AAP committee recommended that federal feeding programs for low-income groups continue to include milk.

Acknowledging that whole milk does contain saturated fats, the AAP committee pointed out that only for children with hereditary hypercholesterolemia should saturated-fat intakes be drastically curtailed. Since milk drinking per se does not lead to obesity and since many children need the calories supplied by whole milk, the AAP committee does not endorse the general use of skim milk by children. Finally, though milk allergy may be a problem for about 2 percent of all American children, this is not a problem for most youngsters.

Having answered the three main arguments of the antimilk spokespeople, the AAP committee admitted that current milk consumption by American children may be above what is necessary for bone and tooth development. Milk intake should probably be cut back for iron-deficient children and for other youngsters who drink most of their calories in milk rather than gaining them from a variety of foods.

*Vegetarians* who do not drink milk or who drink only soy milk must gain their calcium from supplements. While green leafy vegetables do contain calcium, their bulk makes it difficult for young children to obtain sufficient calcium from this source. Supplements may be necessary, even though by the time they reach school age, vegetarian youngsters are usually eating a good many green leafy vegetables.

These vegetables are high in folacin, and folacin may mask the pernicious anemia associated with vitamin $B_{12}$ deficiency. Thus vegetarian children who do not drink milk or take vitamin $B_{12}$ supplements may suffer irreparable nerve damage before this deficiency can be diagnosed and treated. For this reason, $B_{12}$ supplements should be obtained from a physician if a no-milk, no-egg, no-meat diet is undertaken.

Adults who begin a vegan diet without $B_{12}$ supplements may not notice any deficiency symptoms for three to five years, due to their reserves of this vitamin. Children, however, have small reserves to fall back upon and can suffer extensive damage with a relatively short period of deprivation. The nutrient requirements of a vegan child may be met if a vitamin $B_{12}$ supplement is given or fortified soybean milk or fortified soya meat analogs are used.

Lacto-ovo vegetarians should have no vitamin $B_{12}$ problem, since three to four 8-ounce glasses of cow's milk or an equivalent amount of yogurt, cheese, or other dairy products will supply the necessary amounts of this vitamin. Children who enjoy dairy products, eggs, and an otherwise balanced vegetarian diet have low fat intakes, high fiber and water intakes, sufficient vitamin and mineral intakes, and a reduced chance of obesity and heart disease.

## Psychological Aspects

Scholastic success or failure can influence nutritional status. A child who is unhappy or depressed by school activities is not likely to have a good appetite. If his peers ridicule him for his poor performance in the classroom, he is not likely to be able to be relaxed among his tormentors during lunch hour. Conversely, some children who are depressed about social or academic matters at school react by seeking solace in food. Often these children have been offered food as a comfort source from birth.

Peer influence on diet is felt in other ways, from an invitation to eat three candy bars after school to the ridicule of ethnic foods which have long been a child's at-home diet. Often, parents have no direct knowledge of peer influence on nutrition. Instead, they are left to wonder why a child doesn't seem hungry at dinnertime or why she suddenly refuses to eat the beans and rice she has always enjoyed. Unless a child chooses to explain her changing food preferences, parents can only venture a guess as to the reasons behind these changes and offer gentle suggestions concerning good alternatives. Making an issue of a sudden dietary change is usually ineffective and may actually mean delaying any return to "normal" eating patterns.

For example, a first grader who has always loved green beans may announce at the dinner table, "Green beans! Yuk! You know I can't stand green beans!" If a parent can manage to hold himself to a mild "Oh, I thought you liked them," chances are good the child will resume eating the beans within a short time—perhaps at that very meal. More than likely, a favorite friend has just made the same dramatic pronouncement over the green beans on that day's cafeteria menu. The repeated condemnation of green beans may be made out of a simple desire for shock effect, an attempt to be like the bean-hating friend, or a combination of these and perhaps other reasons. Left unnoticed, such a comment will probably have little effect on the child's long-term attitude toward beans. Challenged and debated, the offhand remark may turn into a full-scale battle of wills as the child fights for his right to independent choice and the well-meaning parent fights for his right to influence his child's eating habits.

While some school peers are negative nutrition influences, others may help move a child toward desired nutritional goals. A first-grader who has never eaten broccoli at home may casually remark, "Monty and I ate all our broccoli at school today." If nutrition education of high caliber is being carried out in the classroom, children may become excited about food groups and diet in general. Teachers exert a powerful influence, even when they do not formally teach nutrition. For example, a trick-or-treating six-year-old returned from her teacher's front door to announce, "Mrs. Rumely gave me an oatmeal cookie she made herself. And an apple. I knew she wouldn't be passing out all that candy and junk. She gives nutritious snacks, even at school!"

Grandparents should take heart from this incident. Children are impressed by grown-ups who care about their health. If Papaw brings a bag of grapefruits and oranges as a Christmas treat, that gift is very special to a child who knows that fruit is a delightful and highly nutritious treat. Conversely, a child who knows that candy is bad for his teeth and his overall health is likely to be puzzled by Grandfather's insistence on bringing candy at Eastertime, when books and puzzles would be more welcome gifts. Love and affection should not be bought with food of any kind, but if food gifts are given, certainly they should be gifts which contribute to overall good health.

If children aren't given candy and other undesirable treats, parents are spared the job of persuading them to give up the sweet foods in favor of more acceptable ones. When Halloween's trick-or-treating has garnered a basket of goodies which would send ten children to the dentist, persuading a child to give up those goodies may be difficult. One child suggested her own solution to this yearly problem, "See, mom," she explained after receiving still another lollipop, "we can just take all this junk home to give away again when kids come to our house!"

Of course, parents who do not wish to give their own children sweets should not be willing to give candy to other children, either. Perhaps trick-or-treating for UNICEF is the answer to what to bring home in the box or bag. Sugarless gum can be offered to trick-or-treaters who come to one's own house. A Halloween party featuring popcorn, apples, pumpkin bread with raisins and nuts, and warm apple cider can provide a way to avoid trick-or-treat candies altogether. Partying children could hand bags of popcorn to any trick-or-treaters who ring the bell that evening, and once the party is over, no bag of sweets will be left. If such a party becomes a yearly tradition among school friends, parents can take turns hosting the affair from year to year.

A child who is able to pass through a holiday period and resist most candies is a child who deserves parental praise. Praise, when it is sincerely given and not overdone, is a meaningful way of reinforcing good food choices. Approval, not nagging and reprimands, goes far toward helping a child stay on the path to good nutrition. Mealtimes which disintegrate into petty bickering over a spoonful of beans left on a child's plate or an ounce or two of milk not yet downed are mealtimes which give a child an unhealthy attitude toward food.

Bickering over manners can be equally harmful. Indeed, one nutritionist has theorized that feeding problems for eight- to ten-year-olds are more often behavior-related than food-related. Manners come by imitation, not by coercion. Stressing proper manners at the expense of giving a child pleasant mealtime experiences may lead to the development of unhealthy attitudes toward food. Mealtime should be pleasant, not filled with arguments over petty matters.

Sometimes children six to ten years of age are so involved in their own activities that they are reluctant to eat meals at regular times. By giving a few minutes' warning to a boy engrossed in painting the wings of his model airplane or a girl lost in a Nancy Drew mystery book, a mother can help that child get ready to leave the activity of the moment and come to eat. Often a child who has left an especially interesting activity will rush through his meal, eating just enough to satisfy his hunger pains, then rush back to his project. Later, he may seek a snack to make up for the calories he didn't eat at mealtime. Good snack choices should be made available for such times, though leaving a meal unfinished is hardly a practice a parent wishes to encourage. Setting a minimum mealtime of fifteen to twenty minutes may help a child settle down to the business of eating, despite his interest in the temporarily deserted project.

Television programs can also cause children to be reluctant to come to meals. Occasionally, in the case of a special program, the family dinner hour might be delayed. Basically, television schedules should not control a household, at mealtime or at any other time. Too much television usually means too little exercise and too much exposure to commercials which promote undesirable food items. While some children may not be unduly influenced by such ads, one study indicated that 60 to 80 percent of fifth and sixth graders believed TV ads for drugs and snack foods. Since the average American child watches twenty-five hours of TV per week, and since nearly five hours of that time is spent watching ads, TV influence should not be discounted.

Some children have had no parental guidance in understanding the purpose of commercials and the way in which advertisers omit crucial facts about the products they praise—such as the fact that nearly half the calories from a certain cereal come from sugar. Such youngsters should be given lessons in consumer awareness. The discussion of television ads in the preschooler section of this book should be useful when working with school-age children, too.

While snacks dictated by hard-sell TV commercials are usually best avoided, many young children do need some snacks. As the accompanying chart indicates, morning snacks are relatively rare, as compared to after-school snacks. Since an afterschool snack may provide as much as a quarter of the day's total calories, it should provide high-quality calories. According to the 1974 study from which the two snacking charts below were taken, 21 percent of the snacks consumed by elementary-school children were in the form of sweets. Fortunately, juices, breads, and cereals formed a higher percentage of the snacks they ate, though the inclusion of the term *cookies* under the breads and cereals category makes assessing the food value of the bread and cereal group difficult. For example, sugar cookies provide far fewer nutrients than do whole-grain date cookies.

By providing snack items such as those discussed in the preschooler section, parents can help children make wise snack choices without interfering with their developing sense of independence. In fact, parents may even en-

courage that independence by suggesting that children make their own afternoon treats. Blender yogurt dips for raw vegetables, whole-grain sandwiches, fresh-fruit milkshakes, and even homemade pizza are within the
ability of many youngsters in the lower grades. By encouraging the preparation of nutritious, interesting dishes, parents help mold snacking habits
without using authoritarian tactics.

Generally, all aspects of eating—from manners to snack choices when
company is present—should be approached with a positive, optimistic attitude. If a child is allowed to feel good about himself, he is more likely to
be open to suggestions concerning food choices or behavior patterns. Conversely, if constant criticism is all he has known, he is less likely to be receptive to still further negative comments about his food choices or behavior.
Worse yet, he is likely to associate unpleasant situations with mealtime and

### Frequency of Snacking by Elementary-school Children (Percent)

| Time | Frequency | | |
|------|----------------|--------------|-------|
|      | Almost Always | Occasionally | Never |
| Between lunch and dinner | 86.3% | 13.7% | — |
| After dinner | 43.2 | 25.0 | 31.8% |
| Between breakfast and lunch | 9.1 | 18.2 | 72.7 |
| Before breakfast | 4.5 | 2.3 | 93.2 |

### Percent of Total Snacks Consumed by Elementary-school Children

| Snack Type | Percent |
|------------|---------|
| Breads, cookies, cereals | 29.4% |
| Sweets (candy, pop, dessert) | 20.9 |
| Fruits, juices | 23.2 |
| Milk | 15.7 |
| Noncarbonated flavored drinks | 6.6 |
| Nuts, popcorn, potato chips | 2.4 |
| Vegetables | 1.4 |

SOURCE: Adapted from Nancy R. Beyer and Portia M. Morris, "Food Attitudes and Snacking Patterns of Young Children," *Journal of Nutrition Education* 6 (Oct–Dec 1974),
p. 131.

may have decreased appetite and impaired digestion due to this negative attitude.

# Common Problems

## Dental Caries

Dental caries is rampant among elementary-school children. Over 80 percent of children have caries of permanent teeth by age ten, and over 90 percent have cavities by age twelve. By the time half the permanent teeth are in, the average American child has 6.2 decayed, missing, or filled teeth. Dr. Abraham Nizel, a leading authority in the field of preventive dentistry, believes that the occurrence of cavities in children can be reduced by 60 to 75 percent if the following measures are followed:

1. Children should be taken to the dentist for preventive care by at least age three.
2. Children should be given optimum nutrition, with no high-sugar snacks.
3. Children should receive a fluoride dietary supplement (either flouridated drinking water or a supplement prescribed by a dentist).

A review of the detailed discussion of dental caries in the previous chapter should serve as a reminder that frequent consumption of sugar-containing foods which are retained on tooth surfaces is a primary cause of caries. Thus, both the frequency and the nature of between-meal snacks are important factors in tooth decay. A 1973 study showed positive correlation between the availability of sweets in school canteens and the dental-decay rate in elementary- and secondary-school children. In light of the existing evidence, it would seem that tooth decay cannot be controlled until children's snacking habits are controlled. Early parental guidance can do much to bring about this goal.

## Obesity

Omission of high-calorie, high-sugar snacks can also help combat obesity, another prevalent problem among elementary-school children. In fact, ridding the house of junk food and refraining from eating junk food in the presence of an overweight youngster is an excellent first step toward helping that youngster control her weight. Often the overweight youngster does not appear to be overeating. It is typical for an obese child to gain an extra 4.4 pounds per year by adding an average of only 33 calories per day to what should constitute her optimum calorie level. Gain may be slow but it is constant, so that a weight excess of only 4.4 pounds at age two becomes one of 40 pounds by age twelve. If such slight variations can be this significant, deciding whether an obese child is overeating may be extremely difficult.

Generally, obesity which begins in childhood has become evident by the time a child is in first or second grade. At that point, depending upon the method used to assess obesity, from 3 to 20 percent of school-aged young-sters are overweight. Why these children became overweight is sometimes hard to determine. Overfeeding during infancy and preschool years may be a factor. However, since one study showed that 57 percent of obese ten-year-olds did not become obese until after the age of five, overfeeding in infancy and preschool years is obviously not the only factor involved.

An interesting set of risk factors, based on observation of many obese youngsters, may be useful to parents who are concerned about this problem. According to a recent survey in Great Britain, two or more of the following risk factors are present in 60 percent of obese children.

## Risk Factors in Childhood Obesity

1. Obesity in first-degree relative
2. Elderly mother (over age thirty-five at birth of child)
3. Only-child status
4. Absence of one parent

SOURCE: Adapted from P. W. Wilkinson, J. Pearlson, J. M. Parkin, P. R. Phillips, and P. Sykes, "Obesity in Childhood: A Community Study in Newcastle upon Tyne," *Lancet* I (1977): 350.

In addition to these factors, others may contribute to obesity. Overeating may be triggered by hospitalization, separation from a parent, a move to a new neighborhood, family loss of another child, or any number of other traumatic events. When that overeating is not observed and discouraged by parents or observed and offset by increased exercise, obesity is likely to occur.

However children become obese, statistics indicate that an alarmingly high percentage of obese children become obese adolescents and obese adults. According to one recent study, three-fourths of those persons obese as children (ages six to eleven) are obese as adolescents (ages twelve to sev-enteen). Thus, while infantile and preschool obesity may not be such strong indicators of the likelihood of adolescent obesity, obesity during childhood is a reliable predictor of adolescent obesity. Since this seems to have proven true, independent of such factors as physiological growth, sexual matura-tion and economic status of the children and teens observed, some re-searchers are advocating screening six-year-olds for signs of obesity. In fact, only 15 percent of obese children become normal-weight adults. Retro-spective studies show that 30 percent of obese adults had a history of juve-nile obesity.

Dr. Jerome Knittle, a leading proponent of the increased-fat-cell-number theory, points out that nonobese youngsters show little growth in adipose (fatty) tissue mass between the ages of two and ten. Around age ten, adipose-cell size and number of fat cells increase to adult levels. If a child gains excessive weight during the preschool or elementary years, her number of fat cells in childhood may exceed normal adult levels. Once the ultimate number of fat cells has been attained, that number, according to Dr. Knittle, apparently remains stable, though the size of the cells may be decreased by dieting. Though this fat-cell-numbers theory is not definitive, most nutritionists agree that, for whatever reason, childhood obesity, if it is unchecked, is likely to become lifetime obesity.

Besides the danger of being vulnerable to diseases directly related to obesity, the fat child is plagued by shortness of breath, clumsiness, and skin irritation due to friction and heat. In addition, he is psychologically damaged by the poor self-image and deep-set feelings of inferiority which usually accompany obesity. He may be teased, ridiculed, and left out of games. Cruel and humiliating taunts are hurled at the fat child. Studies show that emotional problems are more prevalent with obesity originating in childhood than with obesity originating in adulthood. The emotional problems of adults who became obese as children are more clearly linked to obesity than are those of adults who became obese in later life. Poor body image and bizarre eating habits are more frequently seen in obese adults who became obese as juveniles.

Once obesity is a reality, parents and child must share a determination to combat it. With a doctor's help, they can devise a realistic plan of attack. Except in extreme cases, where excess weight presents an immediate health hazard (as in Pickwickian Syndrome, where the child is in danger of suffocation), controlled weight gain, not weight loss, should be the goal. Gradually, with careful attention to the tips that follow, an overweight child should be able to reenter the normal ranges of height and weight. At that point, weight-control efforts should be adjusted to allow a "holding pattern" at the desired rate of gain.

Parents should avoid the clean-plate syndrome and should avoid using food as a bribe or a reward. By helping a child take portions appropriate to her calorie needs, helping her cut foods into smaller pieces and take smaller bites, and limiting second helpings and desserts, parents can guide a child toward becoming her own food-intake monitor. Keeping the child's mind busy during mealtime, avoiding letting her eat alone, and limiting her eating to a fixed, designated place can help her keep food from becoming a substitute for socialization. By planning parties which feature foods that an obese child can eat with a clear conscience, a parent can give that child an opportunity to feel at ease with her peers. Finally, by teaching the child the principles of the exchange plan for eating, a parent imparts the blueprint for a lifetime of freedom from obesity.

While most of these suggestions involve ways of decreasing calorie intake, most authorities agree that increasing calorie expenditure of obese youngsters may be an even more important way to help them control weight gain.

Excess pounds are accumulated when inactive children choose television over playing tag or reading over running. Obese children are significantly less active than their normal-weight peers, and they often manage to drop out of physical education classes and any active sports. Since preteens are usually less sensitive about being seen in gym suits than are adolescents, there is no psychological basis for curtailing physical-education activities. Because these children need more, not less, activity, parents should not give in to their pleas to avoid P.E. class. By encouraging active participation in such classes and in YMCA, scouting, and other afterschool activities, parents can help move an inactive child toward the physical exercise in which she should be engaged.

In a society where little physical work is done and where there is an abundance of food, obesity is an inevitable occurrence unless parents make a conscious effort to increase their children's physical activity. Parents who lead a sedentary life usually influence their children to do likewise. Often parents dismiss any suggestion that an obese child should exercise, saying, "If he exercises more, he will just get hungrier and eat even more." According to a study of Boston schoolchildren, a moderate increase in the physical activity of fat, inactive children is not followed by an increase in food intake but is followed by a loss of fat. Nonobese children who increase physical activity moderately automatically increase dietary intakes and thereby maintain their weight at normal levels.

In that same study, 350 obese elementary school children and adolescents were placed in a voluntary exercise program from 1964 to 1967. Physical education classes were increased from two days a week to five days, with two of the forty-five-minute sessions being spent in general P.E. class and three of them spent in special activities for the obese youngsters. These activities included team sports such as soccer and volleyball, and races against the clock in which self-improvement, rather than competition, was emphasized. The children were encouraged to be active over weekends and during vacations as well as during school days. No low-calorie diets were advised, since the researchers believed that obese children need sufficient energy for growth and are not usually overeating. However, nutrition education efforts were made, with suggestions being given for diet improvement.

Operating on the assumption that underexercising is more of a problem than overeating for the obese child, summer camps for the obese offer increased activity, well-balanced diets, and an opportunity for private counseling. Exercise programs at camp or at school work well, with about 60 percent of the children showing reduced rates of gain. Once exercise programs stop, however, most children fall into the old pattern of inactivity. Exercise must be a day-to-day endeavor if it is to make a significant contribution to weight control. Parents who plan family hikes and swimming outings, encourage children to walk to school, and otherwise show the worth of exercise by encouragement and example can help the obese child repattern his activities. The earlier such repatterning begins, the more likely the long-range success of the program.

As the overweight child begins to see that he can control his rate of gain by increasing his activity level and avoiding empty, high-calorie foods, he should gain confidence in his ability to continue to control something he probably believed was beyond his control. Though modifying a child's eating and activity habits may be difficult now, waiting until adulthood will make changes even harder to effect. Unless a child is led to believe he can control his own weight, he may fall into the vicious circle which traps so many obese youngsters. Under the condemnatory remarks of peers and elders, an obese child may become obsessed with his own self-image and develop an expectation of rejection. Self-imposed social isolation may lead to actual rejection and decreased opportunity for experience outside the home and increased exposure to food available within the home. As food becomes a substitute for the social contacts he lacks, the obese child moves toward even greater obesity.

## Hyperactivity

Over the past few decades, much attention has been focused upon the "hyperactive" child. In fact, the term has become one to be dropped at cocktail parties where parents discuss the "impossible" behavior of their youngsters in a one-upmanship recounting of various misadventures. Often these parents are controlling the behavior of their children by means of drugs, much as they themselves use tranquilizers to calm their own nerves or amphetamines to curb their own appetites. While drugs sometimes do cure the symptoms classed under the term *hyperactive behavior,* they do not "cure" whatever may be causing that behavior.

Children diagnosed as hyperactive usually display one or more of the following symptoms: (1) poor power of concentration, (2) shortened attention span, (3) temper tantrums and other impulsive behavior, (4) inability to delay gratification, (5) diminished ability to experience pleasure, (6) altered cognition and perception, (7) altered muscle coordination, and (8) normal IQ but underachievement in school. Estimates of 3 to 10 percent have been given for incidence of hyperactivity in American children, with some researchers estimating incidence as high as 25 percent.

Diagnosis of this "disorder" is often based on parental or teacher reports, which are not always reliable or unbiased. For example, in one study, older teachers tended to rate more children "hyperactive" than did younger ones, perhaps because the older teachers found the activities of certain children harder to accept. Parental tolerance of the increased noise and activity levels associated with child-rearing may also vary from family to family. A child one mother would accept as active but normal, another mother might class as impossible and hyperactive. After all, a parent is somehow less responsible for a child's behavior if that child is abnormal and under a doctor's care. Ironically, parents run from other labels of abnormality, yet seem eager to embrace the label of hyperactivity.

Theories abound as to the cause of hyperactivity, from low-level lead poisoning, carbon-monoxide poisoning, and oxygen deprivation at birth, to exposure to fluorescent lights, milk-drinking, and food additives. These theories are unproven, but their very diversity is indicative of the fact that no easy answers have yet been found. Hyperactive behavior may have physical causes such as hypoglycemia (low blood sugar) or oxygen deprivation due to abnormality of the heart or circulatory system. Dietary factors such as food allergy, low calcium intake, or inability of the body to use calcium may also cause symptoms associated with hyperactivity. Frustration over failure to read due to dyslexia or other learning disabilities may cause a child to "act up" often enough to earn the label "hyperactive."

Hunger from lack of breakfast or from inadequate nutrition in general may be a cause of inability to pay attention to school lessons. A child with these symptoms is not likely to respond to educational stimuli. As he gets further and further behind, he fails to learn because he is missing essential links, essential lessons upon which he has been unable to concentrate. He may wear the label "hyperactive" when the label "hungry" would be more appropriate.

Since drugs such as Ritalin (methylphenidate) and Dexedrine (dextroamphetamine) reduce the symptoms associated with hyperactivity, use of these drugs usually removes the immediate need to look further for the underlying cause of the maladaptive behavior. All too often, teachers and school administrators care less about finding the cause of the behavior than they do about stopping the inappropriate behavior. Consequently, many schools apply pressure to parents, urging them, "Have your family doctor prescribe drugs for Timmy so he can learn to read and stay out of trouble."

Doctors who concur with school and parental diagnosis of a hyperactive child without attempting to find the basic cause of hyperactive behavior may prescribe the drugs they ask for, record the child's improved behavior on subsequent visits, and think no more about why the child had problems in the first place. In the case of relatively difficult-to-diagnose medical problems, such as oxygen deprivation due to cardiac abnormality or low blood sugar due to hypoglycemia, masking symptoms may mean delaying treatment until the condition has considerably worsened. If the cause is perceptual learning problems, psychological difficulties, or social or family problems, taking the prescription drug does nothing to alleviate the real cause of the hyperactive behavior.

Even in cases where no apparent physical cause of hyperactive behavior exists, use of drugs may not be without long-term repercussions. Though thirty years of drug treatment of hyperactive children has not shown that treated children are predisposed to drug abuse, this remains a possibility. Though they are safe enough in small amounts, the amphetamines usually used to treat hyperactivity can be habit-forming and addictive. Ritalin is a more potent hallucinogen per unit of weight than LSD, though when it is taken in the dosages prescribed for hyperactive children, the drug does not act as an hallucinogen. Taken over long periods of time, amphetamines can cause constriction of blood vessels of the brain, increase the likelihood of convulsive seizure, affect carbohydrate metabolism in unknown ways, and alter growth hormone outputs.

Temporary loss of appetite has long been seen as an expected side effect of stimulant drugs given to hyperactive children, but recent studies indicate that long-term use of these drugs may cause a highly significant suspension of growth in height and weight. An average loss of twenty percentile points in weight and thirteen in height has been shown to occur in children on dextroamphetamine. The characteristic growth rebound which occurs when drugs are discontinued during the summer months does not make up for the loss.

Historically, pediatricians have attributed growth lag for medicated children to a loss of appetite alone. However, a 1977 study indicates that use of dextroamphetamine and methylphenidate affect secretion of growth hormone in the children who use these drugs. Doctors have been warned that these risks make long-term use of these drugs unwise in adult weight-reduction programs, yet no such warning has been issued concerning the use of these stimulants in the treatment of hyperactive children.

A 1979 University of Arkansas study of growth suppression of hyperactive children treated with drugs points to the possibility that the drugs may be adversely affecting cartilage and bone development. In that study, methylphenidate, methamphetamine and pemoline were all linked to growth retardation.

Despite the risks involved in using such drugs, many doctors appear convinced that drug therapy is vital in the treatment of hyperactive children. According to a Berkeley research project, seventeen out of forty-eight doctors interviewed felt that depriving a hyperactive child of stimulants (amphetamines) was like depriving a diabetic of insulin. Only ten of the forty-eight doctors disagreed with this view, while twenty-one gave no opinion. Since many parents seem to have no objection to anything that alters the unsatisfactory behavior of hyperactive children, and since amphetamines "work" (at least in one-half to two-thirds of the cases in which they are tried), doctors generally see nothing wrong with delegating children to years of drug therapy.

In the early 1970s, a Vermont psychiatrist reportedly said that drug treatment of school children would be worthwhile if this resulted in reduced classroom tension and peace of mind for family members, even if the drugs failed to benefit the children themselves. While most physicians would surely not share this extreme point of view, too many doctors tend to see drugs as the only solution to this complex behavioral problem. As of 1974, 500,000 to 2,000,000 youngsters were receiving prescription drugs for hyperactive behavior. One wonders how many of those prescriptions were given without thorough exploration of the causes behind the symptoms.

Even though abuse or misuse of drug therapy may occur, there are no doubt many cases in which amphetamines are the only practical means of helping a child function in school and in society. When all other avenues have been explored, drug therapy may, indeed, be the best route for a particular child.

The nondrug option for treatment of hyperkinetic children which has perhaps received the most attention in the past decade is a restrictive diet developed by Dr. Ben F. Feingold. According to Dr. Feingold, many hyperactive patients improve if they avoid foods that contain artificial colors and flavors and foods containing natural salicylates. Other allergists have realized that several of the tension symptoms associated with food allergy (e.g., overactivity, clumsiness, hyperkinesis, irritability, insomnia) are also associated with hyperactivity. Food allergy may be a contributing factor, if not the main cause, of hyperactivity in many children.

The Feingold diet is not without its problems. Although elimination of foods containing artificial colors and flavors may not cause loss of nutrients, elimination of twenty-one fruits and vegetables high in natural salicylates could certainly mean significant alteration of nutrient intakes. Thus, strict adherence to the diet as it was originally conceived without any attempt to achieve variety using the allowed foods might possibly mean that a child would not meet the RDAs for all nutrients. But if care is taken to see that variety *is* achieved within the foods which are allowed, RDAs can be met with no difficulty.

The Feingold diet should definitely not be undertaken without competent medical supervision, but sometimes parents find it hard to convince a physician to assist them in trying the program. Many physicians feel the family cooperation involved in the diet (for example, making additive-free desserts together) or the fact that the diet is relatively low in carbohydrates may have more to do with patient improvement than does the restriction of additives. Some doctors feel that parents and teachers look hard for improvement, for some reason to believe the diet works, when, in fact, improvement may be slight or even imagined. As long as subjective judgments are the only way of diagnosing the disorder or of assessing improvement, cause-effect relationships will continue to be difficult to judge.

Some doctors have found vitamin or mineral deficiencies in hyperactive children. While supplementation to correct known deficiencies may alter hyperactive behavior in some cases, there is no evidence that indiscriminate megadoses of vitamins will cure hyperactivity. Evaluation of one recent study which seems to show impressive results from use of megadoses of several vitamins is difficult because the children in the study were placed on restrictive diets at the same time they were given the megavitamins. Determining whether diet or vitamins caused improvements in behavior is thus a problem. In one case, a four-year-old child showed symptoms of vitamin A toxicity and had serum vitamin A levels which were 710 times the normal level. Though the child's grandmother denied having megadosed the child, the boy's doctor was fairly certain the grandmother had given vitamin A as a "remedy" for the child's hyperactivity.

Just as the diagnosis of hyperactivity is admittedly highly subjective, the diagnosis of improvement or worsening of the symptoms of this disorder is no less subjective. Blind faith in drugs, diet, or any other "cure" for the hyperkinetic syndrome is probably ill advised at this point. Instead, parents, doctors, teacher, and child (if the child is old enough) should work to discover and eliminate any medical, psychological, social or other factors which might be contributing to the child's hyperactivity. If complete laboratory testing and intensive counseling fail to show any apparent reason for the behavior, drug treatment may be warranted.

Whereas many physicians tend to feel that searching for causes is a waste of time and money, Dr. Sidney Walker, III, a neuropsychiatrist with residency experience in neurology, neurosurgery, and psychiatry, is an exception. Dr. Walker notes "In my medical practice I see many . . . hyperactive children. I have never prescribed stimulants for these patients, and I never will." His strong stand on this issue is based on a firm belief "that the hyperactive child's problem can almost always be identified and treated if the physician is willing to take the time and trouble to run through diagnostic tests and evaluate the resulting quantitative data."

Parents faced with the problem of hyperactivity in their children should seek the aid of a physician who is willing to look for the underlying cause of their child's behavior problems and not just prescribe drugs which mask the symptoms. Of course, they should also be cautious of physicians or others who offer miraculous "cures" for hyperactivity, cures which may be useless, expensive, and detrimental to the overall development of the child.

## Allergies

As noted in the above discussion, food allergies may contribute to hyperkinetic behavior patterns of some children. In addition, unrecognized food allergies may cause headaches, stomachaches, cold symptoms and other physical problems. While past efforts to detect allergies have usually been undertaken because of physical problems such as these, the trend of the future may well be detection of allergies in patients who show mental and emotional disturbances which seem to have biochemical causes. The story of Billy, a bright, personable nine-year-old whose allergies nearly cost him his life illustrates the seriousness of biochemically caused mental and emotional disturbances.

Although never troubled by serious illness, Billy suffered from frequent colds, a constant drippy nose, and numerous stomachaches and headaches. He was known for his wide mood swings, and his mother recalls that he was "always high or low—never in between." At the age of nine, his mood swings became more extreme, bedwetting became a problem, headaches and stomachaches increased in intensity and frequency, and he became cross and irritable. He slept poorly, had little appetite, and had dark circles under his eyes. He began to talk about life's not being worth living and told his parents he thought suicide might be a good idea.

After trying many other avenues, Billy's parents consulted a psychiatrist who specializes in mental disorders which may have a biochemical basis. The physician determined that Billy was allergic to several of his favorite foods, including peanut butter, potatoes, and popcorn. According to the boy's parents, elimination of the offending foods has brought about great improvement in Billy's physical and emotional health. He enjoys school, takes part in extracurricular activities, and is free of the physical symptoms which plagued him for years.

When Billy accidentally eats foods which contain some of the items to which he is allergic, his physical problems reappear. Thus, he's learned to be careful about his meals and snacks and to take the doctor's "restricted foods list" seriously. While this close attention to diet isn't always easy, his parents insist that "whatever the bother, we have a really sharp little boy to remind us that we were very, very fortunate to be sent in the right direction."

Billy's experience is similar to many reported by those physicians, psychiatrists, and nutritionists who believe that biochemical causes may lie behind the mental and emotional problems of some children and adults. Though others still question these relatively new theories, more and more professionals are considering undetected food allergies a possible source of emotional as well as physical disorders. Since skin tests and trial food restriction regimens have not been entirely satisfactory means of allergy detection, physicians look with hope toward new detection procedures now in the research stages. When allergies can be more easily pinpointed, cause and effect relationships will no doubt be more clearly understood.

## Constipation

A child who eats a well-balanced diet which includes adequate amounts of fiber from whole grains; fresh, unpeeled—but well-washed—fruits; high-fiber vegetables; and adequate amounts of liquids is not likely to have problems with bowel movements. Often parents feel that unless bowel movements occur on a regular basis, a child must be constipated. By transferring their own fears to their child, overanxious parents may cause a child to worry so much about what should be a natural, easy process that the worrying interferes with that process.

In general, parents should casually and unobtrusively observe the frequency of at-home bowel movements, assuming that no problem exists unless a child indicates otherwise. At that point, prune juice, prunes, bran cereals, or other high-fiber cereals, fresh fruits and vegetables, and abundant liquids may be offered. Usually the addition of one or two of these foods will help relieve temporary constipation. If it doesn't, a physician's advice should be sought before using any laxative or other medical remedy.

## Hypoglycemia

Hypoglycemia—less than normal amounts of glucose (sugar) in the circulating blood—is a disorder which has recently been blamed for any number of vague symptoms, including anxiety, hunger, weakness, trembling, and sweaty palms. In some cases, these symptoms do mean that blood sugar has dropped below normal levels, but in other cases, the symptoms are probably not related to blood-sugar levels.

Though newspaper and magazine articles have made hypoglycemia the root of all evils—from psychopathic mass murders to drug addiction—doctors and nutritionists have not always been convinced of the validity of the cases presented to prove this. Like hyperactivity, hypoglycemia has become a popular disorder. Frequently, those who talk about it most understand it least.

True hypoglycemic patients are usually prediabetic. Once they are diagnosed by means of a glucose-tolerance test, these persons may be placed on a high-protein, low-carbohydrate diet similar to that used by diabetics. Ironically, though insulin output in the hypoglycemic individual is higher than normal, insulin output is likely to drop below normal eventually, an event which marks the onset of true diabetes. Obviously, control of diet is desirable to ward off the onset of diabetes as long as possible. Children who are diagnosed as being hypoglycemic can adjust to a high-protein diet with relative ease, and parents who use the exchange method of meal planning should find that adjusting exchanges to reflect low carbohydrate levels is relatively easy.

No drastic adjustments of this sort should be made without the direction of a physician. Since alarmist articles have made many doctors justifiably skeptical of parents who blame all Johnny's behavior problems, school failures, and other undesirable characteristics on the child's "hypoglycemia," getting appropriate tests authorized may be difficult. In most cases, a single blood-sugar check after twelve hours without food does not really confirm or deny the presence of hypoglycemia. Since the more reliable glucose-tolerance test requires that a child have blood samples taken every few hours after the ingestion of a glucose mixture, the testing procedure may be a traumatic experience for a young child. With this in mind, parents will want to be fairly certain that they have reason to suspect hypoglycemia before insisting upon a glucose-tolerance test. A family history of diabetes plus the presence of the symptoms usually associated with the disorder should be reason enough to gain a physician's opinion on the matter.

In some cases, the cause of hypoglycemia may be the presence of a tumor or abnormal liver function, and home-prescribed treatment of such children with a high-protein, low-carbohydrate diet is likely to be ineffective and possibly dangerous. In general, parents should refrain from assuming that every vague symptom of discomfort can be attributed to hypoglycemia, but they should be aware that when this disorder does occur, it must be treated by a competent physician.

## Food for Young Athletes

Elementary-school athletic programs should be fun for boys and girls, but, all too often, parents and coaches see these early programs as win-or-die situations in which future stars are trained and through which all the frustrated athletic ambitions of onlooking adults can be fulfilled. In extreme cases, coaches have called upon junior athletes to lose several pounds overnight in order to qualify for midget-league participation. Overzealous parents who take such coaching advice too seriously may starve their children and even give them diuretics (water-loss pills) in order to get them down to specified weights. Use of diuretics can deplete potassium stores and upset the child's fluid-electrolyte balance, making him a prime candidate for heat exhaustion. Use of induced vomiting, rubber sweat suits, laxatives, or any other means of unnaturally rapid weight loss can be equally dangerous.

Coaches of young athletes often advocate fad diets. Parents should protest such diets, since they may cause interruption of normal growth. Coveting a grade-school city-wide championship is no excuse for subjecting youngsters to dietary regimens even a professional football coach might be reprimanded for advocating.

In general, junior athletes should eat the same well-balanced diet that is appropriate for nonathletes. If energy intake is adequate, protein, carbohydrate, and fat distributions are within recommended ranges, and vitamin and mineral intakes are sufficient, a young athlete will have an excellent chance of reaching her full growth potential. The strong bones and firm muscles she is developing in this natural way will be ready to serve her well when she engages in junior high and high school sports activities. Best of all, if she has not been driven to unnatural, uncomfortable dietary extremes in the cause of becoming an athlete, she is far more likely to enjoy her participation in such activities.

Heat exhaustion is one diet-related phenomenon which the junior athlete and her parents should understand. Heat stroke is a very serious reaction, in which the heat-regulating centers of the brain are paralyzed, causing the victim's body temperature to soar to brain-damaging, often deadly, heights. Although most coaches of varsity sports are trained in the mechanics of heat exhaustion and heat stroke, a significant number of young athletes are victims of this killer each year. Since the volunteer coaches of pee-wee or midget football are occasionally more zealous and are often less well informed on such matters than professionally trained coaches of varsity sports, even young children sometimes die from heat exhaustion.

Usually such cases occur in hot, humid areas of the country during late-summer, preseason, high-school practice sessions. Since small-fry teams aren't usually formed until after school starts, team drilling in late August is, fortunately, rare for elementary-school athletes. Still, since hot days do occur in mid-autumn, especially in the Southern states, coaches, parents, and children should understand the mechanics of heat exhaustion.

Body temperature normally stays at 98.6 degrees Fahrenheit (37 degrees Celsius); temperatures above 104 to 105 degrees Fahrenheit should be viewed with alarm. When athletes engage in hard practice drills or in games, abnormal exertion normally drives body temperature up. At this point, perspiration forms on the skin and is evaporated into the air. Normal evaporation exerts a cooling effect, but if the humidity is above 90 percent and temperatures are higher than 85 degrees Fahrenheit, sweat is likely to roll to the ground without evaporating. On such high-danger days, practice sessions or athletic contests should be avoided.

Other factors that inhibit the evaporation of perspiration also present hazards. Athletes who wear too many clothes or are overweight and insulated by too many layers of fat are in danger of heat prostration. The young chubby who would make a perfect middle linebacker if he'd just lose 5 pounds is particularly at risk. After being driven to unusual feats of exercise for several days, during which he has kept his consumption of food and water to a minimum, such a child may pass out during a hot afternoon-practice session—a victim of heat exhaustion.

In this case, formation of perspiration has been hampered by the child's curtailed fluid intakes. As the boy gradually becomes dehydrated, the cells that regulate the delicate electrolyte balance cease to function. At this point, his energy level probably drops and his athletic performance deteriorates, but because he continues to exert himself, his body continues to try to regulate itself. Eventually, water begins to leave the blood plasma in order to dilute the salt that is concentrating in his extracellular fluids, causing a sudden reduction in the circulating volume of blood. Sensing that loss in volume, the body marshals the remaining blood to serve the brain, leaving no reserve blood available for the maintenance of the vital sweating mechanism. Within a few moments of sweat cessation, body temperature soars, leading to brain, heart, and kidney failure characteristic of such tragedies.

Often the most conscientious youngsters are the ones who become heat-exhaustion statistics. Since thirst is not a safe indication of the extent of dehydration, athletes should weigh themselves before and after each day's practice and drink enough water to offset the losses which have occurred through exertion. Since young girls may be less likely to gulp extra water, coaches and parents should be sure female athletes understand that the weight loss due to water loss is neither safe nor desirable. If this fact is not made clear, figure-conscious girls may delight in their apparent weight loss without realizing that dehydration can impair their athletic performance and lead to heat exhaustion.

## School Lunch Programs

According to popular legend, Benjamin Thompson, Count Rumford, an American-born physicist, inventor, and statesman, started the first school lunch program while living in Munich, Germany. Its purpose was to curtail vagrancy among schoolchildren. Later, other lunch programs such as the two-cent meals in French school *cantines* around 1867 were designed to offer a noon meal to children involved in public-school programs. A 1906 English law transferred responsibility for feeding schoolchildren in Britain from charitable groups to the government, and by 1910, many other Euopean countries had similar feeding programs.

American school lunches were the dream of Ellen H. Richards, a founder of the home-economics movement in this country. Before she spearheaded the 1894 Boston School Lunch Program, large cities had periodically experimented with such programs without much success. Mrs. Richards' program worked so well that other cities began to follow her example and use her feeding techniques. More often than not, these efforts were still primarily the work of dedicated volunteers.

Not until the depression years of this century did federal officials see that malnutrition of school-aged children was a reality in America. By 1935, a federal law channeled surplus commodities into school lunchrooms in an attempt to correct malnutrition. From 1944 to 1946, the secretary of agriculture directed school milk and lunch programs, but in 1946, the National School Lunch Act gave federal lunch program grants to local schools: states provided matching funds, and students paid whatever they could afford.

Under current provisions, a class "A" school lunch should meet one-third of a child's RDAs. While most schools comply with this regulation, the foods chosen to meet the government's criteria are not always foods that appeal to the appetites of schoolchildren. Children who are not accustomed to high carbohydrate intakes may react unfavorably to school menus. Boys and girls who do not eat vegetables at home may never try vegetables at school. Others who do eat vegetables at home may dislike vegetables at school due to overcooking or other problems in preparation.

The year 1976 marked the thirtieth anniversary of the passage of the National School Lunch Act. Though American school lunch programs have helped prevent malnutrition during the three decades of their existence, they have not always made optimum contributions to children's nutrition. There is much evidence that many school lunch programs are poorly supervised, even when private companies are given school lunch program contracts. Though food costs have continued to rise, well-run school lunch programs can still provide satisfactory menus at reasonable prices. With proper attention to financial and nutritional aspects of lunch programs, we can afford to offer optimum school feeding programs. Can we afford not to?

Plate waste (food left uneaten) in school cafeterias is a cause of great concern. Should children be offered fast-food items, just to cut down on waste and make sure adequate calories are consumed? Won't offering fast foods reinforce undesirable eating habits? Can school lunches be nutritious, popular, and within the financial range allowed for such operations? Many educators offer a pessimistic "no" to this last question and try to ignore the plate waste evident in their own cafeterias. Parent committees, often with no precedents to cite, too frequently give in to this pessimism and send sack lunches to school.

Yet there are school lunch programs which are nutritious, delicious, and economical. Getting such a program started in a school system demands heavy research, willingness to seek out the help of a competent dietitian, and untiring effort to find and utilize all available financial resources. Such a project is not likely to succeed overnight, yet it is within the scope of concerned parent-teacher groups and should be considered by such groups.

Perhaps the most exciting success story concerning the transformation of school lunches is that of the Nutra Natural Lunch program devised and directed by Sara Sloan, a food-service director in the Fulton County School System in Atlanta, Georgia. Mrs. Sloan has managed to give children nutritious, delicious lunches, without exceeding the budget allocated by the school district. For forty cents, an elementary-school child receives a lunch which a gourmet would be happy to be offered. Sample menus include sesame chicken breast with wheat-germ gravy, brown rice, Waldorf salad, whole-wheat rolls, carob cookies; Reuben sandwich made from sauerkraut and fresh corned beef (without nitrates or nitrites) on a whole-wheat bun, raw vegetable salad, and applesauce cake; whole-wheat lasagna with raw vegetable salad, bran bread, and apple crisp; fresh fruit plate with cottage cheese, cracked-wheat rolls, cheddar cheese rounds; Nutra-Burger (mixture of ground meat, vegetables, and selected herbs) on whole-wheat bun, crispy baked potato, garden salad, and fruit. All meals are served with milk and all surpass the nutritional requirements for federally subsidized Type "A" lunches.

Parents who have found their own kids reluctant to try some of the items in Mrs. Sloan's school menus may be skeptical about how well such meals are received. Lunchroom participation is optional in Atlanta, and 87 percent of the student body *chooses* to take advantage of the cafeteria meals. Plate waste has gone down, not up, since the Nutra Natural Lunches were introduced, and student enthusiasm is high.

The secret? Mrs. Sloan's program links school meals with classroom learning. Teachers in elementary schools schedule a "mini nutrition" time each day, in which the day's cafeteria menu is discussed. The nutritional values of various dishes are explained, and new or different foods are introduced. For example, when whole-wheat lasagna is on the menu, children are shown uncooked bits of lasagna and are led in a discussion of why "brown is beautiful." High-school health and nutrition clubs meet with food-service managers and enjoy guest lectures on topics of special interest.

According to Mrs. Sloan, nutritional enlightenment is vitally important to the success of this program. Apparently, once students learn why certain foods are being served, they are usually willing to try them. In most cases they find the new foods tasty and enjoyable, thanks to positive peer pressure, which the nutrition-education program has helped to bring about.

Parents or food supervisors interested in trying Mrs. Sloan's approach might follow her example: she convinced the school board to let her try her program by serving board members a sample Nutra Lunch! For information on *A Guide for Nutra Lunches and Natural Foods* and other related publications, write to Sara Sloan, Fulton County Schools Food Service Program, Box 13825, Atlanta, Georgia 30324.

Though she buys many of the fresh foods used in her program, Mrs.

Sloan manages to use some commodity foods provided by the government. For example, she drains the sugary syrup from fruits and adds fresh fruit and wheat germ. She adds rice polishings and wheat germ to white rice and adds wheat germ, soy flour, and bran to white flour. She cannot afford to ignore foods which have traditionally made up 20 percent of school lunch content at no charge to the school.

In New York, one woman's interest led to changes in the nature of the commodity foods offered to the schools. Due to Susan Feinstein's visit to New York State's Chief of the Bureau of Donated Food, whole-wheat flour, natural cheddar cheese, light-syrup fruits, and brown rice are now available to school lunch programs. Many schools steer clear of these new items, saying they fear the children won't accept the changes. In actuality, children *have* accepted the new foods, leaving no more plate waste than they did before.

Parents who take the time to find out what foods are being served in school cafeterias, and who go a step further to find out *why* those foods are being served, are well on their way to bringing about desired changes in those menus. Now, while interest in nutrition is at an all-time high, parents have an excellent opportunity to upgrade school lunch programs across the nation. Doing so means tax dollars will be put to better use and American schoolchildren will finally receive lunches which offer optimum, not just satisfactory, nutrition. Best of all, through programs like Mrs. Sloan's Nutra Lunches, students learn that *nutritious* can also mean *delicious!*

## Special Projects

### Cooking

Children in the early grades can put many of their newly acquired academic skills to work in the kitchen. Reading recipes and measuring ingredients can turn abstract concepts into concrete, practical bits of knowledge. Gelatin salads with vegetables or fruits, blender milkshakes and dips, and supersandwiches become extraspecial when the children make them themselves.

Even at this early age, children soon learn that sugar amounts can be decreased in almost all recipes and that wheat germ can be added to nearly everything. Projects in which parents and children work together can provide time for sharing thoughts and feelings as well as cooking skills. Special projects, such as making and decorating gingerbread men for the Christmas tree or creating a whole-wheat gingerbread house decorated with dried fruit, can be highlights of the holiday season—even if the gingerbread men have ragged edges and the house skews to the left a bit and loses its chimney on Christmas Eve. Generally, any food a child prepares himself will be a food he enjoys.

### Vacation Projects

The basic travel-food tips we gave for toddlers and preschoolers apply to young school-aged children as well. By taking along favorite sandwich fixings, especially peanut butter, families can have familiar, easily digested food available for quick lunches or snacks. For short excursions, you can bring fruit from home, but vacation travel should provide opportunities for sampling fruits of the regions you are touring.

For example, a trip through southeastern Colorado during melon season yields delicious, peak-of-ripeness watermelons, honeydew melons, and cantaloupes. Some fruit stands provide ice-cold melons. If you buy a warm melon, place it in a stream to cool while the family takes a hike. Somehow, eating cherries in the northwest, apples in Virginia, strawberries in Louisiana, avocados in California, citrus fruits in Texas and Florida, and peaches in Georgia makes these fruits seem especially delicious. In many areas, you can visit the orchards and the family can pick its own fruit.

Through such experiences, children and adults can gain inside knowledge of the region they are visiting. However, many vacationing families are not even aware of the fresh-fruit opportunities available in a particular area, choosing, instead, harried stops at fast-food franchises which offer the same foods served by look-alike restaurants back home.

Restaurants, when they are well chosen, offer learning experiences similar to those available through exploration of regional produce. Across the country, there are restaurants locally famous for their regional specialties. Instead of stopping at the first available cafe, a family can ask service-station attendants, post-office clerks, or motel personnel to recommend an eating place. For example, citizens in Louisiana's Bayou country can direct visitors down along country lanes to Himel's, a tiny restaurant where boiled shrimp, crayfish, and crab are served on long tables covered with newspapers. There the musical accents of Acadian French mingle with the soft drawls of other area residents, making the meal an atmospheric as well as a culinary delight.

A visit to Pennsylvania Dutch country provides an opportunity to sample that famous regional cooking; a tour of San Francisco should include a meal in Chinatown; a day in Mississippi makes possible lunch in Vicksburg's Old Southern Tea Room; a Texas visit gives the family a taste of Tex-Mex food, while crossing the border brings an opportunity for authentic Mexican food. By sampling regional specialties from coast to coast, children meet new foods in their own settings. Tasting unusual meats and vegetables becomes a part of the total experience of absorbing an unfamiliar culture. Since the memories associated with such dining experiences are usually rich ones, chances are excellent that the children will remember the foods with fondness and request them again, once the family returns home.

A Deep-South Thanksgiving dinner, Shrimp Creole, Chinese Egg Rolls, and Sweet and Sour Pork recipes included in Appendix C of this book are regional favorites which may be prepared at home. Families who do not travel across country may wish to plan vicarious vacations during which family members gather books, records, magazine articles, and maps from the region to be "visited." After a discussion of the chosen route, parents and children can plan evening meals characteristic of the area. In some cases, such as a Hawaiian luau, special costumes may be designed and worn during the dinner hour and guests may be invited to join in the fun. Whenever possible, special props, such as chopsticks, can be provided. When foods of different cultures become a total adventure, they are likely to be greeted with excitement and anticipation, rather than distrust.

## Practical Meals and Snacks

Studies have shown that children have a better attitude and improved school performance when they eat breakfast than when they skip it. Children who skip breakfast tend to be careless and inattentive in the late-morning hours. Recognized improvement in scholastic performance and general behavior has been observed when breakfast is eaten by children who customarily skip this meal.

As we mentioned earlier, American households tend to view breakfast as a do-it-yourself meal. By elementary-school age, many children are faced with the responsibility of getting their own breakfast, and most turn to convenient, ready-to-eat cereals. When those cereals are whole-grain, low-sugar products, cereal plus milk and a citrus fruit juice can get a child off to an excellent nutritional start. If a third-grader prefers a breakfast of peanut butter on whole-wheat bread, milk, and an apple, parents should accept that choice and be pleased that the nutrient content of this unorthodox meal approaches that of toast, an egg, a slice of bacon, and milk.

Preventing hunger seems to be the most important benefit of eating breakfast, since hunger leads to irritability, disinterest, and apathy, all characteristics that lessen a child's chances of a happy, productive school morning.

According to one Swedish study, a breakfast of less than 400 calories adversely affects school performance, but children who consume at least 400 calories before school hours seem to fare well.

Eating too much can reduce the benefit of eating breakfast, since children who eat a high-quality breakfast of moderate size are apt to feel better all morning than children who eat an abnormally large breakfast.

Since approximately one-fourth of the schoolchildren in America tend to arrive at school without having eaten breakfast, government breakfast programs have been tried in some areas of the country. As early as 1931, experiments with mid-morning snacks showed that a milk snack decreased the nervousness of schoolchildren and that milk plus a food-supplement concentrate improved persistence, sociability, and general behavior of 85 percent of the children. A more recent study showed that a mid-morning glass of orange juice reduced irritability, relieved fatigue, and decreased "negative behavior" in schoolchildren, while a glass of water brought about none of these changes.

Since most schools do not provide the time or the means for a nutritious midmorning snack, a good breakfast is doubly important. A breakfast cereal which children make themselves can be more appetizing than one from a box, and a homemade breakfast shake containing eggs, milk, and fruit can be more appealing to some youngsters than a scrambled egg, milk, and orange juice. Recipes for homemade granola and nutritious super-shakes appear in the recipe section.

Preparing sack lunches is a task many parents face whose children do not enjoy eating lunchroom food. Make-ahead sandwiches which are frozen the night before make mornings less rushed. Suggestions for sandwiches of this sort, along with several suggestions for making sack lunches inviting, are included in the recipe section. Children who help build their own sand-wiches and choose the fruits and vegetables which go into lunchbox or bag are probably more likely to enjoy lunch than those who have no say about what they take to school.

As the table on page 168 indicates, many children of elementary-school age enjoy afternoon snacks. When those snacks are well planned, they can add nutrients not gained in the day's meals. Without adequate planning, afternoon snacks too often only provide empty calories and quick energy. Young children can plan and make many of the snack ideas on pages 295 to 299. Items such as child-made Pat-a-Pizza and supershakes can provide pro-tein, calcium, and other nutrients in addition to energy.

By following the chart of Exchange Minimums given in Appendix A, chil-dren of elementary-school age should be able to meet or exceed the RDAs for protein, vitamins, and minerals. By adding extra portions of equally nutritious fare, they can also meet the RDAs for energy.

# 8
## Adolescent Years— Eleven to Nineteen

At 6:45 Saturday morning, with the other family members still in bed, twelve-year-old Nora rummaged for her own breakfast—a bowl of high-protein cereal with milk. By 8:30, she was on her way to the gym for a fast-break basketball game, part of the junior high intramural sports program in which she was an active participant.

Home again, she snacked on an apple. Around 12:30 P.M. she had a peanut butter and honey sandwich, an orange, and a soft drink. That afternoon she walked several blocks to collect money from subscribers on her paper route. At 4:30, she went out with the family, returning home around 6:00.

At 6:30, she joined her parents, brothers, and sisters in a formal family meal, the first of the day. One serving of roast turkey, one of carrots and peas, double helpings of dressing and mashed potatoes, and two glasses of milk satisfied her appetite until 9:00 P.M. At that point, she polished off three handfuls of red licorice, dressed for bed, brushed her teeth, and watched TV till bedtime—10:00 P.M.

Five feet and one-half inch tall and weighing 101 pounds, Nora is a healthy, energetic teen. She's intellectually sharp, widely involved in ex-tracurricular activities such as dramatics and sports, and still inclined to enjoy being with family as well as friends. Though she is the youngest of six children, she defies any stereotyping as the spoiled baby of the family.

Her dietary habits, though they are not ideal, are basically adequate. This was an unusually good fruit-and-vegetable day for her—two fruits, including one vitamin-C-rich fruit, and three vegetables, including one vitamin-A-rich vegetable. She easily met her protein requirement through her high-protein cereal, peanut butter, and turkey, and she consumed an adequate number of servings from the bread group. Ideally, she could have used an-other serving of milk, but by not taking it she followed the teen tendency to be slightly low in calcium. Though dentists may shudder at her licorice evening snack, the calories in it helped Nora meet the energy needs of a busy, active day, and the sugar, eaten all at once and followed by nighttime brushing, did less harm to her teeth than would have been the case had she nibbled licorice all afternoon and evening.

With the help of the licorice, she consumed about 1954 calories during the day. According to the RDA chart, a girl of twelve with light to moderate activity levels needs approximately 2200 calories per day. Allowing for the extra calories lost to an hour of basketball, her ideal intake should probably have been around 2400 calories. At 1954 calories, she meets three-quarters of the RDA for calories, coming close enough to the optimum figure to avoid being classed as calorie-deficient.

For now, the fact that her iron intake fell below the 18 milligrams recommended for eleven- to fourteen-year-old girls has no serious consequences, though at only nine milligrams, the intake may be low enough to cause subclinical deficiency symptoms. Once she reaches full maturity, the consequences of suboptimal iron intake could become serious.

Overall, the picture is encouraging. A healthy, active teen chose and prepared two of her Saturday meals by herself, ate one prepared by her mother, enjoyed two snacks of her own choosing, and managed to acquire two-thirds or more of the Recommended Dietary Allowances for all nutrients except iron. Her health is excellent, her hair glossy, her skin clear and fresh, her eyes bright, her muscles well toned. She is definitely not suffering from the effects of severe malnutrition.

However, as a preadolescent girl, she is about to become a member of the sex-age group with the poorest overall diet pattern in America. And, as a later look at her food diary for the other six days of the week will indicate, she doesn't always do quite as well nutritionally as she did on this particular Saturday. So far, she has managed to walk the tightrope of barely adequate nutrition carefully, thus escaping such signs of borderline malnutrition as apathy, irritability, loss of appetite, anemia, gastrointestinal disturbances, and failure to grow in height. Or, more likely, she's possibly been annoyed by one or more of these minor disturbances at one time or another without even dreaming that her less-than-perfect state of health could possibly be related to her diet.

As the American Medical Association has noted, "A person can be well nourished and still not be physically fit, but he can never be physically fit without being well nourished." For Nora, a girl who wants to be always at her best physically, mentally, and emotionally, realizing the weaknesses in her diet proved to be a turning point in her nutrition pattern.

Once she became aware of the basic food groups and their importance, she found it fairly easy to give a little extra thought to her meals and snacks. Since she was physiologically a moderately late maturer just entering the pubescent growth period, she was able to make these dietary changes in time to avoid serious deficiencies during her rapid-growth years. Since good nutrition, even in the years before puberty, may play an important role in establishing a girl's capacity to reproduce satisfactorily in later life, her dietary changes might ultimately be of importance to the health of her children.

Whether the diets of adolescent boys and girls meet their nutrient needs will depend, in large part, on whether teens are given an opportunity to understand more fully the vast physical changes they are undergoing and the nutritional implications of those changes. As in Nora's case, many teens are free to choose their own breakfast, lunch, and snacks, with only dinner remaining under parental direction. Even at dinner, of course, they must make choices—between more bread or an extra helping of dessert, between skipping the salad or taking it because of the nutrients it offers, between drinking milk or tea, between adding sugar to tea or taking it plain.

These choices, plus all the other food choices teens make during the course of the day, can and should be based on sound premises. Too many parents seem ready to give up in despair on nutrition for teens. They assume, usually falsely, that a nutrition pattern like Nora's—one that features no eggs for breakfast and ends with red licorice—cannot possibly be adequate. They may nag or even beg kids to eat better, but they aren't likely to see any changes taking place until teens are given credit for being able to face the facts and make sound decisions themselves. Parents who read and discuss this chapter with their adolescents rather than using its contents as ammunition for nutritional nagging should find the teens ready and eager to learn more about food intakes and overall health, and then to put what they've learned into practice.

Don't expect miracles. The boy who has been a breakfast-skipper since age nine isn't likely to join his parents for scrambled eggs, bacon, toast, milk, and orange juice. But if he's not pushed, if he's not prodded, he just might start off to school munching an apple or a banana and with a bag of granola hidden away in his book pack.

Teens need room to grow, to be themselves, and to learn to like the selves they are becoming. Given this room, plus an opportunity to gain valid information concerning nutrition, they are quite likely to put at least some of that information to good use.

Basically, those adolescents who've been taught good food habits from birth aren't likely to toss them completely out now, even if all their friends prefer candy to carrots and sundaes to spinach. If food training has been a pleasant affair over all the prior years, it's not likely to be an area in which a teen will rebel. Parents who offer gentle guidance through the early years and exhibit unfailing openness and trust during the teen years are likely to find their youngsters continuing basically sound dietary habits, though eating patterns and menu choices may be a far cry from those of the mother-dominated preschool years.

Parents and teens together should study the RDA notes for adolescents, read and discuss the section on physical and psychological changes of these rapid-growth years, look carefully at the special nutrition-related problems teens encounter, plan to try a few of the projects suggested, and then close with a look at the discussion of meals and snacks, a discussion which revisits the Nora whose Saturday meals opened this chapter and introduces four of her five siblings, with their varied meal and snack patterns. By the time readers reach that section of this chapter, teens as well as adults should be able to pinpoint the strong and weak points of the seven-day diet recalls listed there. Better yet, they should be able to assess and improve their own diet patterns, thereby proving that teens are not only able to ask for new freedoms but are also willing and able to accept the responsibilities which come with those freedoms.

# Meeting Nutrient Needs

In order to understand the nutritional needs of adolescents, one must first understand more fully the various changes taking place during these years of rapid growth. Strictly speaking, the years of adolescence have their roots in the prepubescent years, with the start of altered endocrine (hormonal) activities around age eight for girls and ten for boys.

This period of early, hidden changes is followed by pubescence, the years when major recognizable physical events move a boy or girl from childhood to the start of adulthood. These events start, for most girls, at ten to twelve years of age and, for most boys, at twelve to fourteen years of age. Very rapid growth and marked sexual development occur during this period.

With postpubescence, teens settle into a "finishing off" period, which lasts from two to three years after their peak growth period ends. During this time, orderly but highly variable changes still occur as growing bodies complete the transition to adult maturity. During these years, growth in height slows and, in most cases, terminates, yet muscle growth continues, as does sexual maturation.

Since the most marked sexual changes occur about nine to twelve months after the peak growth period has passed, a girl who has had her first menstrual period can be fairly well assured that her height increase is just about completed. Likewise, a boy who has reached full sexual development has probably also passed his peak of rapid physical growth. Conversely, teens who have not yet reached these landmarks of sexual development have probably not reached their growth peaks.

This rule of thumb, while far from absolute, can be helpful to both early and late maturers, since it gives them some insight into the workings of their newly strange bodies and some assurance of where all the changes are leading. In a society which groups students by chronological rather than physiological age, having a bit of inside knowledge can make acceptance of different rates of development a little easier.

Teens do worry about their growth rates. According to one early study, one-third of all boys and one-half of all girls worry enough about at least one aspect of their growth to question a physician or school counselor about it. For teens, being different often seems to mean being somehow inferior, yet teens of the same chronological age may be as far as six years apart in physiological age. Some of the psychological problems associated with such vast differences in growth rate and sexual maturity will be discussed later. For now, a careful look at average growth-rate patterns is in order.

Rapid growth in height may begin quite early, especially for girls. Sixteen percent start their growth spurt at age 9, and half have begun by age 10 ¾. By 12 years of age, half the girls will have crested in growth, with 84 percent having crested by age 13. Those girls who start their growth spurt by 9 and end it by 11 ½ or 12 will also begin breast development and menstrual periods earlier than their peers. The growth spurt and sexual changes of early maturers tend to be faster than those of late maturers. The beginning of the menses marks a rapid decline in growth rate, with most girls growing no more than two inches taller than they are at the time of their first menstrual period.

### Age at Start of Adolescent Growth Spurt (Age Ranges in Years)

|                    | Boys     | Girls   |
|--------------------|----------|---------|
| Early maturers     | 11–13    | 9–11    |
| Moderate maturers  | 13–14    | 11–12   |
| Late maturers      | over 14  | over 12 |

Generally, if an early maturer is worried because she's taller than the other girls in her class, she can find reassurance in the fact that her growth spurt is nearly over, while theirs has yet to begin. Late maturers who grow taller than their classmates will not, of course, have another period in which their friends spurt past them once more. For the tall, late-maturing girl, tallness is likely to be a permanent characteristic.

Fortunately, the torments of the tall are not what they once were. Indeed, fashions favor the tall teen of today, and she can take delight in the fact that weight control is less likely to be a problem for her than for her shorter peers. Ten- and twenty-year class reunions usually bring home this fact rather graphically, though all short girls don't tend to become overweight women, nor do all tall girls manage to remain slender. Diet and exercise in post-high school years will determine weight levels, just as diet and exercise determine weight levels and growth patterns during high-school years.

If tall girls won't be surpassed by their female classmates, at least they can look forward to the gradual, if painfully slow, catching up of the boys in their class. Though twelve-year-old Marla may bitterly lament her tallness because classmate Norris comes only to her nose—a decided disadvantage for cheek-to-cheek dancing—she should take heart in the fact that poor Norris feels just as inadequate as she does. Indeed, their lives may be, at that moment, in such inner turmoil that they'd far rather be working off some of their frustrations by shooting baskets than be aggravating them still further by trying to be dance partners. For those courageous enough to admit this fact, basketball may be more socially rewarding than dancing, though Marla's superior reach may make Norris as uncomfortable in the gym as in the ballroom!

Norris's catch-up time is coming. However, it may not start until he's 14, leaving him plenty of time to be miserable if he becomes too preoccupied with being different. Sixteen percent of boys start their growth spurt as early as 11 ¾ years and half start by 12 ¾ years; the rest may start even later. By age 14 ½, the early maturers are cresting, with only another inch or so in height likely, and by 15 ½, 84 percent of the boys have crested. That still leaves the Norrises, many of whom don't crest for another year or so.

The Norris mentioned here grew to 6 feet 2 inches by age seventeen, while Marla stayed at 5 feet 9 inches. Once they survived the awkward years, they were able to accept their mature heights and cease being preoccupied with their differences. But the agonies of those early years were very real to them both. Had Marla known that onset of her menses at eleven meant she was practically through growing, and had Norris known that his lack of sexual development meant he had plenty of time left for growth, perhaps their adjustment could have been easier.

Perhaps not. After all, sexual changes are often either taboo subjects or just another area in which early maturers may tend to feel uncomfortable and late maturers may tend to feel inferior. With adequate conseling, some of these problem areas could be smoothed over. Without such counseling, teens often spend several confused, unhappy years.

Their health and overall attitude is likely to be even poorer if inadequate nutrition becomes a way of life. The adolescent years of rapid growth are years which bring an increase in blood volume, red blood cells, hemoglobin, blood alkaline phosphatase, systolic blood pressure, heart rate, muscle strength, and sex hormones. All these increases make demands upon the body. All these increases require adequate nutrients, so that getting enough calories (from fats, proteins, and carbohydrates), vitamins, and minerals to insure optimum development and overall good health should be a primary concern of the adolescent.

As the above discussion indicates, height-weight ranges for adolescents vary even more widely than do those for other age groups. Since "norms" given in the accompanying graphs are for average maturers, early maturers like Marla and late maturers like Norris will not likely fall into "normal" ranges for their ages. However, if Marla's height and weight percentiles remain constant, then her growth is probably proceeding normally. If in doubt about growth patterns, teens can and should consult a physician. A few minutes of reassurance can often prevent months and even years of worry.

Parents also play vital roles in reducing teenage anxieties concerning height. If the 6-foot-2-inch coed who is the tallest girl in her class and the 5-foot-5-inch boy who is the shortest male in the group have received love and acceptance from their parents from birth through teen years, they will probably hold their heads high and step proudly on high school graduation day. They will have learned from early childhood that one's place on a height-weight chart need not determine his or her place in life. They will carry with them a strong self image, an acceptance of self that will help them meet and conquer whatever challenges life may bring their way.

Teens whose weight falls 10 percent or more below the ranges given in the charts on pages 196 and 197 are generally classed as underweight. Many slightly underweight persons receive well-balanced, perfectly adequate diets but have either a genetic predisposition to slimness, a preference for low-calorie foods, a love of exercise, or some combination of these traits. Teens who fall 15 percent or more below these standards should be checked by a physician. They may suffer from undernutrition due to a long-term inade-quate diet. On such a diet, tissue structures cannot be replaced, and growth and cellular functions are impaired. Even when a child gets what would normally be an adequate diet, a malabsorption problem or some other bod-ily malfunction may cause undernutrition.

Generally, if no medical problems are to blame, undernutrition and im-paired growth are most often seen among teens of lower socioeconomic brackets, those with emotional problems, or those under excessive pressure at home or at school. Such teens are more susceptible to illness, from colds to tuberculosis, especially if they are also anemic. They are absent from school more often than their well-nourished peers and tend to lack interest in intellectual pursuits or physical activities.

If girls like Marla start their growth spurt earlier than age eleven, their nutrient needs at the time their growth spurt begins should be considered as equal to that of an eleven-year-old. This is because the RDA chart takes age eleven as the average age by which most girls have started their rapid-growth years. Conversely, if the Marlas have completed their growth spurt by age twelve or thirteen, they probably do not need as many calories as their female chronological peers who are just beginning their own height leaps.

This unkind quirk of nature often causes problems in social situations. Marla, already stabilizing in height at 5 feet 9 inches, can daintily nibble at her cafeteria food, while Nora, just beginning her own growth spurt, may feel like wolfing down everything in sight. Hopefully, she will do just that, thus obtaining her needed number of calories. More than likely, she will feel a bit embarrassed by her appetite, especially if boys are around. If this un-easiness makes her decide to be a lunchtime nibbler, too, she's played a cruel trick on her appetite and on her growing body.

## Calories

Several studies have examined the years of the beginning, peak, and end of teen growth spurt. Most indicate that the calorie requirements of teens rise to a peak just before puberty, then drop slightly. This peak coincides with the growth spurt mentioned earlier. If teens increase their calorie intake to meet the needs of the rapid growth years, then fail to adjust downward once those needs have passed, obesity may be the ultimate result. Thus parents who worry because a daughter's appetite seems to be less than it has been should consider whether or not the decrease in appetite came after her growth spurt was over. If so, and if her meals remain well balanced, this appetite decrease is something to be pleased about, not something to fret over.

As the following RDA chart indicates, the calorie needs of the sexes are different because the estimated ages of peak development differ for girls and boys. Even these age-calorie notes should not be taken as absolutes, for physiological, age makes the real difference. If in doubt, teens should ask a doctor's advice in determining their approximate physiological age. Then that age may be used when nutrient needs are being considered.

### Recommended Dietary Allowances: Energy and Protein—Adolescents

|  | Age (years) | Weight kg (lbs) | Height cm (in) | Energy (cal) | Protein (g) |
|---|---|---|---|---|---|
| **Boys** | 11–14 | 45 (99) | 157 (62) | 2700 (2000–3700) | 45 |
|  | 15–18 | 66 (145) | 176 (69) | 2800 (2100–3900) | 56 |
| **Girls** | 11–14 | 46 (101) | 157 (62) | 2200 (1500–3000) | 46 |
|  | 15–18 | 55 (120) | 163 (64) | 2100 (1200–3000) | 46 |
| Pregnant* |  |  |  | +300 | +30+ |
| Lactating* |  |  |  | +500 | +20+ |

SOURCE: Adapted from *Recommended Dietary Allowances,* Ninth Edition (1980, in press), with the permission of the National Academy of Sciences, Washington, D.C.

*For most women past adolescence, adding these extra units to a normal well-balanced diet should cover protein and energy needs during pregnancy find lactation. Determinations of individual needs of pregnant and lactating adolescents should be made by a physician.

# Growth Charts for Adolescents—Ages Ten to Eighteen*

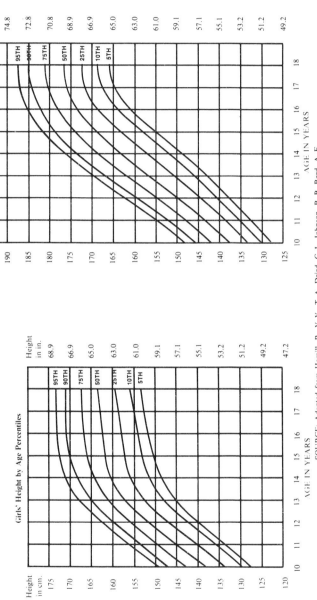

SOURCE: Adapted from Hamill, P. V. V., T. A. Drizd, C. L. Johnson, R. B. Reed, A. F. Roche, *NCHS Growth Curves for Children, Birth—18 years.* National Center for Health Statistics Publications, Series 11, Number 165, November 1977.

*In general, weights and heights that fall within the 5th and 95th percentiles are considered normal. Ideally, height and weight should be within a few percentile points of each other. See pp. 193-194.

## Growth Charts for Adolescents—Ages Ten to Eighteen

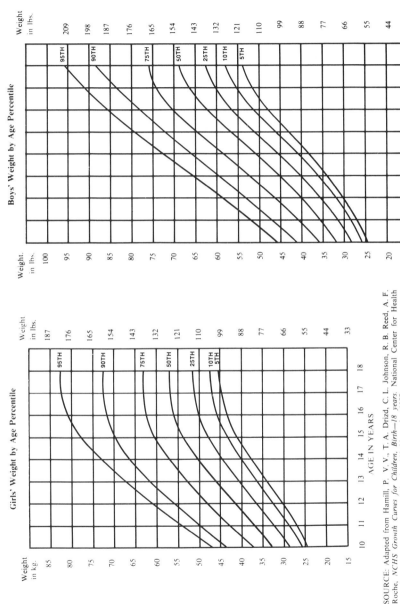

SOURCE: Adapted from Hamill, P. V. V., T. A. Drizd, C. L. Johnson, R. B. Reed, A. F. Roche, NCHS Growth Curves for Children, Birth—18 years. National Center for Health Statistics Publications, Series 11, Number 165, November 1977.

*In general, weights and heights that fall within the 5th and 95th percentiles are considered normal. Ideally, height and weight should be within a few percentile points of each other. See pp. 193-194.

One other major point should be made concerning growth differences and calorie needs. At the start of adolescence, girls begin to lay down the fat stores which will eventually give their figures the roundness of maturity. Girls who have heretofore been thin are likely to panic over the appearance of new "fat" unless they are helped to realize that this "puppy fat" will begin to be better distributed by the end of their growth spurt and should no longer be seen as fat by the time sexual maturity is reached. The most likely exception to this general rule is the girl who has been fat from early childhood. Most girls add fatty deposits in the abdominal area, broaden in the hips, and develop a "pelvic girdle" of subcutaneous fat appropriate for their possible roles as mothers. Boys, too, put on "puppy fat," though this fat may be less cause for concern to them. Eventually, as lean muscle mass and height increase, the little-boy pudgy look disappears.

## Protein

Because boys gain more muscle mass and lean tissue than do girls, they tend to need more protein than girls. Since their calorie levels are considerably higher than are those of girls, the extra protein is automatically a part of their diets, assuming the required extra calories are added across the board, not in the form of low-nutrient, high-sugar treats.

Protein in adequate amounts is vital to growth and development of all teens. In excessive amounts it is, at best, a poor and expensive energy source. Most teens in America meet or exceed the RDAs for protein, though strict vegetarians who do not use eggs or dairy products must be careful to observe the principles of protein complementarity in order to insure sufficient intakes of high-quality protein.

## Fats

Vegetarians generally do not have to worry about excessive fat intakes, for their diets are usually low in fats, especially saturated fats. Meat-eaters, on the other hand, must assess the American Heart Association's warning that excessive intakes of lipids (fats) and cholesterol may lead to atherosclerosis and coronary disease. Before teens assume that hardening of the arteries is a disease only grandparents need worry about, they should realize that autopsies performed on young American Korean War casualties showed fatty streaks in their coronary arteries. The average age of these soldiers was twenty-two.

Even older children and teenagers have shown the beginnings of fatty streaks in the arteries. Fifteen- to twenty-year-old Boston schoolboys already have serum cholesterol levels similar to those of men in their forties and fifties in areas of the world where heart disease is rare. American affluence leads to a diet of more animal protein, more fat, more calories, and fewer natural cereals, whole grains, and leafy vegetables, along with more stress and less physical activity. According to some authorities, this combination may lead to higher serum-cholesterol levels and higher heart-attack rates.

Before becoming fearful of early death from coronary arrest, a teen should realize that high serum-cholesterol levels don't have to be an inevitable consequence of being an American. Diet and heredity, not nationality, make the difference, and some people may be able to lower serum cholesterol and triglyceride levels, if necessary, by altering the "diet of affluence."

Teens who have reason to be concerned about cholesterol intake can easily make the switch to low-fat milk and polyunsaturated margarine, and increase their dietary fiber intake. They can ask their moms to cook with safflower, corn, cottonseed, or soy oil, rather than animal fats. They can cut eggs down to three a week, or use the low-cholesterol egg substitutes now available at the supermarket. They can choose veal, fish, chicken without skin, and other meats from the low-fat section of the meat exchange lists.

By following these suggestions, they will also lower their calorie levels. If the levels are still within recommended ranges, welcome weight loss will probably occur without risk to health. If lowering fat intake causes calorie levels to fall below the RDA, additional complex carbohydrates can be enjoyed to make up the deficit.

## Carbohydrates

Complex, not simple, carbohydrates are the best choices for extra energy with maximum food value. Delicious whole-wheat rolls, baked potatoes, and whole-grain cereals provide valuable vitamins and minerals as well as added energy. If animal-protein sources are being cut to lower cholesterol levels, plant sources of protein such as beans and rice can provide calories, protein, and several valuable vitamins and minerals as well.

While simple carbohydrates, such as candy bars, red licorice, and soft drinks, can help meet energy needs, they offer no other food value and may cause serious dental problems. In fact, excessive consumption of simple sugars is probably the primary reason tooth decay is a leading disease of American teens. Ironically, diet of affluence tends to lead to the dentist's chair, just as it may lead to the coronary-care unit. Though the status of overall nutrition in the United States is higher than in most countries, per capita use of sugar also ranks among the highest in the world. With excessive sugar intakes come excessive numbers of cavities.

Sugar does give quick energy in a form popular to most teens. Thus, an occasional candy bar or soft drink is not to be condemned, provided the tips given in earlier chapters for minimizing the chances of tooth decay are followed carefully. In this way, a teen can keep his or her sweet tooth moderately satisfied, yet cavity-free.

Maybe one outgrows a sweet tooth—nine- to fifteen-year-olds tend to eat more high-sugar products than do most adults. On the other hand, maybe weight-conscious adults tend to give up sweets as lowered physical activity makes them unable to eat empty calories without gaining excess pounds. Since eating habits are harder to break the longer they're reinforced, teens would do well to start limiting empty, high-sugar snacks and treats during their high-school and junior-high years.

## Vitamins and Minerals

Generally, if teens gain the recommended number of calories from all the major food groups, their overall nutrient intake will probably meet or exceed the RDAs and include those essential nutrients for which no RDAs have yet been established. Since teenage boys tend to need 500 to 700 calories per day more than teenage girls, their chances of gaining adequate amounts of other nutrients are increased accordingly. Both male and female athletes, requiring 5000 to 6000 calories a day during sports seasons, should find getting adequate amounts of vitamins and minerals a very simple task —provided their meals and snacks are well balanced.

As can be noted by comparing items on this chart to those on the elementary-school-years chart in the preceding chapter, most increases in vitamins and minerals are in line with increases in calories. However, the increases in RDAs for calcium, phosphorus, iron, and vitamin A are slightly greater than those which occur as a natural result of adding more calories from a variety of foods to an already well-balanced diet. After the rapid-growth years, calcium and phosphorus requirements will drop to prepuberty levels for both sexes. The needs of females will rise again during pregnancy and lactation. Iron needs for boys drop to prepuberty levels at the end of the teen years, but iron needs remain at 18 milligrams or more per day for young women throughout the child-bearing years. As the following discussion indicates, some of the vitamins and minerals which are in greatest demand during the teen years may be the ones found to be in insufficient supply in teen diets.

Perhaps because of the difference in caloric intakes we noted earlier, girls and young women in all age groups above age nine were found to have low intakes of more than one vitamin or mineral in a 1965 U.S. Department of Agriculture (USDA) dietary survey. In that same survey, boys between the ages of twelve and seventeen were also low in more than one vitamin or mineral. While these figures do not mean that Americans in these age-sex categories are seriously undernourished, it does mean that the diets of these groups could be improved.

A closer look at the specific nutrients which appear in insufficient amounts should be helpful. Dietary surveys taken over the years show that most teens meet or exceed the RDAs for all but a few vitamins and minerals. Remember that two-thirds of RDA is considered within the normal range, so the deficits spoken of here generally mean the diets analyzed provided less than that.

Furthermore, since many of the surveys from which the following data

# Recommended Dietary Allowances: Vitamins and Minerals— Adolescents

| | Boys | | Girls | | Pregnant Women† | Lactating Women† |
|---|---|---|---|---|---|---|
| Age (years) | 11–14 | 15–18 | 11–14 | 15–18 | | |
| Weight (kg) | 44 | 66 | 46 | 55 | | |
| Weight (lbs) | 99 | 145 | 101 | 120 | | |
| Height (cm) | 157 | 176 | 157 | 163 | | |
| Height (in) | 62 | 69 | 62 | 64 | | |
| **Fat-soluble vitamins** | | | | | | |
| Vitamin A[a] ($\mu$g* R.E.) | 1000 | 1000 | 800 | 800 | +200 | 6000 |
| Vitamin D[b] ($\mu$g) | 10 | 10 | 10 | 10 | +5 | 400 |
| Vitamin E[c] (mg T.E.) | 8 | 10 | 8 | 8 | +2 | 15 |
| **Water-soluble vitamins** | | | | | | |
| Ascorbic acid (C) (mg) | 50.0 | 60.0 | 50.0 | 60.0 | +20.0 | 80.0 |
| Folacin ($\mu$g) | 400.0 | 400.0 | 400.0 | 400.0 | +400.0 | 0.6 |
| Niacin[d] (mg N.E.) | 18.0 | 18.0 | 15.0 | 14.0 | +2.0 | +4.0 |
| Riboflavin (mg) | 1.6 | 1.7 | 1.3 | 1.3 | +0.3 | +0.5 |
| Thiamin (mg) | 1.4 | 1.4 | 1.1 | 1.1 | +0.4 | +0.3 |
| Vitamin $B_6$ (mg) | 1.8 | 2.0 | 1.8 | 2.0 | +0.6 | 2.5 |
| Vitamin $B_{12}$ ($\mu$g) | 3.0 | 3.0 | 3.0 | 3.0 | +1.0 | 0.004 |
| **Minerals** | | | | | | |
| Calcium (mg) | 1200 | 1200 | 1200 | 1200 | +400 | 1200.0 |
| Phosphorus (mg) | 1200 | 1200 | 1200 | 1200 | +400 | 1200.0 |
| Iodine ($\mu$g) | 150 | 150 | 150 | 150 | +25 | 0.15 |
| Iron (mg) | 18 | 18 | 18 | 18 | +18†† | +18†† |
| Magnesium (mg) | 350 | 400 | 300 | 300 | +150 | 450.0 |
| Zinc (mg) | 15 | 15 | 15 | 15 | +5 | 25.0 |

SOURCE: Adapted from *Recommended Dietary Allowances*, Ninth Edition (1980, in press), with the permission of the National Academy of Sciences, Washington, D.C.

* $\mu$g is the standard abbreviation for microgram, or 1/1000 milligram.
[a] Recommendations for vitamin A are expressed in $\mu$g of R.E. (micrograms of retinol equivalent). One retinol equivalent is equal to 1$\mu$g of retinol or 6 $\mu$g of carotene.
[b] Vitamin D is expressed as $\mu$g of cholecaciferol, with 10$\mu$g cholecalciferol being equal to 400 IUs of Vitamin D.
[c] Vitamin E appears as mg $\alpha$T.E. (milligrams of alpha tocopherol equivalents).
[d] Niacin appears as mg N.E. (milligrams of niacin equivalent), with 1 N.E. being equal to 1 mg of niacin or 60 mg of dietary tryptophan.
†For most women past adolescence, adding these extra units to a normal well-balanced diet should cover vitamin and mineral needs during pregnancy and lactation. Determinations of individual needs of pregnant and lactating adolescents should be made by a physician.
††Since increased iron requirement of pregnancy cannot be met by ordinary diets, the use of 30 to 60 mg of supplemental iron is recommended by the National Research Council. Though iron needs during lactation are similar to prepregnancy needs, continued supplementation of the mother for two to three months after the birth of her child is advisable in order to replenish iron stores depleted by pregnancy.

were drawn were based on twenty-four-hour-recall diet questionnaires, and since nutrient intakes vary greatly from day to day, especially among teens, one should not assume that all boys and girls within certain age and sex groups get insufficient amounts of these nutrients.

On the other hand, the nutrients discussed here have been proven time and again to be the most likely to be deficient in teen diets. Certainly, then, teens should be aware of the possibility that these same deficiencies are likely to crop up in their own diets and take steps to see that they do not.

The 1965 USDA Food Intake Survey mentioned before showed thiamin intakes low for many adolescent girls, with vitamin A, riboflavin, and vitamin C intakes also low for some adolescent females. Fifteen percent of the teen girls in a 1967 Berkeley survey showed low intakes of vitamins A and C. Ten percent of the boys in that survey were low in vitamin A, and 30 percent were low in vitamin C. Other surveys have revealed similar findings. (The benefits and hazards of the therapeutic use of vitamin C are discussed in the preceding chapter.)

Since most studies of teen diets show that fruit and vegetable intakes are usually low, it is predictable that vitamin A and C intakes are likely to be low. Unless breads, legumes, and whole-grain cereals are consumed in sufficient quantities, thiamin intake is likely to be insufficient. On the other hand, low intakes of these and other vitamins are not likely if a teen manages to include foods from all the basic food groups in his diet and if he manages to achieve variety within those food groups.

As in other age groups, *vegetarian* teens who use no dairy products or eggs in their diets are at risk for vitamin $B_{12}$ deficiency, which can lead to pernicious and megaloblastic anemias.

Typical teen diets also fall below RDAs in certain minerals. Ironically, the deficient minerals are especially vital to optimum growth and development, and significantly low intakes might well alter growth rate or otherwise impair health.

According to the 1965 USDA survey, calcium intakes were well below two-thirds of the RDA for women and girls. A 1979 article noted that boys aged nine to nineteen drink only two-and-a-half glasses of milk a day, yet they need approximately four glasses to meet RDAs for calcium. Girls from age nine to eleven average only two cups of milk a day, and by age eighteen they reduce milk intake to one and-a-half cups, far below the recommended intake for that age group. Half the girls in the Berkeley survey had calcium intakes of less than one-third of the RDA. Even with their higher calorie intakes, boys, too, sometimes consume inadequate supplies of calcium. Since all teens need this vital mineral for tooth and bone development and general good health, dairy products should be a part of each day's food plan.

Strict vegetarians who avoid all dairy products will find it very difficult to gain the recommended amounts of calcium from other dietary sources. Calcium supplements may be necessary for teens on such a diet. If you are in doubt, consult a physician.

Though it is not often cited as a deficiency item, iodine should be a concern of teens, since iodine must be present to aid in the increased thyroid activity characteristic of the rapid-growth years. Iodized salt is the safest and easiest way to insure adequate intake of iodine, and supplements should be avoided.

Iron, the one nutrient most often lacking in teen diets, is one of the most vital for the rapid-growth years. Boys between the ages of eleven and eighteen need 18 milligrams of dietary iron daily to help meet their increased need for hemoglobin and to help bring about the 85 percent of their growth which comes in the form of lean muscle mass. Girls need that amount from age eleven to the onset of menopause, due to monthly loss of iron in menstrual blood.

The USDA Food Intake Survey of 1965 noted that iron intakes for most women and girls were less than two-thirds of the RDA. The more recent Ten-State Nutrition Survey showed mean iron intakes of three-quarters to less than one-half of the RDA for both sexes, with means for women falling to 44 to 55 percent of the RDA. The 1967 Berkeley Survey revealed that half the teen girls in that group received less than half the RDA for iron. One researcher reported overweight girls ages eleven to seventeen with iron intakes of less than 50 percent of the RDA, and another recent survey of 118 teens showed low iron as the most serious nutritional problem of both sexes.

The average adult diet contains around 6 milligrams of iron per 1000 calories, but surveys show that diets of many teens contain less iron than that. Since girls' calorie levels are lower than those of boys, meeting or exceeding the RDA for iron is a more difficult task for them. For this reason, many authorities recommend iron supplements for girls from twelve to seventeen years of age. After that age, a carefully chosen diet with relatively few empty calories will probably mean that adequate iron supplies can be gained without further use of supplements.

Though teen girls tend to take in less iron than do their male peers, they lose more iron, at least once their menstrual periods have begun. The average iron loss for a teenage girl is 20 milligrams per menstrual cycle, but some girls may lose twice this much. Girls who feel they may have heavier than average menstrual flow should consult their physicians about the advisability of using iron supplements. Obviously, if iron levels before the onset of the menses have been less than optimum, there will probably be no iron stores available to offset the iron lost during menstrual periods.

Though boys' diets tend to be somewhat higher in iron, many young male teens fall well below the RDA for iron. Boys, too, may need to consider taking iron supplements, especially during the period of their most rapid growth and development. For both boys and girls, low iron stores can mean loss of endurance, increased susceptibility to disease, irritability, weakness, anxiety, depression, and restlessness.

Since it is possible to be iron deficient without being anemic, and since some of the above symptoms appear in subclinical iron deficiency, teens cannot afford to ignore the effects which low iron intake may have on their overall health and sense of well-being. If it is continued, low iron intake leads to severe anemia, and classroom performance and general health are likely to be seriously affected. The need for supplemental iron can be determined by a simple blood test that is often done routinely during a general physical examination.

In view of the prevalence of iron deficiency in America and other countries, many foods are now iron-fortified. Cereals often contain added iron, and some researchers wish to extend iron fortification to other products as well and to increase the levels in foods that are presently fortified. Others fear that wider fortification of foods would mean increased iron intake for 20 percent of the population, while only 2 percent show advanced anemia. Would such intake have adverse effects? In Sweden, where fortification programs are already under way, a larger than normal percentage of adult males have developed early hemochromatosis or "bronze diabetes," a progressive disease in which excessive amounts of iron are stored in bodily organs such as the liver and pancreas. Though this disease is basically hereditary, it apparently occurs earlier when those who are susceptible to it receive diets highly fortified with iron. Though researchers in the United States are working to find new ways to fortify common foods with iron, they are not rushing to employ their findings until more is known about the ramifications of overfortification.

Iron in large doses is toxic. Iron poisoning ranks high among poisonings of infants and toddlers, and teens who obtain iron supplements should do so only with a doctor's help and should keep supplements out of reach of younger siblings. As in the case of most other nutrients, enough is enough and more doesn't necessarily mean better. Megadoses of iron won't work miracles, though they can lead to tragedies. Whenever possible, RDAs should be met through food intake. You can consult the following chart to find foods rich in iron, then add these foods to the diet as often as possible.

## Sources of Iron

| Food | Serving Size | Iron (mg) |
|---|---|---|
| *Liver (pork) | 3 ounces | 17.7 |
| *Liver (lamb) | 3 ounces | 12.6 |
| *Liver (chicken) | 3 ounces | 8.4 |
| *Oysters, fried | 3 ounces | 6.9 |
| *Liver (beef) | 3 ounces | 6.6 |
| Dried apricots | ½ cup (12 halves) | 5.5 |
| *Turkey, roasted | 3 ounces | 5.1 |
| Prune juice | ½ cup | 4.9 |
| Dried dates | ½ cup (9 dates) | 4.8 |

| | | |
|---|---|---|
| *Pork chop, cooked | 3 ounces | 4.5 |
| *Beef | 3 ounces | 4.2 |
| Dried prunes | ½ cup (10 prunes) | 3.9 |
| Tostada (bean) | 1 | 3.2 |
| Kidney beans, cooked | ½ cup | 3.0 |
| Baked beans with pork and molasses | ½ cup | 3.0 |
| *Hamburger | 3 ounces | 3.0 |
| Soybeans, cooked | ½ cup | 2.7 |
| *Beef enchilada | 1 | 2.6 |
| Raisins | ½ cup | 2.5 |
| Lima beans, canned or fresh-cooked | ½ cup | 2.5 |
| Refried beans | ½ cup | 2.3 |
| Dried figs | ½ cup (4 figs) | 2.2 |
| Spinach, cooked | ½ cup | 2.0 |
| *Taco (beef) | 1 | 2.0 |
| Mustard greens, cooked | ½ cup | 1.8 |
| Corn tortilla, lime-treated | 8-inch diameter | 1.6 |
| Peas, fresh-cooked | ½ cup | 1.4 |
| Enchilada, cheese, and sour cream | 1 | 1.4 |
| **Egg | 1 large | 1.2 |
| Sardines canned in oil | 1 ounce (2 medium) | 1.0 |

SOURCE: Copyright © Bull Publishing Co., 1976. Reprinted (with adaptations) by permission of the publisher from *Food for Sport*, by Nathan J. Smith, M.D., published by Bull Publishing Company, P.O. Box 208, Palo Alto, California 94302.

*Foods of animal muscle origin. Iron in foods of animal muscle origin is absorbed twice as efficiently as iron in foods of plant origin.
**The iron in eggs is thought to be not readily available.

## Psychological Aspects

The nutrient needs of the teen years can be met—provided that teens know and understand these needs and have a thorough knowledge of the foods that can help meet those needs. As the following discussion should indicate, knowing what foods to eat and managing to eat them as often as they are needed may be two very different propositions.

The psychological upheavals which accompany the physical changes of adolescence have a direct bearing on the quality of teen diets. These psychological rough spots are not always as dramatic as tradition would declare, however. In fact, one mother of four teens remarked to a friend with toddlers, "I enjoyed my children as babies, but I'm enjoying them even more as teens." Such a remark should encourage parents who may wait with fear for the adolescent rebellion they have been taught to expect. Teenagers, like children and adults of all ages, generally reward parents with whatever they expect. If parents assume rebellion to be on the way, it will probably materialize. If they expect cooperation and family rapport, these will probably become realities.

This is not to minimize the deep-seated emotional upheavals that many teens experience. Such upheavals, however, usually have their roots in infancy and early childhood, and do not appear without warning simply because a child turns thirteen. On the other hand, some psychological problems are directly related to the physical changes which occur at this point in development. A discussion of these problems and their relationship to eating habits should be of help to parents and teens who wish to make the years of transition from childhood to adulthood as smooth and as healthy as possible.

First, sexual and other physical changes come to a teen at the very moment when he wants to be like his peers. Due to varying developmental timetables, a teen may be years ahead or behind a close friend or favorite member of the opposite sex. Hiding a 6-inch growth spurt isn't easy. Though slouching and poor posture are often reactions to new height, they accentuate, not conceal, the new growth. Disguising a changing voice is nearly impossible, though some boys go into long weeks of classroom silence and are crushed when they are forced to recite or answer questions in their squeaky, unpredictable voices. Concealing the fact that one does—or does not—have well-developed breasts or that one is—or is not—40 pounds overweight can be difficult when physical education classes require one to shower in open stalls.

Both early and late maturers have problems, and though these problems differ, they are equally important in the eyes of the teens who must deal with them. Since American schools group youngsters by chronological age, early-maturing boys are usually stronger and better coordinated, with a decided advantage in sports. They are usually more self-confident and older-looking than their peers, so they are sometimes put under more pressure to perform than they can easily handle. If they are ahead of their classmates only in physical growth and not in social and intellectual pursuits, they may have still more problems.

Early maturers may complain that their parents still treat them as children, though their classmates recognize their maturity. In many instances, parental assessments may be more accurate than peer judgments, though early maturers do often assume and fulfill leadership roles. They also tend to hold a decided edge in heterosexual activities, since their height and increased interest in girls often make them more desirable dates than their shorter, less sexually mature classmates.

Late-maturing boys usually manage to keep up in sports and social events until the junior-high years. At this point, they are often crowded out by their more physically advanced peers. They are usually outclassed as athletes, leaders, and Romeos, and, if they dwell on their inability to catch up, they are often miserable. Some late maturers manage to find a niche for themselves outside the three key areas in which they have been outclassed, and those who do often become more sensitive to and understanding of others, probably owing to their own experiences in coping with inadequacies. Late maturers need to be encouraged to find areas in which they can excel and should be reminded that their time of growth, though it is delayed, will soon give them the height advantage they now lack.

Early-maturing girls may be liked and dated by older boys, yet older girls may view them as competition and younger girls or later maturers may shy away from them because they seem somehow "different." Early maturers are usually more interested in clothes and jewelry, dating, and daydreaming than they are in games or strenuous athletic activity. Because they prefer and are preferred by older boys, they may be seen as promiscuous by their mothers and their peers.

Late maturers may be less interested in boys and dress and may be less attractive sexually to older boys. If they become depressed over delayed sexual development, they may end up with such a negative body image that even the long-awaited development of breasts and onset of menses does not make them able to accept themselves. Generally, the late-maturing girl is able to avoid such preoccupation with her inadequacies, perhaps because she often takes such an active part in sports and extracurricular activities that she has little time to feel sorry for herself.

During these ambivalent times, teens look back to the "knowns" of childhood with nostalgia, weather the unknowns of today through sheer willpower, and long for the imagined freedoms of full adulthood. Impatient with long-range plans, they tend to live—or die—for the moment at hand. Whether or not they have a date on Friday looms as the key to future success rather than as an eventuality not even likely to be remembered ten years from now.

Teens need to like themselves and their bodies, yet they need to practice restraint as they take on the responsibilities which sexual maturity brings. They have many adjustments to make and need family and peer support as they strive to make them.

The struggle between dependence and independence is reflected in the eating patterns of adolescents. Many teens are involved in so many extracurricular activities that eating meals at home with the family becomes a rarity. They may gulp breakfast (or skip it), eat lunch hurriedly because of a student council meeting, and eat dinner late, owing to football practice. Yet the very nature of the hectic schedule most teens keep means that they need better, not worse, nutrition if they are to achieve optimum growth and development.

Parents who wish to help teens gain optimum nutrition must be willing to lay aside preconceived notions of what constitutes acceptable meals. Indeed, surveys indicate that the teens who have the best overall nutrition usually do not eat in a conventional three-meal-a-day pattern. They are more likely to eat five or even six small meals, with no more than one featuring a "normal" menu.

A look at the diet pattern of Nora's siblings, given at the close of this chapter, should show that snacks are a vital part of the teen dietary regimen. Parents who condemn snacking and discourage it may be unduly limiting nutrient intakes. Having a hamburger and a malt with the gang after school can mean gaining from a third to a fourth of the day's calories and nutrients in snack form, and not having that snack doesn't guarantee that a teen will be hungry enough at the scheduled dinner hour to eat enough of mom's cooking to make up for the lost snack.

On the other hand, if that afternoon snack consists of a Coke and a candy bar, the calories contribute nothing but energy to the teen's stores and may, therefore, rob him of valuable nutrients later. Wise snacking can help teens meet their nutrient needs, while poor snacking can hurt their chances of gaining adequate protein, vitamins, and minerals and increase their chances of becoming obese. When teens include low-fat milk and cheese or fresh fruits and vegetables in snacks, their diets can be dramatically improved, for these three items are usually quite low in adolescent diets.

Though most teen snacks are low in vitamin A, thiamin, calcium, and iron, the majority of them do meet or exceed the RDAs for protein, riboflavin, and vitamin C. Far from being "empty," such snacks often do make major contributions to teen dietary intakes.

Parents who wish to help teens make snacks an even more valuable part of the day's food intake can do so by making excellent snack foods available at home and by avoiding the purchase of less desirable snack items. Though teens are independent enough to buy such items on their own, they need not be further tempted by them at home. A review of the snack discussions in the two previous chapters should clarify which snacks are best—in view of dental, coronary, and weight-control factors.

Though snacks can help fill out the day's food needs, an afternoon snack can't completely make up for a skipped meal. Why? Because the effects of meal skipping, especially if that meal is breakfast, will be evident immediately. Protein and calcium at 4:00 P.M. won't make an 11:00 A.M. class any easier to sit through. One Massachusetts survey of 3500 high-school students showed that 11 percent of the boys and 19 percent of the girls had no breakfast, and that 40 percent of the boys and 50 percent of the girls who did have breakfast had a poor or inadequate one. These figures are probably typical, and they lead to the question, why do teens skip breakfast? The answers are varied: "I prefer to spend morning time dressing," "I got up too late," "I'm not hungry before eight," "Mom doesn't cook breakfast," "My bus comes early," "I want to lose weight."

This last answer is interesting, in view of the fact that more often than not, obese breakfast-skippers do not tend to lose weight when they skip the first meal of the day. Of further interest is the fact that breakfast is more popular with boys than with girls, again perhaps related to the mistaken idea girls have that skipping breakfast will bring about desired weight loss.

Actually, skipping breakfast brings about a drastic drop in blood sugar. This is particularly serious among teens, since studies indicate that blood-sugar levels of adolescents can drop below fasting levels even when breakfast has been eaten. To risk even more drastic drops is to invite a less than optimum morning.

Could there be one other factor at work when teens skip breakfast? In some cases, this may be one small, but important, way to assert independence, break clear of the rules and habits of childhood, and feel a bit more like an adult. Since a breakfast-skipper is likely to feel like a very tired adult, such motivation should be reexamined!

Teen food intakes are often influenced—either directly or indirectly—by the psychological and social problems of the moment. Parents should try to find out the whys behind certain less-than-ideal eating habits. If they then offer, but do not force, suggestions for improving those habits, they can probably influence a teen's diet for the better. Any iron-handed "eat-that-breakfast-because-I-said-to-eat-it" approach is as unwise now as it was in infancy and early childhood. Acceptance, openness, and understanding are more important at this stage of the parenting game than are strictly enforced dietary regulations.

After all, the years of laying a good nutritional foundation are not likely to be completely destroyed by the erratic meal patterns of the teen years. By late adolescence, most teens who have been brought up with a sound knowledge of the principles of nutrition are putting those principles into practice on their own.

Mom and dad can't accompany the teen to college. Or on his first out-of-state job. Or into his first home. If an adolescent doesn't learn to be his own keeper during his teen years, when will he learn this vital lesson? His attempts to provide for his own nutrition needs may seem awkward and inadequate, as did his first attempts to feed himself with a spoon, but he must make the attempts. Gradually, with some parental guidance—but without nagging—the adolescent will learn to apply on his own those principles of good eating which his parents have tried to teach him from birth. This is his testing ground, and chances are good that he'll pass the test and finish out his teen years as a healthy and well-nourished individual.

## Common Problems

Most of the problems concerning adolescent dietary intakes are related to body image and, ultimately, to an intense need for social acceptance. Special foods are not miracle workers guaranteed to solve all the problems which preoccupy teens. Grapefruit diets don't transform unsightly bulges into pleasing curves. "Natural" foods don't transfer one into a world better than the "getting and spending" one which most adults seem to occupy. Avoiding chocolate doesn't assure one of a peaches-and-cream complexion. Nonetheless, eating habits can have some effect on these and other problem areas of adolescence. Teens who gain a thorough understanding of what foods can and cannot do for them are likely to avoid getting caught up in fad diets which promise much but offer far less than do the well-balanced diets described throughout this book.

## Obesity

Often listed as the number one diet-related problem of American teens, obesity plagues thousands of boys and girls across our nation. As in all other ages of life, obesity in adolescence occurs when calorie intake exceeds calorie output. It's a simple, straightforward formula, but it's often ignored when teens seek to overcome obesity.

Often ignored, too, is the fact that fatness is relative. What passes for obesity to one girl would be seen as the ideal state by her fatter classmate. Indeed, so obsessed is the American public with the image of slimness and the ugliness of obesity that fairly slender young girls may embark on rigorous starvation diets to rid themselves of extra pounds and ounces. Often they are trying to lose the innocent "puppy fat" described earlier, fatty deposits which nature will eventually rearrange as a girl reaches sexual maturity.

Since so many teens seem to fear obesity, they may need professional aid in assessing their own body composition. Self-conscious about appearance and eager to blend with the crowd, teens tend to feel unattractive, too thin, or too fat. Bombarded by ads which contend that thin is beautiful, adolescent girls often starve themselves in an attempt to become more like the glamour girls who adorn magazine covers. Unaware of the fact that even starvation cannot make some body structures look willowy thin, many of these girls feel only frustration and failure, even after strict adherence to extreme weight-loss diets.

An understanding of body type should help teenagers set more realistic height-weight goals. Although extremely subjective, classification into endomorph, mesomorph, and ectomorph does serve as a useful way of looking at body types, provided one realizes that this system is not an absolute and fool-proof way of analyzing body structure. Furthermore, these generalizations primarily apply to body types of teens and young adults, for in middle age, even ectomorphs may become pudgy or actually obese, primarily due to decreased activity levels.

According to this theory of classification, there are three basic body types: endomorph, mesomorph, and ectomorph. *Endomorphs* are born with a body which tends to lay down fat unless a less-than-average diet or more-than-average physical activity becomes a way of life. Not all endomorphs become obese, but the tendency is there, and a teen with this body build is better off recognizing her tendency toward weight gain early on than falling into obesity unaware.

While they are less likely to become obese than are endomorphs, many *mesomorphs* do tend to lay on fat easily. On the other hand, *ectomorphs,* persons with long, slender hands and feet and a naturally slim build, very seldom become obese. These generalizations primarily apply to body types of teens, for in middle age, even ectomorphs may become pudgy or actually obese, largely as a result of decreased activity levels.

Since body build, tendency to overeat, and tendency to underexercise are products of a teen's hereditary and environment, an overweight, slow-moving, constantly hungry endomorph might feel justifiably discouraged at his odds against winning the fight against fatness. Surely his work will be harder than that of many of his friends, but if his goals are realistic and his motivation is good, he, too, can return to normal weight. It won't be easy. It won't be something he can achieve today and relax and forget about tomorrow. But it is not impossible.

For parents and friends of obese adolescents, a word of caution is in order. In dealing with obesity, you are dealing with a *person* underneath that excess fat. Very often this person has already heard countless unkind remarks about her laziness, gluttony, lack of willpower, and general unworthiness. In fact, studies have shown that obese girls tend to show personality characteristics similar to those of ethnic and minority groups who are victims of intense prejudice. They feel rejected, isolated, and totally undesirable. Worse yet, while blacks and Chicanos are winning increased favor and recognition in the light of slowly changing social attitudes, obese boys and girls cannot stay fat and expect acceptance. Add obesity to the normal who-am-I? crisis of adolescence, the normal conflicts with family and peers, and normal physical and sexual changes, and one is able to see why so many obese teens live lives of quiet desperation.

This rejection pattern haunts the obese even as they try for college entrance. Though college application rates are about equal for obese and nonobese high-school seniors, nonobese adolescents are accepted in significantly greater numbers. Until a court decision forced it to abandon the practice, one private university placed obese students under threat of expulsion unless they lost weight at a specified pace throughout the year. Though this seems extreme, it is really not a harsher pressure than society at large exerts upon the obese teen.

Though Bill Cosby's Fat Albert character has done much to show young people that obese teens can be acceptable—even likeable—people, the truth is that an obese teen often feels so hostile toward himself that he is, indeed, not a very likeable individual.

Parents, teachers, and friends should encourage teens who wish to lose weight, but they should be careful not to make loss of weight a criterion for love and acceptance. In some cases, obese teens do not seem to be able to change their body composition, a fact thinner persons can never quite understand because they find weight loss, exercise, and even dieting easier than do many obese persons. Certainly, in terms of overall health and well-being, weight loss is desirable. However, if that loss fails to occur, the obese teen still needs love and understanding as much as—and perhaps more than—the slender teen.

Evidence of what can happen when slimness and weight loss become a total obsession is seen in cases of *anorexia nervosa,* a disorder usually related to deep-seated psychological problems that are manifested as an obsession with thinness. It has been reported that one out of every hundred girls between the ages of sixteen and eighteen shows signs of this disorder. Some of the girls who embark upon the program of self-imposed starvation characteristic of this disorder have been obese at some younger age and remain horrified at the prospect of a return to obesity. Others have never been fat but have always thought of themselves as fat. Still others diet to extreme thinness, yet continue to worry because they still see themselves as having fat thighs, stomachs, or buttocks.

These girls often alternate binge eating with self-induced vomiting and heavy use of laxatives and diuretics. On the surface, they appear to know much about nutrition, and they hide their odd eating and weight-losing behavior very carefully, often until they are in a highly dangerous state of near-starvation. Any weight loss that drops weight to 70 pounds or less after adolescence, or to 40 percent below ideal weight, requires immediate medical intervention. A dramatic weight loss of 25 percent or more may be an indication of trouble and should be discussed with a physician; preferably, a doctor should be consulted much earlier, since waiting for the terminal stages makes treatment of this disorder risky and complicated.

Usually, *anorexia nervosa* girls become hyperactive—jogging, playing tennis, or doing vigorous calisthenics in every spare moment. They deny hunger, deny fatigue, and deny their thinness, even when all three facts are set before them in indisputable form. Since their distorted body image does not allow them to be reasonable about diet, they are usually very difficult to treat. Doctors often must force a correction of their poor state of nutrition through tube feeding, but such force-feeding seldom solves the problem. It is ironic that while so many teens lack the willpower to lose 5 pounds over as many weeks, *anorexia nervosa* patients are capable of starving themselves to death. The mortality rate has remained 5 to 10 percent, and fewer than two-thirds are likely to respond to treatment readily and remain cured. Even when they've been brought out of a starvation ritual, many of these girls are quite likely to enter upon another one some months or years later.

Often *anorexia nervosa* patients have no confidence in their ability to control their own lives. They diet to excess because they feel they will overeat unless they force themselves into a highly restrictive diet regimen. Often these girls are good to excellent students who exhibit this same fear of loss of control in their study habits. They spend long hours doing homework because they feel that only by such forced effort will they have enough will power to achieve their goals in the classroom. They approach physical exercise with the same attitude—they must go to extremes or else they will be tempted to exercise too little. Their compulsive dieting, studying, and exercising usually leave them little time for social contacts.

Psychologists attempt to convince these young women that they need not resort to extreme dietary regimens in order to maintain weight control. Often the entire family must be counseled in order that family members can help the *anorexia nervosa* patient gain a sense of autonomy, gain confidence in her ability to control all aspects of her life.

Awareness of the suffering which *anorexia nervosa* patients undergo in the name of thinness tends to make one more reluctant to impose standards of slimness on an obese adolescent. However, since starvation dieting by an *anorexia nervosa* victim is usually only an outward manifestation of severe psychological disorders, parents need not fear that advising an overweight teen to diet will make her a victim of this dramatic disease.

For most overweight teens, death or damaged health from *anorexia nervosa* is a far less likely occurrence than death or damaged health from continued obesity. If parents, teachers, and peers can help an obese adolescent realize what she can do to lessen her weight problem, help her embark on that course of action, praise her for her successes and not condemn her for her failures, they may help her avoid a lifetime of obesity. This may be her last chance to avoid that fate, since the obese adolescent has a 75 percent chance of adult obesity and since obese persons who haven't moved to normal weight by age twenty face odds of twenty-eight to one against successful weight reduction after age twenty.

Often the obese adolescent has plenty of company at home, since 40 percent of obese adolescents have obese siblings, and 60 to 70 percent at least one obese parent. They have company at school, too, yet they don't tend to find comfort in the companionship of obese peers and family.

Often, determining obesity on the basis of height-weight charts is nearly impossible, since such charts cannot allow for all variations in body build. Doctors often use a triceps skin-fold test, which measures the thickness of the skin at the midpoint of the back of the upper arm. A normal adult skin fold (double thickness) should measure ½-inch to 1 inch at that point. A fold markedly greater than 1 inch indicates excessive body fatness, while one markedly less than ½-inch indicates abnormal thinness. Since ideal skin-fold thicknesses vary with age, and since accurate measurement is crucial to accurate evaluation, this test is best performed with special calipers and analyzed by a physician.

A test that is easy to perform at home is the mirror test. If a person looks fat when he is standing naked before a full-length mirror, he probably is fat. However, as we noted before, teens may be so obsessed with slimness that they see fat where none exists. Before they undertake a drastic diet, they should seek a physician's advice.

One recent estimate noted that 16 percent of the American population under age thirty belongs in the "unquestionably obese" category. These persons generally know they are overweight, yet don't always know what to do about the situation. Again, obesity is the result of caloric intake that exceeds caloric output. It is not a disease of overeating alone. In its milder form, it may not be related to overeating at all.

While many obese girls and boys blame their obesity on overeating, underactivity is more often the real culprit. In fact, obese girls are often so guilt-ridden over what they see as their own gluttony that they refuse to believe they aren't having more snacks or eating more at mealtimes than their thinner peers, even when they are confronted with food records which prove this to be true.

In study after study, obese teens are shown to eat no more than their peers and often to eat less. They often eat less frequently and skip meals more often than their thinner peers. They tend to eat fewer fruits and vegetables than do nonobese teens. In one study, obese and nonobese seventh-graders all preferred sweeter foods of higher caloric density, though this preference posed weight-gain problems only for the obese.

When obese teens do overeat, they often do so out of boredom and tend to have favorite times and places for eating binges. When they are away from the environment that stimulates their binges, they are less likely to overeat. Furthermore, teens who work as a group to lower food intakes and overcome obesity often have a higher success rate than those who try to lose weight on their own.

Seascape, a camp for obese girls, reports a fairly high success rate for those who spend summers there. They set caloric intakes at the lowest level considered consistent with continued optimum growth and development. Despite evidence that underexercising is probably as great a contributer to adolescent obesity as is overeating, Seascape leaders encourage exercise but do not force it. Penelope Peckos, the camp director, feels that decreasing caloric intake is more realistic than increasing caloric output, since the girls aren't likely to continue team sports and other exercise activities after camp has ended. The girls are told to cut down on high-calorie foods but not to feel they must eliminate them. Frequency and quantity are key words at Seascape, since girls are led to see that these two factors determine the extent to which certain foods can be tolerated without danger of losing control of one's weight.

There is no Pollyanna approach at Seascape. The girls are cautioned that control of obesity will be a lifelong project for most of them, a project which will require high motivation, persistence, and hard work. Realistic as to the limitations of any weight-loss program, Director Peckos accepts the fact that there are some girls who lack sufficient motivation to bring their weight under control. She warns these girls not to allow obesity to rule their lives and not to use being overweight as an excuse for lack of achievement in all other areas.

While others agree that calorie-restriction diets can be successful in helping teens lose weight, all nutritionists and doctors stress that these diets must be nutritionally adequate and well-balanced. Suggested caloric minimums for the rapid-growth years are 1200 calories per day for girls and 1400 calories per day for boys, with a doctor's supervision of the diet program. If an overweight teen is still growing, his diet goal should be to allow his height to catch up with his weight. A loss of 1 percent of body weight should allow for continued growth and development, but losses in excess of that are not recommended for teens still in their growing years. A sensible, safe goal for loss is one pound per week, a goal which calls for a 500-calorie-per-day reduction in food intake, or for a daily 4-miles-per-hour walk of one hour and fifteen minutes.

For many obese teens whose caloric intakes are already low, the walk is the better choice, since lowering caloric intake by an additional 500 calories per day would mean risking the loss of valuable nutrients. This plan is especially appropriate, considering that many studies have shown that under-activity is the primary cause of adolescent obesity. While all the suburban girls in one study were seen as fairly inactive, the obese girls in that study were much more inactive. Indeed, the obese girls spent less than half the time spent by the nonobese in any sort of activity. Often, when obese girls claim embarrassment from ineptitude at sports and unsatisfactory appearance in gym clothes, they are able to obtain letters from cooperative family doctors excusing them from physical education classes, thus compounding the problem of inactivity still further. In this particular study, the food intakes of the nonobese were significantly greater than those of the obese, and because the activity level of the nonobese was twice that of the obese, food intake did not pose problems for the nonobese.

Other studies have shown that even when obese girls swim, play tennis, or hike, they tend to do so with less physical movement than do their leaner counterparts. For example, while thin girls are in motion 90 percent of the time during a tennis match, obese girls move only 50 percent of the time. Even so, since the movement of the larger body mass requires the use of more calories, the obese do tend to lose weight through exercise. A 175-pound teen who should weigh 110 pounds does far more work when she runs after a tennis ball than does a 110-pound teen of the same age, height, and bone structure.

In an attempt to put this finding into action, researchers began a voluntary exercise program for obese youngsters which produced good to excellent weight-loss results for 60 percent of the youngsters involved. Incorporating such special programs into public-school physical-education structures would allow P.E. classes to be an obese adolescent's route to freedom from fat. Separating obese from nonobese students would allow for exercises geared to aid in fat reduction and help avoid the embarrassment obese teens feel in front of their slimmer classmates.

Many obese teens believe that more exercise will lead to overeating and no weight loss, but the opposite has been shown to be true. An obese teen who spends most of the day in low to moderate activity can add up to an hour of exercise without increased appetite. Many overweight teens underestimate the caloric cost of exercise, assuming they could never do enough exercise to work off all their fat. In actuality, as a look at the following chart should make evident, any number of activities well within the reach of obese teens can help them lose the 500 calories a day needed to effect losses of one pound per week.

## Energy Expenditure for Selected Recreational Activities

| Activity | Output per Minute* (in calories) |
|---|---|
| Sitting | 1.5–2 |
| Walking, on level (3 mph) | 2.8–5.2 |
| Walking, on level (4 mph) | 3.3–7 |
| Canoeing (4 mph) | 3–7 |
| Volleyball | 3.5–10 |
| Playing with children | 3.5–10 |
| Biking (13 mph) | 4.5–11 |
| Golf (walking, not carting) | 5 |
| Archery | 5.3 |
| Dancing | 4.2–7.8 |
| Swimming | 4.3–11.3 |
| Tennis | 7–10 |
| Squash | 10.3–20 |
| Cross-country running | 10.5–15 |
| Skiing | 10–20 |
| Climbing | 10.5–12.3 |
| Running (10 mph) | 19–20 |

SOURCE: Derived from P. O. Astrand and K. Rodahl, *Textbook of Work Physiology* (New York: McGraw-Hill, 1970), p. 439

*Most of these activities would not utilize maximum energy for all minutes within an hour of participation. Downward adjustments should be made when figuring per-*hour* output (i.e., three-fourths hour might be at peak rate, with one-fourth hour at diminished rate).

The following chart should be useful to teens who wish to know how much energy output will be needed to work off a calorie splurge such as a 421-calorie milkshake. Those inclined to be content with less extravagant splurges, such as a modest helping of potato chips, should be encouraged to note that a brisk walk of approximately twenty minutes should burn off that little snack.

## Activity Required to Expend the Calories Gained by Eating Various Foods

| FOOD | CALORIES | Walking[a] | Riding bicycle[b] | Swimming[c] | Running[d] | Reclining[e] |
|---|---|---|---|---|---|---|
| Apple, large | 101 | 19 | 12 | 9 | 5 | 78 |
| Bacon, 2 strips | 96 | 18 | 12 | 9 | 5 | 74 |
| Banana, small | 88 | 17 | 11 | 8 | 4 | 68 |
| Beans, green, 1 cup | 27 | 5 | 3 | 2 | 1 | 21 |
| Beer, 1 glass | 114 | 22 | 14 | 10 | 6 | 88 |
| Bread and butter | 78 | 15 | 10 | 7 | 4 | 60 |
| Cake, 2-layer, 1/12 | 356 | 68 | 43 | 32 | 18 | 274 |
| Carbonated beverage, 1 glass | 106 | 20 | 13 | 9 | 5 | 82 |
| Carrot, raw | 42 | 8 | 5 | 4 | 2 | 32 |
| Cereal, dry, ½ cup with milk, sugar | 200 | 38 | 24 | 18 | 10 | 154 |
| Cheese, cottage, 1 tbsp. | 27 | 5 | 3 | 2 | 1 | 21 |
| Cheese, cheddar, 1 oz. | 111 | 21 | 14 | 10 | 6 | 85 |
| Chicken, fried, ½ breast | 232 | 45 | 28 | 21 | 12 | 178 |
| Chicken, TV dinner | 542 | 104 | 66 | 48 | 28 | 417 |
| Cookie, plain | 15 | 3 | 2 | 1 | 1 | 12 |
| Cookie, chocolate chip | 51 | 10 | 6 | 5 | 3 | 39 |
| Doughnut | 151 | 29 | 18 | 13 | 8 | 116 |
| Egg, fried | 110 | 21 | 13 | 10 | 6 | 85 |
| Egg, boiled | 77 | 15 | 9 | 7 | 4 | 59 |
| French dressing, 1 tbsp. | 59 | 11 | 7 | 5 | 3 | 45 |
| Halibut steak, ¼ lb. | 205 | 39 | 25 | 18 | 11 | 158 |
| Ham, 2 slices | 167 | 32 | 20 | 15 | 9 | 128 |
| Hamburger | 350 | 67 | 43 | 31 | 18 | 269 |
| Ice cream, 1/6 qt. | 193 | 37 | 24 | 17 | 10 | 148 |
| Ice cream soda | 255 | 49 | 31 | 23 | 13 | 196 |
| Ice milk, 1/6 qt. | 144 | 28 | 18 | 13 | 7 | 111 |
| Gelatin, with cream | 117 | 23 | 14 | 10 | 6 | 90 |
| Malted milkshake | 502 | 97 | 61 | 45 | 26 | 386 |
| Mayonnaise, 1 tbsp. | 92 | 18 | 11 | 8 | 5 | 71 |
| Milk, 1 glass | 166 | 32 | 20 | 15 | 9 | 128 |
| Milk, skim, 1 glass | 81 | 16 | 10 | 7 | 4 | 62 |
| Milkshake | 421 | 81 | 51 | 38 | 22 | 324 |
| Orange, medium | 68 | 13 | 8 | 6 | 4 | 52 |
| Orange juice, 1 glass | 120 | 23 | 15 | 11 | 6 | 92 |

| | | | | | | |
|---|---|---|---|---|---|---|
| Pancake with syrup | 124 | 24 | 15 | 11 | 6 | 95 |
| Peach, medium | 46 | 9 | 6 | 4 | 2 | 35 |
| Peas, green, ½ cup | 56 | 11 | 7 | 5 | 3 | 43 |
| Pie, apple, 1/6 | 377 | 73 | 46 | 34 | 19 | 290 |
| Pie, raisin, 1/6 | 437 | 84 | 53 | 39 | 23 | 336 |
| Pizza, cheese, 1/8 | 180 | 35 | 22 | 16 | 9 | 138 |
| Pork chop, loin | 314 | 60 | 38 | 28 | 16 | 242 |
| Potato chips, 1 serving | 108 | 21 | 13 | 10 | 6 | 83 |
| Sandwiches | | | | | | |
|   Club | 590 | 113 | 72 | 53 | 30 | 454 |
|   Roast beef with gravy | 430 | 83 | 52 | 38 | 22 | 331 |
|   Tuna-fish salad | 278 | 53 | 34 | 25 | 14 | 214 |
| Sherbet, 1/6 qt. | 177 | 34 | 22 | 16 | 9 | 136 |
| Shrimp, fried | 180 | 35 | 22 | 16 | 9 | 138 |
| Spaghetti, 1 serving | 396 | 76 | 48 | 35 | 20 | 305 |
| Steak, T-bone | 235 | 45 | 29 | 21 | 12 | 181 |
| Strawberry shortcake | 400 | 77 | 49 | 36 | 21 | 308 |

SOURCE: Adapted by permission of the publisher from F. Konishi, "Food Energy Equivalents of Various Activities," *Journal of the American Dietetic Association* 46 (1965): 186. Used by permission.

[a] Energy cost of walking for 150-pound individual = 5.2 calories per minute at 3.5 miles per hour.
[b] Energy cost of riding bicycle = 8.2 calories per minute.
[c] Energy cost of swimming = 11.2 calories per minute.
[d] Energy cost of running = 19.4 calories per minute.
[e] Energy cost of reclining = 1.3 calories per minute.

A brief look at the members of one family is a graphic way to summarize this discussion of the interaction of diet and exercise in obesity control. In this particular family, the mother has been overweight since childhood, the father has always been slim, and two of the three daughters are overweight. The father's activity level is moderate to heavy, with farming chores taking up many of his hours. The mother's activity load is light to moderate, and the two obese older sisters, having been overweight since childhood, tend to avoid P.E. classes, dances, and other strenuous physical activities. The youngest girl, a junior-high all-city basketball forward, was not obese as a child and shows no signs of obesity as a teen. Though she and her father tend to eat more than the obese members of the family and though all eat a moderately high-starch diet, slimness prevails in the two active family members, while obesity has claimed the three more sedentary members of the household.

Teens who realize the importance of equalizing caloric intake and output in order to stabilize weight gains or effect weight losses might keep a food-and-activity record to help them monitor the changes they choose to make. In programs where such records are coupled with weight-loss graphs and regular counseling with a nutritionist, encouraging results have been reported.

For the mildly or severely obese adolescent, the message is clear. There are no magic, quick-loss diets to take off excess pounds speedily, safely, and permanently. There are no weight-loss drugs which doctors currently feel work well enough to warrant their prolonged use. There is only the basic formula: Weight gain and obesity occur when caloric intake exceeds caloric output. And its corollary: Weight loss occurs when calorie output exceeds caloric intake.

Putting these formulas to use can mean moving from obesity, with all its physical and psychological problems, to normal weight. As Penelope Peckos tells the dieters at Seascape:

**Heredity + Food You Eat + Motivation + Physical Activity = You**

## Diet Alterations—Pros and Cons

Some teenagers may significantly alter their diets for one reason or another. For those who want to lose weight, hundreds of diets exist. Some diets are sensible, but others can only be called fad diets—those resorting to extreme measures or promising magic or overnight results. Other teens change their diets in the belief that they will improve their health, their lives, and the world around them. A discussion of several common teen diet alterations follows.

### Group Membership Weight-Loss Diets

Such self-help groups as TOPS, The Diet Workshop, Weight Watchers, and Overeaters Anonymous have helped many teens and adults lose weight. Most of these programs advocate a sound, well-balanced diet, though a low-calorie one. Results obtained by joining such groups may be impressive, since the organizations usually employ diet and exercise plans similar to the ones advocated in this book.

Teens should carefully evaluate the proposed diet plan before joining any group. Not all such groups offer equally valid diets. Also, teens should be careful not to reduce caloric intakes below the level approved by their physicians and should realize that they could follow a similar diet and exercise plan without becoming dues-paying members of a diet group. For some, the group support is well worth the extra cost of the diet. For others, the money saved could be applied to purchase of fruits, vegetables, and meats to enhance a well-balanced diet.

### Fad Weight-Loss Diets

A good many overweight teens are not interested in the facts outlined in the preceding section. They prefer to avoid the sound principles of diet and exercise and to rely, instead, on magic diets that promise instant weight loss with a minimum of effort. They are prime targets for those who promote the various fad diets which sweep America from month to month.

Fad diets, whether they are aimed at weight loss or other goals, tend to have certain telltale characteristics, such as exclusion of an entire food group (e.g., breads and cereals) or a major nutrient (e.g., carbohydrates or fats) from the diet; dependence on a limited number of foods; a hint that the diet is somehow mystical or magical in its ability to cure obesity, arthritis, or other disorders; the offering for sale of certain foods or supplements (e.g., liquid protein compounds) which are crucial to the success of the diet; and claims that the medical profession's objections to the diet stem from a fear that people will follow the diet, be cured of their ills, and no longer need the services of doctors.

A look at several types of fad diets aimed at weight loss shows that these diets all share one or more of the above characteristics.

*Restriction Diets.* Typical of food-category restriction diets are all the variations of the low-carbohydrate diet. Such diets claim that if a designated food category is excluded—in this case, carbohydrates—then other foods may be eaten at will. If such a diet is followed for only a short time, it may produce an initial weight loss at no great sacrifice to health. Followed for longer periods of time, especially by athletes and other active teens, it could cause serious problems.

The low-carbohydrate diet depends on the burning of stored body fat to replace the energy normally gained through carbodydrates. As this body fat is burned, excessive ketones, which are the end products of fat metabolism, are produced and collect in the blood. Ketosis can be a dangerous state, especially if a teen becomes pregnant while she is on this diet. Gout, extreme fatigue, irregular heartbeat, calcium depletion, intolerance to alcohol, and increased serum-cholesterol levels are possible side effects of the low-carbohydrate diet.

No low-carbohydrate diet (including such popular ones as Dr. Atkin's Diet Revolution and Dr. Stillman's Quick Weight-Loss Diet) should be used for longer than two to three weeks except under a doctor's supervision.

For teens, adhering to any restrictive diet means that some nutrients essential to optimum growth and development will be lost. Furthermore, since eating habits aren't being altered in a meaningful way during the weeks of dieting, weight gain is likely to occur as soon as the fad diet is left behind.

*Magic Food Diets.* An interesting variation of the restriction diet is the Grapefruit or Magic Mayo Diet. Not magic and not endorsed by the Mayo Clinic, this diet restricts starches and sugars, encourages the use of meat, fish, and eggs, and insists that a half grapefruit or a half cup of grapefruit juice be taken with every meal. Though its proponents insist that the grapefruit activates fat burning, its chief benefit is the addition of vitamin C to the diet. High in saturated fats and low in carbohydrates, this diet is also not recommended for prolonged use.

Similar diets, including Mary Ann Crenshaw's Lecithin, $B_6$, Apple-Cider Vinegar and Kelp Diet, and Simeons HCG (Human Chorionic Gonadotropin) Plan, base their "success" on the magic ingredients which set their diets apart from all others. Researchers tend to deny the effectiveness of such diets, and most feel that money spent on the special ingredients could be put to better use by purchasing fresh fruits and vegetables to supplement a well-balanced weight-loss diet. Furthermore, excessive intake of some of these items might, over a period of time, produce signs of toxicity, especially when the individual is also limiting himself to 500 to 1000 calories per day.

*Monotony Diets.* Monotony diets, such as the Banana-Milk Diet and the Peel-a-Pound Diet, rely on the premise that a steady diet of only one food will result in boredom, loss of appetite, and subsequent weight loss. Fortunately, most people eventually become so bored with such a diet that they drop it altogether. If they did not, signs of nutritional deficiencies would soon appear, since no one food is able to supply all the essential nutrients. Though these diets recommend vitamin and mineral supplements, such supplements usually contain no protein, carbohydrates, or fats and cannot possibly contain all the vitamins, minerals, and trace elements essential to good health.

*Liquid or Formula Diets.* Used to take the place of only one meal per day, some liquid diet formulas might be acceptable for use by over-weight teens. However, used on an exclusive basis for a prolonged period of time, these formulas could lead to serious deficiency symptoms. Carried to its extreme, the liquid formula diet becomes the liquid protein diet, a regimen so widely attacked by medical authorities that its popularity has waned. No teen should embark upon this diet.

Again, as in the case of other one-food diet schemes, drinking a formula does nothing to help a teen move toward the overall alteration of eating habits which will be necessary to achieve safe, long-term weight loss.

*Starvation Diets.* These diets depend upon fasting for losses of up to a pound a day. When they are closely supervised by a physician, fasting diets can be of help to morbidly obese teens, once their rapid-growth period has passed. When they are used without medical supervision, however, they can lead to ketosis, dehydration, nausea, fatigue, dizziness, and loss of vital minerals such as potassium, calcium, and magnesium.

Ironically, starvation diets are often used by athletes who want to "make weight" for wrestling or boxing events. One look at the side effects should convince both coach and athlete that top performance is not likely to follow a starvation diet. Since ultimate growth and development may be hampered by such dieting, no athlete should be directed to take such drastic steps toward weight reduction.

*Meal-skipping Diets.* These usually end up making no contribution to weight loss and often contribute to health problems and nutritional deficiencies. Skipping breakfast and enjoying a heavier than usual evening meal work against the principles of weight loss.

## Other Dietary Alterations

Many of the other diets popular with today's teens are not chosen for weight loss but for other reasons. *Vegetarian* diets, whether they are adopted to save our dwindling resources, to lower serum-cholesterol levels, or to avoid exploitation of animal life, can be excellent. If they are taken to extremes, as in the case of the Zen Macrobiotic regimen, they can be highly dangerous, especially for the growing teen.

Three other diet categories popular today are *natural food diets,* which contain no foods contaminated by antibiotics, preservatives, additives, or excessive processing; *organically grown food diets,* which exclude all foods produced with commercial fertilizers or pesticides; and *health food diets,* which rely on vitamins, minerals, or foods purported to add years to life, cure various "incurable" diseases, and produce magical results such as increased sexual potency.

*Natural food diets* usually emphasize foods with a minimum of processing. Such diets recommend whole-grain instead of white breads, and fresh vegetables and fruits rather than highly processed ones. Some followers of natural foods diets use only raw milk and fertile eggs. Most try to avoid products containing chemical preservatives; some avoid all products with additives.

While natural foods can be excellent, all processed foods aren't necessarily bad. For example, enriching milk with vitamin D adds a valuable extra dimension to that food. Conversely, some raw milk may carry nature's undesirable "additives," brucellosis or tuberculosis organisms. While fertile eggs from a small farm are certainly tasty, infertile eggs produced by a commercial egg farm offer essentially the same nutrients. By shopping around, one can even find infertile eggs with bright yellow egg yolks.

Honey and brown sugar differ from white sugar in taste, but once the body has begun its digestive work, these three sugars are very much alike. Natural vitamin capsules and synthetic ones make identical impressions on the body, though the natural ones make a heavier dent in the pocketbook!

Many adherents of natural food diets are quick to acknowledge the pitfalls which await those who are not wary consumers. "Natural" has become one of the most powerful words in advertisements for food products, and many foods labeled "natural" may not be worthy of that title. For example, some "natural" cereals are higher in sugar—usually brown sugar or honey —than are cereals which make no claim to be natural. *Caveat emptor*—"let the buyer beware"—is certainly an appropriate warning for proponents of natural food diets.

The same warning also holds true for those who prefer to eat *organically grown* foods. Since no government regulations as yet impose stringent labeling laws on those who claim their fruits and vegetables are "organic," many fruits and vegetables may be falsely labeled. Thus, the problem with paying higher prices for organically grown foods is that you may not get what you pay for. Even if a customer does get an organically grown apple, it may be wormy or inferior to the apples available in the supermarket, since no quality controls or grading standards are as yet in effect for such products.

One very positive result of the natural food and organic food movements is that teens who follow those movements become more interested in fruits, vegetables, and whole grains and less interested in soft drinks, candy, and other junk foods. Thus these movements are helping to accomplish what decades of nutrition education have failed to accomplish.

Furthermore, even though organically grown produce may never become a widespread reality in this century, those who have demanded organically grown foods have done much to remind all of us that we must stop poisoning our environment with *overuse* of pesticides and fertilizers of uncertain content. If people continue to question the products which are used to enhance the growth of fruits, vegetables, and grains and to reduce the toll taken by insects and other pests, perhaps more attempts will be made to consider the overall impact of products used to increase the world's food supply.

Proponents of *health food diets* are sometimes willing to continue enjoying highly processed foods and foods which are not organically grown, provided they are able to supplement their diets with various vitamin and protein preparations which manufacturers claim will magically restore or maintain the user's good health. Unfortunately, those who manufacture, advertise, and sell health foods often make claims which cannot be substantiated, and belief in such claims can be dangerous or even fatal. For example, a consumer may depend on a certain food preparation to cure an illness, putting off seeking a doctor's advice during his weeks or months of experimentation with the "magic" food cure. During the long delay, the disease or disorder may become more severe and more difficult to treat by conventional means. While there are instances in which disorders may be directly related to diet (as in the case of food allergies and hyperactivity), as a general rule, psychosomatic illnesses are the only ones likely to be cured by the "magic" foods pushed as panaceas for a multitude of ills.

Health food stores usually offer special vitamin preparations as well as special foods. In such stores, megadoses of certain vitamins are often sold with promises of "renewed vitality," "increased sexual potency," or "restoration of lost head hair." Such claims are not usually based on scientific fact, and overdoses of many of these vitamins have been known to produce toxicity states in some people. Furthermore, many of these "magic" vitamin compounds differ from other multivitamin preparations only in cost.

Adopting an unusual diet may be some teens' way of rebelling against the establishment and finding a comfortable place for themselves among a counterculture group. Rather than actually leaving home and joining the group they admire, they simply adopt the group's dietary patterns. As long as adolescents take a commonsense approach to the new diet and do not carry it to undesirable or dangerous extremes, parents should probably view the dietary alteration as a part of teens' search for independence. If they are not berated for their actions, they will probably eventually come around to a happy medium between the foods of their adopted culture and the more familiar foods of home.

## Skin, Teeth, Hair, and Nails

For most teens, physical attractiveness means a complexion that is clear and smooth; a smile which reveals sound, white teeth; and a hairstyle which shows to best advantage hair that is glossy and healthy. All of these attributes are more likely to be obtained if one follows sound eating habits.

Some of them have direct ties with the food a teenager chooses to consume.

*Acne,* a skin disorder which often plagues adolescents, has long been tied, by doctors and laypeople alike, to the foods a teen consumes, and, more recently, health-food stores have claimed that acne is somehow related to vitamin consumption. Concern about acne has lead some teenagers to take extreme measures. For example, one teen, hearing that megadoses of vitamin A would clear up her pimples, took dietary supplements equal to thirty-seven times the Recommended Dietary Allowance over a three-year period. She developed numerous physical disorders; most of which were more serious than the acne she had set out to cure. Worse yet, there is no record that her acne even improved.

Acne is caused by overactive oil glands, not by vitamin deficiency. Most dermatologists now agree that treatment should be aimed at preventing infections and minimizing skin damage through cleanliness, antibiotics (under a doctor's care), ointments, and topical applications. They generally do not advocate treatment with hormones.

Though teens have been warned for decades to give up chocolate, french fries, and other foods, most dermatologists now say that there is no reliable evidence that food restriction is important in the treatment of acne. Alan Shalita, assistant professor of dermatology at College of Physicians and Surgeons, Columbia University, observed, "Although chocolate, peanuts, milk, fried foods, etc., have long been forbidden to acne patients, there is no evidence that dietary factors have a *direct* role in the pathogenesis of acne." (Authors' emphasis.) Other doctors seem to be in agreement with Dr. Shalita's views, though most point out that some teens may have undetected food allergies which can cause other complexion problems.

Most dermatologists also agree that general health, a well-balanced diet, and sufficient sleep and exercise are important in keeping skin healthy; and that fatigue, anxiety, tension, and emotional disturbances are probably more important factors than diet in aggravation of acne.

*Dental caries* has been listed as one of the most serious diet-related health problems of America's teens. As we mentioned earlier, high-sugar foods promote cavities, and snacks should be chosen with dental health, as well as other factors, in mind. A review of the dental health sections of the previous chapters should help teens plan their snacks wisely and thus avoid sugar-related damage to permanent teeth.

Some teens try to improve the appearance of brittle, thin *hair* by drinking gelatin. There seems to be some basis for belief in the effectiveness of this treatment, since researchers report that hair diameter increases with daily ingestion of ½-ounce (14 grams) of unflavored gelatin. There's no evidence that hair grows faster with this regimen, but an increase in diameter means increased strength of hair fibers and less susceptibility to breaking and splitting. Females with fine, fragile hair seem to benefit most from use of gelatin, with males and females who already have coarse, strong hair showing lesser changes in hair diameter. The smaller the hair diameter originally, the greater the increase.

Perhaps this increase is due to the fact that gelatin increases blood flow to the hair, thus leading to greater growth. Apparently, this same principle applies to *fingernail* growth, since nails are usually strengthened when gelatin is consumed. These changes diminish once gelatin treatment is stopped, with hair diameter returning to original measurements within six months of discontinuance of gelatin therapy.

While some teens may help their hair and nails by drinking gelatin in fruit juice for limited periods of time, all teens can improve their overall personal appearance by eating a well-balanced diet every day. When the entire body is well nourished, skin, teeth, hair, and nails are all likely to be in top condition, too.

## Contraceptives

Statistics show that today's teens tend to mature sexually and physically several months to a year sooner than teens of past generations, though the reasons for this are not clearly understood. Ironically, though they become capable of reproduction at an earlier age, society has programmed them for long years of continued schooling and, usually, of continued dependence upon parental financial support. Early marriages still occur, but more and more young people are postponing marriage to allow time for completion of their education or establishment of their careers.

Twenty to thirty years ago, postponing marriage meant what our parents called "delaying gratification," postponing sexual union until specified educational and career goals had been met and the time for marriage had arrived. To postpone marriage today may mean setting up a "live-in" arrangement with a girl- or boyfriend, thus postponing the legalities of wedlock but not the sexual intimacies. Such arrangements are made possible, of course, only because twentieth-century people have admitted that sexual intercourse can be enjoyed in and of itself, not just as a means of procreation, and such a declaration is made possible only because modern contraception devices usually prevent unwanted pregnancies.

It is to be hoped that increased openness between parents and children on the subject of sexual activity will mean that fewer and fewer adolescents will have to decide on a means of contraception without parental guidance. The prevalent attitude of the past has been that pregnancy is the worst thing which could possibly happen to a sexually active, but unmarried, adolescent girl. With increasing evidence that oral contraceptives and intrauterine contraceptive devices (IUDs) may pose severe health risks for some women, a teenager should consider *all* health risks when deciding how to guard against pregnancy.

For example, use of a diaphragm and spermatocide, or a condom, while less convenient and slightly less effective, has no harmful side effects for either the boy or the girl. They may be the best choice for those teens for whom the pill and the IUD pose unusual health risks. All teens, boys and girls, should at least be made aware of the possible side effects of contraceptive pill and the intrauterine device.

The "pill," usually cited as the most effective means of contraception, presents certain health hazards. The most notable of these, thromboembolic phenomena (blood clots), stems from the estrogen content of the oral contraceptive being used. Theoretically, oral contraceptives with lower estrogen levels do not pose the same dangers as those with higher levels. Though it is not related to diet, this side effect is one which should be seriously considered by young teens. Since prolonged use increases the likelihood of blood clot development, teens who begin using the pill in their junior-high days and use it continually for six to eight years may be at risk for such problems.

Users of the pill who have mild folacin-malabsorption problems, marginal intake of folacin, or excessive alcohol intake, as well as girls who become pregnant shortly after discontinuing use of contraceptive pills, may suffer from folacin deficiency. One young woman discovered her folic-acid deficiency and the macrocytic anemia it brought on because she became concerned over an uncontrollable compulsion to eat ice. She worked in a restaurant at the time, and chewing ice was her constant pastime. When she told her doctor of this habit, he explained that her abnormal craving for ice, called pica by nutritionists, was probably owing, in part, to a natural craving for trace elements missing in her diet. In some instances, dirt, starch, clay, and other possibly harmful substances are consumed in an instinctive attempt to gain missing nutrients.

In this case, the young woman was anemic, despite her good dietary iron intake. When iron tablets alone failed to correct this problem, her doctor prescribed iron with folic acid. Folic-acid deficiency can cause macrocytic anemia, a disorder in which red blood cells decrease in number, increase in size, and are low in hemoglobin. The iron-folic acid supplements corrected both forms of anemia, and the young woman gave up her compulsive ice eating.

For some women using the pill, vitamin $B_{12}$ metabolism is greater than normal. Since the average diet supplies adequate amounts of $B_{12}$, this slight increase in need is not a problem for most women. Vitam $B_{12}$ deficiency may, however, be a problem for strict vegetarians (vegans) who do not use supplements and who already have abnormally low levels of this vitamin before they begin to use oral contraceptives. Low levels of vitamin $B_6$ (pyridoxine) seem to result from use of the pill. While some girls adjust to changes in pyridoxine levels, others do not and may feel depressed unless supplements are used. If a girl's riboflavin level is already low, use of the pill may lower it still further. Vitamin C and zinc levels may appear lower in pill users, but this is probably the result of a bodily redistribution of these elements caused by hormonal changes brought about by the pill. Vitamin A levels are usually higher than normal in pill users, and iron levels are also higher, owing to reduced menstrual flow.

One supplement which claims to be compounded especially for pill users is actually little more than a multivitamin with relatively high folic-acid and

$B_6$ levels, and a very high price tag. While this pill and much cheaper general multivitamin and mineral compounds do not contain the folic acid and $B_6$ which pill users might need, they alco contain iron and vitamin A, two nutrients not likely to be needed by users of the contraceptive pill. Except in the case of malabsorption problems, most teens should be able to prevent $B_6$ and folic-acid deficiencies by giving extra attention to foods which supply these vitamins.

The young woman who developed an urge to eat ice later became concerned that long-term use of the contraceptive pill might cause circulatory problems. At her doctor's suggestion, she abandoned the pill in favor of an intrauterine contraceptive device (IUD). This time her main concern was iron loss due to increased menstrual blood flow. Since this is a common side effect of IUD use, a young woman who chooses this means of contraception should make every effort to increase her dietary iron intake or should have her doctor prescribe an iron supplement.

## Pregnancy

Pregnancy among adolescents usually carries far more health risks than does use of oral contraceptives or IUDs, and in pregnancy, the health risks involve two lives—that of mother and baby. While birth rates in general have fallen over the past several decades, birth rates among teens have risen. In 1960, sixteen teens per thousand became mothers, while in 1971, that number rose to twenty-four per thousand. One of every fourteen mothers bearing a first child in the United States is under the age of twenty.

Teen mothers are often alone, may lack funds for prenatal care, have no access to nutritional guidance or psychological counseling, and try to keep their weight gains abnormally low in order to disguise the fact of their pregnancy. With such poor prenatal care, maternal mortality rates rise, so that 6 percent of all deaths among eighteen- and nineteen-year-old girls result from complications of pregnancy and childbirth.

Poorly nourished teens are poor obstetric risks. Many have not yet completed their own growth at the time their bodies must suddenly support a new life. Especially if fad diets have been followed for weight-loss purposes, nutrition prior to conception may have been very poor, so that no stores are available with which to meet the added stresses of pregnancy. Iron, folic acid, vitamins A and C, and the B vitamins may be especially low, yet adequate amounts of these vitamins are essential to the health of both mother and child.

Teens tend to have low-birth-weight infants (under 5.5 pounds) with higher neonatal and postneonatal infant-mortality rates. Infant-mortality rates for teenage mothers grow proportionally higher for every year of the mother's age below seventeen.

Since 10 to 12 percent of pregnant adolescents begin pregnancy in an obese state, many young mothers-to-be may be tempted to diet. Especially if they are bothered by morning sickness, they may consider this the perfect time to lose weight. Such action is extremely unwise, for, as the National Research Council in its publication, *Maternal Nutrition and the Course of Pregnancy*, has warned,

> *When the nutritional demands of pregnancy are superimposed on those of adolescence, there should be no stringent caloric restriction. Even for the obese young adolescent, a modest weight gain should be permitted during pregnancy, and any attempt to reduce maternal weight by caloric restriction or drugs should be postponed until after delivery. The standardized diets commonly used in prenatal clinics are especially unsuited to the special nutrition needs of the young adolescent.*

Doctors and health-care experts agree that adolescent pregnancy demands a sophisticated program of care, and an important part of that care is nutrition education. Old rules of thumb such as "Cut out the salt" and "Don't gain more than twenty pounds" are no longer looked upon as valid by authorities such as the American College of Obstetrics and Gynecology. For the sake of her own health and that of her unborn child, a teen needs to seek the help of a competent physician who is aware of the latest trends in the childbirth field.

As a look at the RDA nutrient chart for teens reveals, pregnant girls require more calories, protein, vitamins, and minerals than do nonpregnant girls. If teen mothers choose to breast-feed their babies, additional nutrients will be needed to meet the stress imposed by lactation. If a mother-to-be or new mother feels unsure of her own dietary needs or those of her baby, she can seek help from such organizations as National March of Dimes Foundation or WIC (Women's Infant's Children's Program of USDA). The WIC program can be of special help to the teen whose financial resources are limited. Helpful guidebooks for nutrition during pregnancy are also available.

Use of hallucinogens, heavy smoking, and immoderate use of alcohol can all increase the chances of complications of pregnancy. The shocking news that fetal alcohol syndrome was responsible for the birth of many mentally retarded infants should serve as a warning that we do not yet know all the possible ways in which what a pregnant woman consumes affects the mental and physical state of the child she carries. Prescription drugs can be dangerous too, especially if a doctor prescribes medication without realizing a teen is pregnant.

In summary, the responsibilities of motherhood start when a child is conceived, not at the moment it is born. As more and more unmarried young women are choosing to have their babies and bring them up alone or to have them and give them up for adoption, prenatal care for adolescents becomes an increasingly important area of concern.

One beautiful young teen was asked by a friend why she decided to attend childbirth classes, to have her illegitimate child by the Lamaze method, and to nurse the infant for the first week of life, especially in view of the fact that she planned to give the baby up for adoption. The young mother's answer came quickly: "From the moment I decided this baby had a right to be born, I knew that she had to be well born in order to have a good start in life. I had good prenatal care and an excellent diet from that moment on. When I heard about childbirth without drugs, I realized that was the perfect way to give one last bit of love and care to my baby. Breast-feeding her was a hard decision, because I knew I'd want to keep her once I'd nursed her. Still, I knew giving her the nutritional head start was important. I gave her up because I wanted more for her than life with a high-school-dropout mother could provide. Now both of us have a chance for better things. I made a mistake but my daughter will never suffer because of it."

That baby girl, beautiful and healthy from birth, now lives with parents and siblings who love her dearly and will be forever grateful that the child's mother cared enough to leave her baby one of life's most precious legacies —a head start on good health.

## Drugs

Other teen mothers-to-be aren't so conscientious. They lack the self-discipline necessary to make the nine months of pregnancy a time of excellent health practices. They may use hallucinogens, tobacco, and alcohol during pregnancy, often increasing this use if depression or apprehension occurs as the time of delivery approaches.

Excessive use of drugs can pose problems even for nonpregnant teens. Teens who smoke excessively often lose keenness of smell or taste, so that foods seem less appealing. Hallucinogens, tobacco, and alcohol all tend to dull appetite and may lessen a teen's chances of getting enough calories and other nutrients.

Teenage alcoholism is on the increase. Aside from the very strong likelihood that heavy drinkers may cause auto accidents or otherwise jeopardize their lives and the lives of others, teens who drink to excess are highly vulnerable to certain nutritional disorders. Some alcoholics derive as many as 1800 calories per day from alcohol. By consuming so many of their calories in the form of alcohol, they limit their intake of foods, which offer more than calories alone. Deficiencies in thiamin, pantothenic acid, niacin, and pyridoxine are likely to occur.

Alcoholics are frequently victims of Wernicke-Korsakoff's syndrome, a disorder involving paralysis of eye muscles, rapid movement of eyeballs, uncoordinated gait, inability to learn new things, and failure to associate past events in proper sequence. Patients are usually confused, fearful, and delirious. Vitamin therapy restores attentiveness and alertness, but restoration of lost memory is rare.

Obese teens who have a drinking problem are likely to find weight control by calorie restrictions almost impossible. All teens should be aware of the many ways in which excessive use of alcohol can effect their health, now and in the future. When inadequate nutrition and alcoholism occur simultaneously, damage to health is likely to be even more severe.

## Food for Athletes

Early Friday morning, Panther quarterback Kevin Stevens ate two scrambled eggs and three strips of bacon with orange juice. At noon, his father came by to take him and his favorite wide receiver, Rick Evans, to lunch at a steak house. This game-day lunch of 8-ounce T-bones had become a cherished father-son ritual which they observed to provide plenty of good red meat for Kevin's strength during the evening game. Rick and Kevin drank ice water with their steak to prevent the "cotton mouth" feeling which the coach had warned them drinking milk on game day would produce. Back at school, Kevin managed to get through afternoon classes, though his mind was on the big game with his crosstown rivals, the Istruma High Indians.

By four P.M., his stomach had begun its weekly pregame churning, so he stopped all food and water intake and starved out the hours until it was time to enter the dressing room, get taped and uniformed, and hear a message from his coach. By eight P.M., he had forgotten his hunger in the excitement of last-minute game plans.

From kickoff time on, thoughts of food were far away. For two quarters, Kevin played like the all-state quarterback he deserved to be, passing for two touchdowns so that the Panthers led 13 to 0 at the half. After the half-time pep talk, he returned to lead the team once more, but his third-quarter passes seemed a bit shaky. Though tired and thirsty, he was careful to follow coach's rules—absolutely no drinking of water during a game. The opposing team scored once that quarter and made their point after. Throughout the fourth quarter, the Panther defense fought hard to hang onto their 13 to 7 lead, but the offense continually bogged down and Kevin couldn't seem to get his passes going again. The game ended 13 to 7, with the Indians stalled on the Panther 17-yard line. A close squeak, at best.

"Another good half a game," grumbled Kevin's father on the way home. "You were lucky the defense held. Why don't you ever seem to be able to last past the third quarter?" Then, seeing that his son already felt gloomy enough about his poor second-half performance, he reached across the car and gave the boy's shoulder a punch. "Never mind, Kev, next week I'll buy you two T-bones for lunch!"

Ironically, Mr. Stevens would probably have served his son better by buying him two baked potatoes instead. Though red meat has long been considered a prime food for athletes, evidence shows that high-protein meals are not the ideal pregame fare, since carbohydrate foods provide a more readily usable energy source. However, tradition does not die easily.

This is especially true if the tradition is centuries old! Until the fifth century B.C., the diets of Greek athletes were predominantly vegetarian, with pregame meals consisting of items such as porridge, meal cakes, figs, and fresh cheese. Shortly after the Persian wars, Dromeus of Stymphalus, two-time winner of the long race at Olympia, introduced a meat diet for the wrestlers he was training. In 460 B.C., since wrestlers were not separated according to weight, heavy wrestlers had a decided advantage over their opponents. A meat diet helped the wrestlers who trained with Dromeus gain that weight advantage, but Hippocrates, the famous Greek physician, denounced the trainees' new diet as likely to produce "a dangerous and unstable condition of body."

Whether or not Hippocrates' early health warning was valid, today's athletes who overload on steaks may raise their cholesterol levels and, in most cases, lower their endurance potential! Though protein is needed for muscle growth and development, excessive intake of protein does not build bigger, better muscles, and the fat content of beefsteaks is more likely to produce soft bulges than hard biceps.

The protein needs of the young athlete can easily be met by a well-balanced diet. An excessive intake of protein, whether in foods or in protein supplements, not only deprives an athlete of calories from more efficient energy sources but can also lead to dehydration, loss of appetite, diarrhea, and frequency of urination, none of which is likely to enhance athletic performance.

Though researchers disproved the notion of protein as a prime source of muscular energy over one hundred years ago and thus made the beefsteak ritual of the training table a nutritional fallacy, many coaches, both college and professional, find it hard to change such a deep-seated tradition. Steak is not magic to a tackle. Raw eggs won't enable a distance runner to set a new state record. Pizza won't make a guard sink 100 percent of his free throws. There's no scientific reason to believe in the power of any of these foods. Yet, to a certain extent, an athlete plays well on foods he believes will help him play well. If he believes he can't possibly win without steak, then, psychologically, he may have to have steak in order to play his best game. Physiologically, he may play well in spite of, not because of, his pregame eating habits.

If steak is not the key to athletic success, then what food is? All foods! The best nutritional insurance policy a player can have is a well-balanced daily dietary intake. If a boy or girl has enjoyed optimum nutrition from birth, chances are good that early nutritional practices have helped produce a healthy, well-muscled body. Continuing to take well-balanced meals and snacks throughout the sports year increases an athlete's chances of being in peak physical condition for competition.

Calorie needs during training and competition months may increase drastically, depending upon the energy demands of the sport in which an athlete participates. For example, while the RDA chart lists 2800 calories per day for the average American boy age fifteen to eighteen, one study revealed that 38 percent of Australian Olympic performers require 3000 to 4000 calories per day, 23 percent utilize 4000 to 5000 per day, and 6 percent use 6000 or more calories each day. To be an effective performer, an athlete must adjust her caloric intakes to meet her new calorie output. The approximate energy cost of various exercises and sports which follows should help a young athlete decide approximately how many extra calories she needs each day. If an athlete gains her extra calories by adding additional foods from all the major food groups, chances are excellent that she will receive all the nutrients she needs to be at her best in competition.

There may be an increased need for B-complex vitamins due to their role in the various biochemical reactions which make energy available for muscular work, but including foods containing these vitamins should insure sufficient intakes. While serious deficiencies in these vitamins would probably decrease performance quality, an athlete who receives a well-balanced diet of sufficient quantity is not likely to suffer B-vitamin deficiency symptoms. There have been claims that megadoses of vitamin C improve endurance, but research has not supported these claims. By drinking one 6-ounce glass of orange juice, an athlete can meet the RDA for vitamin C. Some people claim that vitamin E and wheat germ oil build endurance quickly, but these claims are also debatable. Despite claims to the contrary, consumption of wheat germ and wheat germ oil does add calories to the diet, a fact which athletes concerned with weight control should certainly be aware of.

Since there's no evidence that excess intake of any other vitamins will improve performance, most researchers don't advocate the use of megavitamin supplements by athletes, the testimonies of Bobby Riggs and others notwithstanding. Those coaches and players who believe in megadosing say, "What can it hurt?" The pocketbook, for one thing. American athletes are said to have "the world's most expensive urine"—due to all the expensive excess water-soluble vitamins excreted by the kidneys. However, there may be far more serious losses to consider than money.

Though vitamin C is water soluble and can be excreted in the urine, excessive intake of this vitamin may cause kidney stones in susceptible individuals and may destroy vitamin $B_{12}$. Fat-soluble vitamins are not excreted in urine but are stored in the body. Since vitamins A and D have both been proven toxic in large doses, an athlete would be better off to rely on natural or fortified dietary items for these vitamins.

Minerals, too, should be obtained from dietary sources, not megavitamin-mineral capsules. Sodium, potassium, and iron are used more quickly by teens who engage in strenuous sports activities, but normal amounts of table salt or a cup of bouillon can restore sodium losses, bananas and oranges can replenish potassium stores, and raisins and other dried fruits can provide needed iron. Minerals obtained from foods pose no risk of overdose and offer all the advantages of supplements, plus the double bonus of added nutrients and added calories. Occasionally, female athletes find that menstrual blood losses are heavier than usual during sports participation. In that case, there may be a reason to ask a physician to prescribe iron supplements.

In general, if an athlete adds the extra calories he needs through consumption of more foods from the basic food groups we discussed earlier, he will also be adding all the extra protein and other nutrients he needs. Of course, if he ends football season in late November and continues to take in an extra 3000 calories a day, he's likely to acquire a few pounds of undesirable fat before spring training! Fall football players who join the wrestling team as soon as they turn in their pads and helmets are made acutely aware of this problem because they must often "weigh in" in early December in order to receive weight classification. If this fateful meeting with the scales falls just after Thanksgiving turkey time, problems are compounded. Since most coaches seem to operate on the as-yet-to-be-proven assumption that a wrestler performs best in his lowest possible weight class, crash diets, sweat suits, and self-induced vomiting are often advised for weigh-in week.

Even if a wrestler manages to qualify for a low weight class in the late fall, his problems usually aren't over. In fact, by forcing himself into a lower-than-normal division, the athlete is faced with the necessity of continuing to keep his weight down. Often dietary patterns for wrestlers are a nutritional nightmare! For several days before a match, food and water intakes are cut to a minimum (often 500 calories or less), sweat suits are worn, and "water pills" (diuretics) and laxatives are taken. In short, everything possible is done to squeeze every extra ounce from the athlete's body. Such dietary abuses cause dehydration, so that the major weight loss achieved is water loss. As the discussion of diet for elementary-school athletes shows, dehydration can lead to many ill effects, including heat stroke and death. Despite these risks, coaches continue to encourage unsafe reducing regimens that have led doctors to label wrestling as "the internal water sport," since it often leads to dehydrating and rehydrating its participants at least once every week. Such practices are so dangerous to overall health and optimum growth and development that at least one medical group has called for the abolition of junior-high and high-school wrestling.

Such a drastic step would mean a great loss of athletic opportunity, but the strong feelings of the doctors who advocated it underscore the importance of raising serious questions about the current means of handling "making weight." How can a youngster who has lost valuable minerals through use of water pills really be at his peak? How can a boy who is dehydrated possibly wrestle at his best? Often he does well early in the match, only to be outpointed in the late periods. If he manages to win, neither he nor his coach is likely to realize that he was at a low ebb toward the close of the match. Even if he loses, no one is apt to connect his loss of strength with the fact that his body is operating under far less than optimum circumstances. If he has lost over 5 percent of his body weight within a twenty-four-hour period, he has probably significantly decreased his ability to perform and placed undue stress on his cardiovascular system.

What, then, is the ideal wrestling weight? When a competitor has achieved a healthy and effective level of hydration and optimal muscle mass and has brought his body fat to approximately 7 percent of his overall weight, he is probably at his peak for wrestling. Even if these guidelines mean he is in a slightly higher weight class, he should perform better there. Bringing body fat to the 7-percent level, and not losing water, should be the athlete's goal if he wishes to move to a lower weight class. Fat can be lost by lowering caloric intake slightly (but never below 2000 calories per day during the active season) while increasing physical activity in order to burn up excess calories. Gradual, steady loss is in order, not prematch crash diets that take off pounds, only to be followed by post-match eating binges that put them on again.

One medical group has recommended checking the specific gravity of the urine of wrestlers before competition so that dehydrated contestants might be barred from participating in wrestling events. Such a practice would discourage dieting practices which generally hurt the performance of teenage wrestlers. Research has proven that better hydrated wrestlers tend to perform better. In one instance, the average hydration of first- and second-place competitors was higher than that of wrestlers with lower scores.

Junior-high boys who want to make a bantam football league or girls who want to make the gymnastic team or the ice-skating squad may also be pressured to lose pounds quickly. By exercising an additional hour a day and by keeping the diet well balanced, with calorie intake steady, most teens can lose a pound or two per week. Losses of more than two pounds per week should be attempted only under a doctor's supervision. Losing too quickly usually means losing vital stores of protein, glycogen, vitamins, minerals, and water, and may have long-range ill effects on kidneys, growth, development, and overall health.

The need to gain weight quickly is a problem for other athletes, especially football linemen. To gain 2 pounds a week, one needs to increase the calorie intake by 1000 calories per day. If training has already begun, this extra 1000 calories must be in addition to those calories added to offset the energy lost during practice sessions. An athlete should avoid overloads of saturated, high-cholesterol fats by using vegetable oils and avoiding excess intake of high-fat meats. If an athlete adds over 1000 to 1500 calories a day to his diet for the purpose of weight gain, much of the weight gained will likely be in the form of fat. Continuous training, plus 1000 extra calories per day, should mean that most of the added weight will be in the form of lean muscle mass.

No matter how urgently an athlete wishes to add pounds and muscles, she or he should not use androgen hormones. Though these hormones do seem to work, there's no guarantee that the momentary gains will be worth the possible long-range ill effects. If an athlete takes them before the growth spurt has ended, these steroids stunt growth by premature stoppage of growth of the long bones. Side effects such as deepening of the voice, skin disorders, excessive body hair, and breast enlargement have been noted. When an athlete takes them after the teen growth spurt, the drugs can lead to such serious problems as diminished testicular size, loss of sexual potency, and permanent decrease in sperm production. Adolescent athletes and their parents should make every effort to bring such practices to a halt if they are included in a high-school or college athletic program.

Parental intervention of this sort is often beneficial in other areas, for when a coach is recommending questionable dietary regimens, he may be willing to listen to persuasive evidence presented by concerned parents in favor of a change in policy. For example, any coach who was presented with the facts on water intake and dehydration outlined in the preceding chapter would probably pass this information on to his players and coaching staff. While many coaches seem to fear that their athletes will become "water-logged" if they are allowed more than a mouth-rinse of water during competition, others have begun to allow at-will water drinking because they've been made aware of studies which show that performance is improved when water intake is allowed during a game.

Since a 3-percent loss of water means impaired performance, a 5-percent loss may bring evidence of heat exhaustion, a 7-percent loss leads to potentially fatal heat stroke, coaches cannot afford to ignore the dangers in failure to replace water lost before or during competition. In fact, conscientious coaches should introduce pre-and post-practice weigh-ins and give their athletes some idea of the water loss which should be made up, especially since thirst is not a reliable guide as to how much water has been lost. For every 2 pounds of weight lost during game or practice, 1 extra quart of water should be taken.

There is no basis for restricting water intake of athletes during competition, and, according to Sir Edmund Hillary's testimony, there is every reason to keep water intake high. Sir Edmund's team succeeded in climbing Mount Everest partly because of a valuable lesson learned from the Swiss climbers who were defeated in their attempt a year earlier, owing, in part, to exhaustion during the final days of the climb. The Swiss group took only enough fuel to allow melting of snow for one pint of water per climber per day. Since the low atmospheric humidity and heavy exertion demanded by the climb caused far greater body-water losses than one pint could replenish, the Swiss team became dehydrated and lacked sufficient strength to complete the ascent. Sir Edmund's group, armed with enough fuel to produce snow-melt of 5 to 7 pints of water per climber per day, avoided the fatigue of dehydration and made it to the top.

Finding the key to endurance is the goal of many athletes. In recent years, as the mysteries of muscular energy have become better understood, coaches have become aware that carbohydrate is probably the one food substance which brings the greatest energy benefits to athletes. Though fat supplies 70 percent of the energy needed for prolonged, slow work, and for low-intensity exercise such as fly-casting, an athlete who works at 75 percent of maximum capacity needs carbohydrates for energy.

Adenosine triphosphate (ATP) and phosphocreatine (PC) are two muscle-energy sources which are ready instantly. However, only an athlete such as a 50-yard-dasher or a sprint-swimmer can rely on stores of these sources alone, since they are exhausted very quickly.

Once an athlete burns up his quick energy stores, his system calls on fats and glycogen, a storage carbohydrate made of glucose and found in the liver and muscles. By eating a diet high in complex carbohydrates for several days before competition, and by resting for a few days between the last exhaustive workout and the big event, one can build glycogen stores and thus ward off the exhaustion which comes when glycogen levels are insufficient.

Some athletes have been intrigued by reports that glycogen-storage capacity can be increased to levels far above normal through a process known as carbohydrate loading. For events longer than a half-hour to one hour, and especially for very long events such as marathon running or swimming, carbohydrate loading may be valuable, but this practice is definitely not recommended for use by high-school athletes. The basic pattern used by carbohydrate loaders is as follows: For about a week before competition, an athlete chooses a low-carbohydrate, high-protein diet and engages in heavy workouts or long runs. This dual effort lowers glycogen stores so drastically that performance in mid-week practice sessions may be adversely affected. Then, forty-eight hours before the event, the athlete tapers off exercise and begins a high-carbohydrate diet. This diet is continued through game day, and no strenuous exercise is engaged in for twenty-four hours prior to competition.

Varying amounts of success have been reported with carbohydrate loading. In a mid-1970s Trail's End Marathon (26.2 miles) in Oregon, loaders proved to be 6.0 to 11.5 minutes faster than nonloaders, with the main differences in timing being noted in the final 6.2 miles. Before that point, differences between loaders and nonloaders were slight. The researchers who analyzed this particular marathon attempted to make adjustments for such differences as age, experience, training, and so on, in order to get a true picture of the difference loading could make, and their conclusions seem valid.

To the professional athlete, having that last surge of energy might be important enough to warrant carbohydrate loading for particularly crucial competitions. For the high school or college athlete, the disadvantages and possible risks probably outweigh the advantages. First, excess glycogen stores also mean excess water retention, so that overloaded muscles may seem stiff and heavy, a real handicap for short-distance runners. Second, preloading days call for carbohydrate intakes low enough to impair practice, and profitable practice sessions are probably more vital to a high-school athlete than endurance. Finally, some older athletes who have tried carbohydrate loading for marathon runs have exhibited significant heartbeat irregularities. In view of all these factors, and because of the general lack of knowledge about the long-term effects of this practice, authorities have urged that carbohydrate loading not be undertaken, even by the professional athlete, except for the most important events, and then only under the supervision of a competent physician.

Even if the full regimen of carbohydrate loading is not a technique safe enough for or suited for use by high school or college athletes, any athlete can safely choose a diet high in carbohydrates for twenty-four to forty-eight hours before game time. On game day, small meals high in carbohydrates will be more easily digested than heavy meals high in fats and will provide a more usable energy source than meals high in protein. A cereal and skim-milk breakfast plus a banana mid-morning snack makes for a good start, and there's no evidence that low-fat milk on game day leads to "cotton mouth," digestive troubles, or decreased respiratory output. If the last meal is eaten at least three hours prior to the event, some low-fat protein may be included without posing problems in digestion or elimination. One serving of a starchy vegetable such as potato or macaroni, one serving of another vegetable, one cup of skim milk, one portion of broiled lean meat, poultry, or fish, one piece of fruit, and one piece of plain, low-fat cake (angel food or sponge) might be a typical pregame menu. One to two cups of extra fluid, such as apple juice or bouillon, should be taken so that the body is well hydrated before competition begins.

For some athletes, even this relatively light meal may be too much. Nervous tension can cause decreased blood flow to the stomach and small intestine, and thus interfere with digestion. Especially if an athlete is nervous, eating a full meal may bring on stomach cramps, weakness, belching, diarrhea, nausea, or vomiting. By avoiding fats, gas-formers (such as beans), high intake of protein (which may add to urine output), or bulky foods (which may cause the need for bowel movements during competition), athletes can avoid most problems associated with game-day meals and snacks.

If even a light meal with these restrictions poses digestive problems, a liquid meal such as Ensure, Sustagen, or Sustacal can provide still more easily digested pregame nourishment. These liquid meals are not to be confused with various diet drinks or instant breakfasts, since those foods often contain more protein and fat than would be deemed wise for pregame meals. Athletes should also steer clear of formulas made of predigested protein and other synthetic items. A homemade formula calling for ⅓ cup nonfat dry milk, 3 cups of skim milk, ½ cup of water, ¼ cup of sugar, and 1 teaspoon of vanilla flavoring provides 200 calories per 8-ounce cup. Two cups may be sufficient as a pregame meal, depending on the caloric needs of the athlete.

No athlete should try a new diet regimen just before a big game. A pre-scrimmage meal test should be made before one decides on a pregame meal. During the event, athletes should also stick to tried and true regimens. Water or special glucose-and-water mixtures may be taken, though mixtures too sugar-rich or consumed at a rate in excess of 200 calories per hour may cause digestive upsets which interfere with performance. Some teams enjoy using diluted fruit juices or, if the temperature is high, frozen fruit juice popsicles. Tea and coffee should be avoided, since they tend to stimulate, then depress. Alcohol is likely to impair performance and should not be used at all, either just before or during competition.

After the game is over, food again becomes an issue. Usually athletes need a rest period prior to eating, and often they fare better on familiar rather than exotic foods. If a team is on the road, sandwiches from home (made without mayonnaise or meats that might spoil), hamburgers at a quick-food place, or a soup and sandwich supper at a café which has been notified to expect the late arrival of a busload of players may be good choices. Whenever possible, after-game meals should be a decision left to the team, for they have done their job well and deserve to have a voice in the menu afterward.

## Fast Food

Teens usually enjoy eating where food is good, service is fast, and costs are within their limited means. Fast-food outlets fill these requirements and attract a large part of the teen away-from-home meals-and-snacks market. As in all restaurant situations, the choices a teen makes will determine the nutrient content of his meal. Learning to make sound choices is a crucial part of becoming a wise consumer of fast foods.

Assuming that a full burger snack meal gives an adolescent one-third of his or her total calories for the day, getting the necessary nutrients along with those calories is important. In general, protein, iron, and thiamin levels in hamburger-type meals are all about one-third RDA. If milk in some form is not taken with the meal, then calcium and riboflavin are likely to be below one-third RDA, even though calorie intake reaches one-third RDA. Choosing a cheeseburger rather than a hamburger can help boost calcium intake for the meal or snack.

Unless salads are offered, teens will find it difficult to obtain adequate amounts of vitamins A and C at a fast-food chain whose specialty is hamburgers. Some vitamin C will be gained by choosing fries. Mexican food specials which feature lettuce, tomatoes, and tomato sauce on a taco may bring up vitamin A and C levels, but other nutrients in such a menu may not reach one-third of RDA.

For obese teens on calorie-restricted diets, fast-food establishments provide an exercise in willpower. Choosing a small diet drink or plain milk over a shake and ordering a burger high in beef rather than one which offers three slices of bun mean a weight-watcher is off to a good start. Setting aside one of the two halves of the bun and passing up french fries make for an admirable finish. Choosing a fish sandwich may seem to be a wise decision, but fast-food-chain fish sandwiches are generally higher, not lower, in calories than are hamburgers. They are also higher in fat and sodium and, in most instances, offer fewer vitamins and minerals. There's no reason an overweight teen shouldn't enjoy a burger break after school, provided he remembers his dietary goals and chooses foods that help him stay within those goals.

For teens who eat not more than one meal per week at fast-food establishments, there's no need to worry about whether that meal might be slightly deficient in one or two nutrients. Teens who eat a hamburger lunch without milk several times each week, however, may build up significant nutrient deficits. Even when a fast-food chain features menu choices making it pos-sible to obtain a well-balanced meal, the teen must *choose* those menu items in order to achieve balance and meet nutritional goals.

## College Meals

Once an adolescent goes to college, the novelty of eating away from home may wear off as the monotony of institutional food sets in. Many dorm cafeterias have traditionally served high-starch menus which wreak havoc on the diet plans of the obese and on the overall eating habits of most teens.

Nonetheless, once a meal ticket is paid for, college students usually accept whatever items appear in the cafeteria food line. Fortunately, more and more colleges are offering fairly wide choices. Once he is away at college, a teen's training for independence will be put to a sterner test than ever before. Left on his own, can he choose the foods that contribute to a well-balanced diet?

In general, college students usually display the habits they've acquired over a lifetime of eating. The breakfast-skippers skip breakfast, the vegetable-haters avoid vegetables, the meat-eaters rush to be first in line on steak night. Basically, the nutritional balance of college food-service meals, like the nutritional balance of fast-food meals, depends upon the choices the student makes. If good eating has been a way of life, making such decisions should be relatively easy, even when food choices are fairly limited.

At many colleges and universities, an effort is being made to provide wider choices for students. Skim milk and other nutritious, low-fat items have been added to dormitory menus, and charts are posted to help calorie counters make wise decisions. Such helpful devices not only aid the student now but offer excellent training for food decisions she will be called upon to make once her college career has ended.

## Teens Entertain

At home or at school, teens who plan parties have an opportunity to share favorite dishes with their friends. By choosing to offer fresh raw vegetables as well as chips with a hot-cheese dip, they allow their friends to make choices consistent with their particular needs. By offering low-calorie drinks or water as well as punch, they allow calorie-conscious friends to socialize without overindulging.

When more formal events call for full meals, a teen can set the budget, plan the menu, do the shopping, and, with the help of a friend or two, prepare gourmet fare to please even the fussiest eater. By planning a well-balanced menu, a teen offers friends delicious food that's not only good but good for them. Boys and girls alike can profit from practical food-prepara-tion experiences such as this.

# Practical Meals and Snacks

Some teens gain food-preparation experience even earlier than the junior-high years. Nora, the twelve-year-old whose Saturday menu and activity schedule opened this chapter, was given the opportunity to prepare her own breakfast, lunch, and snacks as an elementary-school student. Her parents, practical and well aware that the logistics of running a household of eight necessitates early assumption of certain responsibilities, allowed their children a great amount of food-choice freedom and food-preparation experience.

Using the knowledge gained through the reading of this chapter, teens and parents should be able to study the food diaries kept by Nora and four of her five siblings and make a fair guess as to their nutritional adequacy. Only five teens are included in this survey because the sixth, a college sophomore, was not available for the study.

Teens can compare their own analyses of the following food intake records to the RDA computer analyses given for these diets. Though the computer analyses were based on 1974 RDAs, in most cases the percentages given would not be greatly changed by using 1980 RDA values instead. Calorie intakes would be somewhat affected. With lower RDAs for energy being cited for 1980, the Smith children whose diets are analyzed on the following pages should all come closer to meeting RDAs in that category. Since the 1980 RDA for vitamin C is slightly higher than the 1974 standard, the teens would be lower in this vitamin than the computer analyses would seem to indicate.

Once the weak areas of each diet have been observed, family members can make suggestions as to ways to strengthen these weak spots. A review of the vitamin and mineral overview charts in Chapter 2 should be of help, along with a comparison of each day's menu with the Minimum Exchanges Chart in that chapter.

## Joe's Seven-Day Dietary Intake Record

**Age:** 17 years   **Weight:** 171 lbs (77.2 kg)   **Height:** 6'4" (197.1 cm)

| Saturday | | Bread | |
|---|---|---|---|
| Cornflakes (2 bowls) | 9:00 A.M. | Milk | |
| Cream of chicken soup (1 can) | 1:00 P.M. | Marshmallows | 12:00 A.M. |
| Milk (2 glasses) | | **Monday** | |
| Cheeseburger | 3:30 | Ice cream sandwich | 12:15 P.M. |
| Fries | | Licorice | 2:30 |
| Milk | | M & M's | |
| Pasta, nibbled intermittently | | Turkey (2 helpings) | 6:00 |
| | | Mashed potatoes (2 helpings) | |
| **Sunday** | | Milk (2 glasses) | |
| Alpha-Bits (2 bowls) | 10:30 A.M. | Chocolate-chip cookies (4) | |
| Milk | | **Tuesday** | |
| Licorice ( ¼ lb) | 12:00 P.M. | Meat loaf (2 helpings) | 6:00 P.M. |
| | | Milk (2 glasses) | |
| Turkey with stuffing (2 helpings) | 2:30 | Ice cream (large bowl) | |
| | | Milk | 7:30 |
| Pasta | 8:00 | Orange juice | 9:30 |

| **Wednesday** | | **Friday** | |
| --- | --- | --- | --- |
| Cookies (4–6) | 4:00 P.M. | Orange juice | 7:30 A.M. |
| Milk | | Sausage sandwich (large) | 5:00 P.M. |
| Peanut butter sandwich | | Milk | |
| Beef stroganoff (2 helpings) | 6:00 | Pasta, nibbled intermittently | |
| Cookie cake (2 helpings) | | | |

**Thursday**

| | |
| --- | --- |
| Pasta (2–3 helpings) | 8:30 P.M. |
| Milk (2–3 glasses) | |

Pasta, nibbled intermittently

| **Computer Analysis (% of RDA)** | |
| --- | --- |
| Calories | 56 |
| Protein | 133 |
| Calcium | 74 |
| Iron | 52 |
| Vitamin A | 38 |
| Thiamin | 66 |
| Riboflavin | 100 |
| Niacin | 75 |
| Vitamin C | 68 |

A quick look at Joe's food diary shows that his meal pattern is highly erratic, partly due to his eight-hour work schedule on Thursday, Friday, Saturday, and Sunday evenings. As a junior chef for a restaurant specializing in pasta, he taste-tests through many of the eight hours of his work. He skipped breakfast four out of seven mornings and had a relatively light breakfast the remaining three days, a pattern typical of many teens. He ate between-meal snacks which favor tooth decay, yet he and his brothers are cavity-free. When he ate meals, he ate heartily, but he had few vegetables and fruits during the week.

As discussed in Chapter 2, achieving two-thirds the Recommended Dietary Allowance in calories, protein, vitamins, or minerals is considered adequate for most persons. Joe's computer nutrient analysis shows his caloric intake at 56 percent, approximately 300 calories below two-thirds RDA. However, since 1980 RDAs for energy are somewhat lower than were 1974 RDAs, Joe is probably closer to two-thirds RDA than the computer analysis shows. Furthermore, the calories from three nights of pasta nibbling, unentered on the computer, would probably have brought his caloric intakes to two-thirds of the RDA. Since Joe's rapid-growth years are over, caloric intakes of that amount will not lessen his chances for optimum growth and development. His weight is nearly perfect for his height and his light-to-medium frame, and his relatively low caloric intake means that obesity is not likely to become a problem. At the time this diet survey was made, Joe's activity level was moderate, but when ski season opens, he will spend at least one day a week on the slopes. As in past years, his appetite will probably increase, so that he instinctively adds enough extra calories to offset those he loses through the extra activity.

Despite relatively few meat servings, Joe's protein level is over 100 percent of the RDA, a typical finding among American teens. Adequate milk consumption is evident in his calcium and riboflavin intakes, and his vitamin C, niacin, and thiamin intakes are acceptable. Since Joe's growth years are coming to an end, the 18-milligrams-per-day iron RDA is probably high. At 9 to 10 milligrams per day, his iron intake is probably adequate. His most serious dietary problem is seen in his vitamin A intake—38 percent of the RDA. This is not surprising, since Joe does not usually eat green leafy vegetables and does not like many yellow vegetables or fruits. Carrots are acceptable to him, and a carrot snack once or twice a week would probably bring his vitamin A level up. Had the computer nutrient analysis included the tomato sauce in Joe's nibbled pasta snacks, chances are excellent that the analysis would have shown his vitamin A level significantly higher than it did.

Joe's diet was a revelation to his parents, and they feared such illogical menu and snack choices must mean total disaster nutritionally. They were pleasantly surprised when analysis revealed that though some nutrient intakes were borderline, the total diet was basically sound. Of course, other essential nutrients for which no RDAs have yet been established may well be missing from Joe's diet. Increasing the variety of the overall diet would lessen the chance of developing deficiencies of these nutrients; making breakfast an established part of his diet could accomplish this and would improve Joe's overall nutrition status. A look at the vitamin and mineral overview charts in Chapter 2 should reveal the foods Joe can add to make his borderline nutrient intakes still more satisfactory. These same charts indicate the health risks he may run if borderline nutrient intakes should move far below two-thirds of the RDA.

## Chris's Seven-Day Dietary Intake Record

**Age:** 16 years   **Weight:** 155 lbs (70.4 kg)   **Height:** 6'2" (189.7 cm)

### Saturday

| | |
|---|---|
| Turkey (1 helping) | 6:00 P.M. |
| Stuffing (1 helping) | |
| Potatoes (1) | |
| Licorice ( ¼ bag) | 8:30 |

### Sunday

| | |
|---|---|
| Doughnuts (2) | 7:00 A.M. |
| Cheeseburger | 1:00 P.M. |
| Fries | |
| Milk | |
| Turkey sandwich (2) | 6:00 |
| Iced Tea (3) | |
| Ice cream cake (4 helpings) | |
| Ice cream | 8:30 |

### Monday

| | |
|---|---|
| Raisin Bran | 7:15 A.M. |
| Pizza | 12:10 P.M. |
| Rolls (2) | |
| Milk | |
| Cookie | |
| Turkey leg | 6:00 |
| Mashed potatoes and gravy | |
| Dressing | |
| Tea (2 cups) | |
| Chocolate-chip cookies | 9:30 |
| Pie (1/3) | |

### Tuesday

| | |
|---|---|
| Hot dog | 12:10 P.M. |
| Tater Tots | |
| Milk | |
| Cake (1 piece) | |
| Roll cake (1 piece) | 4:15 |
| Potato chips (handful) | |
| Chex party mix (3 bowls) | |
| Meat loaf (2 pieces) | 6:00 |
| Potato (1) | |
| Rolls (4) | |
| Tea (3) | |
| Ice cream (2 bowls) | |

### Wednesday

| | |
|---|---|
| Bologna and cheese | 12:10 P.M. |
| sandwich | |
| Carrots (2) | |
| Applesauce | |
| Milk | |
| Beef stroganoff and noodles | 6:00 |
| Rolls (3) | |
| Milk | |
| Celery (2 sticks) | |
| Chocolate chip cookies (3) | 7:00 |

### Thursday

| | |
|---|---|
| Raisin Bran and milk | 7:15 A.M. |
| (1 bowl) | |
| Meat gravy over potatoes | 12:10 P.M. |
| Rolls (2) | |
| Milk | |
| Chicken noodle soup | 6:00 |
| (3 bowls) | |
| Milk | |

### Friday

| | |
|---|---|
| Raisin Bran | 7:15 A.M. |
| Fish sandwich | 12:10 P.M. |
| Apple | |
| Cookie | |
| Milk | |
| Cherry pie (1 piece) | 10:00 |

## Computer Analysis (% of RDA)

|            | %of RDA |
|------------|---------|
| Calories   | 67      |
| Protein    | 135     |
| Calcium    | 66      |
| Iron       | 93      |
| Vitamin A  | 91      |
| Thiamin    | 60      |
| Riboflavin | 83      |
| Niacin     | 85      |
| Vitamin C  | 39      |

Chris's breakfast patterns were about like those of his older brother—no breakfast at all on four of the seven days recorded and a light breakfast on the remaining three. His calorie intake was two-thirds RDA, but since his weight percentile is about 20 percent lower than his height percentile, he could consume more calories without becoming overweight. Protein intakes were high, and much of that protein was in iron-rich meats, a fact which helped give Chris the family high in iron. This is fortunate, since he is currently in the midst of a growth spurt, having added 4 to 5 inches to his height in the past twelve months. His celery and carrot nibbling gave him a high intake of vitamin A, but his thiamin intake was below optimum. Adding whole-grain breads could raise that intake and also increase his calorie intake. Calcium, riboflavin and niacin intakes were satisfactory. Chris's most serious low is vitamin C. Since 1980 RDAs for that vitamin are even higher than were the 1974 RDAs on which the computer analysis of his diet was based, Chris's vitamin C level is cause for concern. By including a glass of orange juice, a citrus-fruit snack, or an ascorbic-acid-rich vegetable in every day's food intake, he could bring his vitamin C level to RDA standards. By adding a few more dairy products to his week's intake, he could raise his borderline calcium intake.

## Steve's Seven-Day Dietary Intake Record

**Age:** 15 years   **Weight:** 105 lbs (47.7 kg)   **Height:** 5'4" (164.1 cm)

### Saturday

| | | | |
|---|---|---|---|
| French toast (6 pieces) | 6:00 A.M. | Chicken (3 helpings) | 5:00 |
| Hash browns | | Corn | |
| Tacos (2) | 1:00 P.M. | Mashed potatoes (1) | |
| Apple | | Salad | |

Coke
Ice cream

## Sunday

| | |
|---|---|
| Pancakes (4) with syrup | 7:00 A.M. |
| Bacon (2) | |
| Orange juice (3 glasses) | |
| Bananas (3) | 12:15 P.M. |
| Doritos | 12:35 |
| Banana | 2:35 |
| Ham and cheese sandwich | 5:30 |
| Chips (3 helpings) | |
| Tea | |
| Cake roll (3 helpings) | |
| Coke | 8:30 |

## Monday

| | |
|---|---|
| English muffin | 7:30 A.M. |
| Hot chocolate (2 cups) | |
| Ham and cheese sandwich | 12:20 P.M. |
| Apple | |
| Chips | |
| Chocolate milk (2) | |
| Banana | 5:15 |
| Mashed potatoes (2) | 6:15 |
| Tea | |
| Milk | |
| Rolls with honey (3) | |
| Pan cookies (4) | |
| Milk (2) | 9:30 |

## Tuesday

| | |
|---|---|
| English muffin | 7:15 A.M. |
| Hot chocolate (2 cups) | |
| Ham and cheese sandwich | 12:20 P.M. |
| Apple | |
| Chips | |
| Chocolate milk (2) | |
| Bananas (2) | 4:20 |
| Meatloaf | 6:10 |
| Baked potato | |
| Milk | |
| Tea | |
| Rolls with honey (3) | |
| Ice cream | |
| Sea toast crackers | 7:10 |

## Wednesday

| | |
|---|---|
| Orange juice | 6:50 A.M. |
| Ham and cheese sandwich | 12:20 P.M. |
| Chips | |
| Apple | |
| Doughnuts (3) | |
| Cola | |
| Iced tea | 5:55 |

## Thursday

| | |
|---|---|
| English muffin | 7:20 A.M. |
| Hot cocoa | |

| | |
|---|---|
| Ham sandwich | 12:20 P.M. |
| Apple | |
| Chips | |
| Chocolate milk (2 glasses) | |
| Meat loaf | 6:00 |
| Tater Tots (2 helpings) | |
| Milk (2 glasses) | |
| Rolls with honey (2) | |
| Ice cream (2 bowls) | 8:00 |

## Friday

| | |
|---|---|
| Orange juice | 6:00 A.M. |
| Grilled ham and bacon sandwich (2) | 10:00 |
| Coke | |
| Fries | |
| Coke | 3:00 P.M. |
| Roll of lifesavers | 3:30 |
| Italian crepes (2) | 10:00 |
| Salad | |
| Coke (2 glasses) | |
| Strawberry crepe | |

## Computer Analysis (% of RDA)

| | |
|---|---:|
| Calories | 86 |
| Protein | 184 |
| Calcium | 103 |
| Iron | 65 |
| Vitamin A | 52 |
| Thiamin | 86 |
| Riboflavin | 140 |
| Niacin | 81 |
| Vitamin C | 178 |

Steve, the only child ever considered a "problem eater," topped the family in meeting calorie RDAs. Furthermore, as a look at his other percentages shows, he gained his calories through fairly well-balanced meals and snacks. His iron intake was a bit below two-thirds of the RDA, probably because his favorite meat, ham, is not high in iron. A moderately late maturer, he will need to keep his iron intake adequate as his rapid-growth period continues.

His vitamin A level needs improvement, as one might guess from the fact that the only green vegetable he ate came in a single tossed salad. If this salad was made of head lettuce only, the vitamin A and folic-acid content was probably minimal. Including other salad greens would have made the salad an excellent source of these two vitamins.

Generally, Steve's dietary intake is better than average, a fact which gave him great pleasure, since his brothers and sisters often tease him about his unorthodox food choices. The monotony of meat choice probably lowered his RDA percentages of several important nutrients and, perhaps, of nutrients for which no RDAs have yet been established. His regular consumption of breakfast probably increased his percentages in nutrients and helped give him the family calorie-intake championship. Steve needs those calories, for he is just entering the adolescent growth spurt and is at his peak for calorie need. The breakfasts Steve chose weren't always balanced, but he always ate something in the early-morning hours, which probably gave him added alertness and endurance for late-morning classes. His snack choices were generally wise, too, with fruit being a favorite item. Steve, the "problem eater," wins the overall family-nutrition award hands down!

# Cissie's Seven-Day Dietary Intake Record

**Age:** 13 years   **Weight:** 120 lbs (54.5 kg)   **Height:** 5'3" (161 cm)

## Saturday

| | |
|---|---|
| French toast (2) | 8:30 A.M. |
| Hot chocolate | |
| Raisin Bran with milk | 2:30 P.M. |
| Turkey | 6:30 |
| Potatoes (2 helpings) | |
| Stuffing (2 helpings) | |
| Water (2 cups) | |

## Sunday

| | |
|---|---|
| French toast (2 pieces) | 8:30 A.M. |
| Orange juice | |
| Hot chocolate | |
| Turkey sandwich | 2:30 P.M. |
| Turkey sandwich | 6:00 |
| Chips | |
| Ice tea | |
| Licorice (lots) | |
| Cake roll (2 pieces) | |

## Monday

| | |
|---|---|
| Hot chocolate | 7:25 A.M. |
| Vegetable soup | 12:30 P.M. |
| Cake | |
| Chocolate milk | |
| Turkey | 6:00 |
| Pan cookies (3) | |
| Mashed potatoes (2 helpings) | |

## Tuesday

| | |
|---|---|
| Hot chocolate | 7:25 A.M. |
| Pizza | 12:30 P.M. |
| Chocolate milk | |
| Cookie | |
| Meatloaf | 6:00 |
| Buns (2) | |
| Iced tea | |
| Ice cream | |
| Bananas (2) | |

## Wednesday

| | |
|---|---|
| Hot chocolate | 7:20 A.M. |
| Chili | 12:30 P.M. |
| Rice | |
| Milk | |
| Cake | |
| Beef stroganoff | 6:00 |
| Water | |
| Bun with honey | |
| Pan cookies (4) | |

## Thursday

| | |
|---|---|
| Hot chocolate | 7:20 A.M. |
| Noodles | 12:30 P.M. |
| Milk | |
| Cookie | |
| Pan cookies (2) | 4:00 |
| Meat loaf | 6:00 |
| Tater Tots (2) | |
| Water | |
| Licorice (handful) | |

## Friday

| | |
|---|---|
| Hot chocolate | 7:20 A.M. |
| Hamburger | 12:30 P.M. |
| Root beer | |
| Grilled cheese sandwich | 6:00 |
| Water | |
| Roll | |

## Computer Analysis (% of RDA)

| | |
|---|---:|
| Calories | 64 |
| Protein | 149 |
| Calcium | 59 |
| Iron | 64 |
| Vitamin A | 58 |
| Thiamin | 50 |
| Riboflavin | 108 |
| Niacin | 84 |
| Vitamin C | 52 |

Though Cissie worries about getting too fat, her calorie intake is only 64 percent of the 1974 RDA, and since her height and weight percentiles are equal, her weight is "ideal" for her height. The "puppy fat" deposits normal for a thirteen-year-old girl are the only evidences of fat, but Cissie worries about her appearance. This is typical, since the slightest evidence of extra pounds usually causes a teenage girl great dismay. Part of her problem is hearing shorter girls with lighter bone structure complain about weighing 105 or 106 pounds. Such conversations make Cissie overly sensitive to her 120-pound weight. Actually, should overweight ever become a problem for Cissie, it will probably be due to her preference for breads, starchy vegetables, and candies over other vegetables and fruits. Adding a variety of vegetables and fruits to her diet should increase Cissie's less-than-optimum vitamin-A and C intakes and decrease the likelihood of deficiencies in nutrients for which no RDAs have yet been established. Her low calcium intake could be improved by the addition of more dairy products to her diet. Since adequate calcium stores will be especially important to Cissie in later years, should she begin a family, adequate intake during the rapid-growth years should be her goal now.

Adding more red meats to her diet would help Cissie move her iron levels upward. The slight boost in iron will become even more important as her iron needs continue to increase throughout the childbearing years. Replacing white bread with whole-grain products could increase Cissie's vitamin-E intake. Whole grains should also help her reach two-thirds of the RDA for calories and some other nutrients.

## Nora's Seven-Day Dietary Intake Record

**Age:** 12 years   **Weight:** 101 lbs (45.9 kg)   **Height:** 5' ½" (155.1 cm)

### Saturday

| | |
|---|---|
| Cereal | 6:45 A.M. |
| Apple | |
| Peanut-butter-and-honey sandwich | 12:30 P.M. |
| Orange | |
| Soft drink | |
| Turkey | 6:30 |
| Stuffing (2 helpings) | |
| Mashed potatoes (2 helpings) | |
| Carrots and peas | |
| Milk (2 glasses) | |
| Red licorice (3 handfuls) | 9:00 |

### Sunday

| | |
|---|---|
| French toast | 8:00 A.M. |
| Orange juice | |
| Cocoa | |
| Peanut-butter-and-honey sandwich | 2:00 P.M. |
| Potato chips | |
| Turkey sandwich | 6:00 |
| Iced tea (3 glasses) | |
| Tortilla chips (4 handfuls) | |
| Cake (3 pieces) | 6:20 |
| Soft drink | |
| Milk | 7:30 |

### Monday

| | |
|---|---|
| Orange | 7:30 A.M. |
| Vegetable soup | 11:30 |
| Peaches (3) | |
| Cake | |
| Milk | |
| Roll | |
| Turkey | 6:00 P.M. |
| Mashed potatoes | |
| Peas and carrots | |
| Popcorn (½ bowl) | 9:00 P.M. |

### Tuesday

| | |
|---|---|
| Pizza | 11:30 A.M. |
| Green beans | |
| Roll | |
| Milk | |
| Potato chips (handful) | 4:10 P.M. |
| Alphabet soup | 7:15 |
| Sea biscuits (2) | |
| Ice cream | 7:40 |

### Wednesday

| | |
|---|---|
| Rice with chili | 11:30 A.M. |
| Cake roll | |
| Milk | |
| King Vitamin cereal (2 bowls) | 4:10 P.M. |
| Milk | |
| Beef stroganoff (small serving) | 6:30 |
| Peas | |
| Chocolate chip cookies (3) | 8:30 |

### Thursday

| | |
|---|---|
| King Vitamin cereal (2) | 7:30 A.M. |
| Orange juice | |
| Cookie | 11:30 |
| Roll | |
| Chocolate milk | |
| Tater Tots (3 helpings) | 6:30 P.M. |
| Peas | |
| Milk | |
| Chocolate chip cookies (2) | |
| Sunflower seeds (½ bag) | |
| Red licorice (4 handfuls) | 8:30 |

### Friday

| | |
|---|---|
| Milk | |
| King Vitamin cereal (2) | 7:30 A.M. |
| Pizza bread | 11:30 |
| Chocolate milk | |
| Tomato soup | 6:15 P.M. |
| Cheese and ham sandwich | |
| Soft drink | 8:00 |
| Crunchios (2 handfuls) | |

| Computer Analysis (% of RDA) | |
| --- | --- |
| Calories | 72 |
| Protein | 131 |
| Calcium | 70 |
| Iron | 48 |
| Vitamin A | 156 |
| Thiamin | 87 |
| Riboflavin | 112 |
| Niacin | 86 |
| Vitamin C | 147 |

Nora's calorie intake is over two-thirds of the RDA, and all her nutrient intakes except iron are adequate to excellent. By eating more whole grains, meats, and green leafy vegetables, she could bring her intake of this nutrient up to desired levels.

Consumption of whole grains could improve nutrient intake levels for the entire family, and since calorie levels for these teens are not excessive, adding high-quality breads to the diet would not be likely to lead to obesity. Upon hearing this news, Cissie, who enjoys cooking, learned to bake whole-grain breads and rolls. Nora, not to be outdone, began to experiment with cheese-and-yogurt dips for afternoon vegetable snacks. In this way, calcium, vitamin A, and B-complex vitamins became available for hungry after-school hours. With these simple alterations, plus more attention to iron-rich foods, the borderline areas of the family's teen diets should be improved.

How did these teens develop the eating habits revealed in the food diaries? Lest this family's nutrition story seem to be based on long years of conscientious attention to diet and exercise, a few facts should be examined. The family was chosen as a typical upper-middle-class family whose food habits might provide interesting insights into the actual menus of real teenagers, insights which cannot always be gained from the study of a thousand statistically "average" teen diets. None of the background information which follows was known to the interviewer at the time the teenagers were asked to keep food records.

From birth to the teen years, family eating habits developed more on the basis of traditions passed down from past generations than on the basis of formal nutrition education. Since family tradition supported breast-feeding, these six youngsters were all nursed until the age of six months. The mother relied on the advice of her mother and her doctor, reading no publications on breast-feeding and attending no supportive group meetings for nursing mothers. Though she was puzzled by an interviewer's use of the term *let-down reflex,* this breast-feeding mother apparently had no need for a scientific explanation of what her body took care of on its own.

By breast-feeding her infants in the 1950s and 1960s, this mother was ahead of her time. Most doctors were telling their patients that bottle-feeding offered all the advantages of breast-feeding, plus added convenience. As we noted in an earlier chapter, doctors today realize that breast-feeding can offer many advantages over formula-feeding and are encouraging their patients to use nature's way of infant feeding. In the area of introduction of solids, this mother followed the advice of her physician, advice which followed the trend of those years but contradicts current advice. She introduced solids very early—at one to two weeks of age—and was feeding cereals, fruits, vegetables, and meats by six months. Fortunately, none of the children suffered from food allergies and none became obese. All six enjoyed healthy infancies.

Food intakes for the children during the preschool and elementary years were probably quite adequate, an assumption based on the long-term excellent growth and development and excellent medical and dental health records of each child, and on the academic and athletic achievements of various siblings. Adequate exercise was a way of life from their early years, since those years were spent in a temperate climate in which the children were free to spend many hours playing in a large backyard. Since the parents enjoyed physical activities and involved their children in family sports, hiking, and swimming activities from early childhood, the children's activity levels were fairly high. Even now, when many families have given up trying to get even two children together for a family outing, this family usually spends one or two summer Sundays a month on mountain hikes. There is nothing mandatory about participation in such outings, yet the teens seldom miss a family hike.

In summary, adequate nutrition has been a natural happening, not a practiced art, for this family. No guidebook was followed, no nutrition courses studied. The family fared well primarily because both parents had been brought up in families with good eating habits, although these habits were also based only on tradition. The parents' scientific knowledge of nutrition was minimal. Though she was college-educated, the mother never took a high-school or college home-economics course and was surprised to learn such nutritional basics as the facts that eggs are an excellent source of protein, calcium can be obtained through cheese as well as milk, and carrots are a good source of vitamin A.

Family meals were probably well balanced because they were varied. A number of foods from each of the major food groups were included in meals and snacks because the family enjoyed these foods, not because the foods were supposed to be "good for the family." However, since the father grew up in a "meat-and-potatoes" setting, the mother tended not to buy and prepare many of the vegetables he did not care for. Lack of variety in this one food group is evident in the current dietary preferences of the teenagers. Consumption of licorice, the father's favorite candy, is further evidence of the impact a father's eating habits can have upon the food choices of his children. Finally, up until the time when five of the six children agreed to keep seven-day food diaries, no family discussions of nutrition had been held and none of the children had taken a home-economics food or nutrition course.

The fact that these teens are making any attempt at all to change deep-seated eating habits should be encouraging to parents who realize that their own children's meals and snacks are not always adequate. Certainly, setting optimum nutrition patterns from birth is easier than altering unsatisfactory patterns during elementary and teen years. However, parents who don't expect too much and who are able to be content with small, day-to-day changes will find that the diets of children of any age can be improved. By making nutritious snack items available, by setting a good example through their own food choices, and by offering gentle guidance rather than heavy-handed insistence, parents can help children move toward meals and snacks which offer optimum nutrition for now and for the years ahead.

# Appendix A:
# Minimum Exchanges Chart;
# Six Exchange Lists;
# Recipe Conversion Chart

As noted earlier, the key to balance is variety. Not only should one choose foods from all the major food groups, but one should also work for variety *within* each food group. The chart on page 000 indicates the minimum number of exchanges from each food group which should be included in any day's dietary intake. The chart gives serving sizes appropriate for children from birth through three years, and the food lists which follow the chart indicate serving sizes appropriate for adults and older children. The food lists also indicate the primary nutrients supplied by the various foods.

If you plan meals that include a wide variety of items from the six food groups represented on the exchange lists, all family members should obtain adequate protein, carbohydrate, fat, vitamins, minerals, and fiber over a seven-day period. Remember, including only the minimum amounts of these foods in the diet will not allow you to meet the full calorie (energy) needs of each family member. Adding extra portions of items from the first five lists is an ideal way to increase calories to the desired level, since foods from these lists supply valuable nutrients as well as energy.

Since most meals include dishes which combine items from several lists, a recipe conversion chart has been included, which makes it easy for you to determine exchange values for your own recipes. Exchanges per serving are given for all recipes included in Appendix C of this book. You should remember that exchange lists and the Minimum Exchanges Chart are intended to be used as *guidelines,* not as absolutes. Relax and enjoy adding variety to your family's diet.

## Family Guide to Minimum Exchanges from Six Major Food Groups

| Age (in years) | Food Groups[1] | | | | | |
|---|---|---|---|---|---|---|
| | Milk[2] | Vegetable[3] | Fruit[4] | Bread and Cereal | Meat[5] (oz) | Fat[6] |
| $1/2$–1 | 2–3 (16–24 oz) | $1/2$–1 (4–8 tbsp) | $1/2$–1 (4–8 tbsp) | $1/2$–1 (4–8 tbsp) | 2 | As |
| 1–3 | 3 (24 oz) | 1 (8 tbsp) | 1 (8 tbsp) | 2 (16 tbsp) | 3 | needed |
| 4–6 | 3 | 2 | 2 | 3 | 4 | to |
| 7–10 | 3 | 2 | 2 | 4 | 4–5 | meet |
| 11–14 | 4+ | 2 | 2 | 4 | 6 | calorie |
| 15–18 | 4+ | 2 | 2 | 4 | 6 | require-ments |

NOTE: To these minimums, one must add extra portions in order to reach recommended caloric levels each day. Once these minimums have been met, added calories may come from any of the above food groups or from the exchange lists for simple carbohydrates or prepared foods.

The recipes given in this book are exchange-keyed to make it easier to determine the exchanges gained from casseroles, breads, desserts, or other dishes. A chart for converting other recipes to exchanges is included in Appendix A.

[1]On this chart, all portions are expressed as *adult*-sized exchanges (see exchange lists). Children's portion sizes are 1 to 2 tablespoons for each year of age to age three; for children under three years of age the minimum tablespoons recommended per day are indicated in the chart, along with the equivalent number of adult-sized portions.

[2]Teens need to add more dairy products such as puddings, ice cream, and cheeses, in order to keep calcium levels high during rapid-growth years.

[3]Include two or three vitamin A vegetables each week. Do not depend on white (head) lettuce to supply vitamin A or folic acid in significant amounts; romaine, red leaf, and green leaf lettuce are all higher in these nutrients than head lettuce and contribute significant fiber.

[4]Include one vitamin C fruit or vegetable each day. Also include dried fruits to help raise iron levels.

[5]Include pork at least once a week for thiamin value. Rotate meats, including chicken, pork, beef, fish, as often as possible in the diet. This should insure iron and other mineral intake of sufficient quantity, plus intake of vitamins such as $B_6$. Peanut butter or peanuts can add $B_6$ to the diet.

[6]Include fat as a natural part of the diet in amounts suited to help meet calorie needs. If desired, polyunsaturated fats may be used to avoid excessive cholesterol intake.

# Exchange Lists

## Milk Exchanges

These exchange lists have been adapted from *Exchange Lists for Meal Planning*, a booklet prepared by Committees of the American Diabetes Association, Inc. and the American Dietetic Association in cooperation with the National Institute of Arthritis, Metabolism, and Digestive Diseases and the National Heart and Lung Institute, National Institute of Health, Public Health Service, U.S. Department of Health, Education and Welfare. Though the lists in *Exchange Lists for Meal Planning* were devised for diabetics and others with health problems, OUR ADAPTATIONS OF THE LISTS ARE NOT SUITABLE FOR USE BY DIABETICS because they include many items which diabetics must usually avoid. Our modified version of these lists is intended to give a realistic picture of the foods available for consumption by nondiabetic persons who wish to have a varied, well-balanced diet.

Milk products, humans' leading source of calcium, also provide protein, phosphorus, vitamin A, magnesium, and some B-complex vitamins (including riboflavin and $B_{12}$). Fortified milk products provide vitamin D. Fortified nonfat and 2-percent milk products provide the above nutrients at a lower calorie cost than do whole-milk products.

|  | Amount Equal To One Exchange |
|---|---|
| **A. Nonfat fortified** | |
| Skim or nonfat | 1 cup |
| Powdered | ⅓ cup powder |
| Canned evaporated skim | ½ cup |
| Skim-milk buttermilk | 1 cup |
| Skim-milk yogurt (plain) | 1 cup |
| **B. Low-fat fortified** | |
| 1% | 1 cup |
| 2% | 1 cup |
| 2% yogurt (plain) | 1 cup |
| 2% chocolate milk (commercial) | 1 cup |
| **C. Whole** | |
| Whole canned evaporated milk | ½ cup |
| Buttermilk | 1 cup |
| Yogurt (plain) | 1 cup |
| Malted milk* | 1 cup |
| Cocoa* | 1 cup |

NOTE: Except for nonfat milk products, milk products provide fat exchanges as well as milk exchanges: 1-percent products, add ½ fat exchange; 2-percent products, add 1 fat exchange; whole-milk products, add 2 fat exchanges.

*Contains sugar.

## Vegetable Exchanges

Leafy green vegetables contain vitamins A and E, and pyridoxine, folic acid, and riboflavin. They also contain magnesium and potassium. Other vegetables supply varied amounts of B-complex vitamins, vitamin E, magnesium, and phosphorus. Carrots and summer squash are rich sources of vitamin A.

**Each exchange equals ½ cup, cooked.**

Alfalfa sprouts
Artichoke
Asparagus*
Bamboo shoots
Bean sprouts
Beets
Bok choy*
Broccoli*
Brussels sprouts*
Burdock root
Cabbage*
Carrots
Cauliflower
Celery
Collard greens*
Cucumbers
Dandelion greens*
Eggplant
Kale*

Mushrooms
Mustard greens*
Nori seaweed
Okra
Onion
Peppers (green, red, chili)*
Rhubarb
Rutabaga
Sauerkraut
Scallions (green onions)
Spinach*
String beans (yellow or green)
Summer squash
Swiss chard*
Tomatoes and tomato juice*
Turnip greens*
Turnips
Vegetable juice cocktail*
Zucchini squash

*High vitamin C content.

**The following vegetables may be eaten raw as desired.**

Chicory
Chinese cabbage
Endive
Escarole

Lettuce (red leaf, green leaf, iceberg, romaine)
Parsley
Radishes
Watercress

NOTE: Starchy vegetables are found in the bread exchange list.

## Fruit Exchanges

Fruits may be used fresh, frozen, canned, dried, cooked or raw, as long as no sugar is added. Fruits provide significant amounts of vitamins, minerals, and fiber. Apricots, bananas, berries, grapefruit, grapefruit juice, mangoes, cantaloupes, honeydews, nectarines, oranges, orange juice, and peaches are all rich in potassium. Oranges, orange juice, and cantaloupe provide folic acid. The vitamin-A-rich fruits are marked with an asterisk. Vitamin-C-rich fruits appear in the second list given.

**One exchange equals the serving size shown.**

A.  **General fruits and juices**
    Apple, 1 small
    Applesauce (unsweetened), ½
        cup
    Apricots (fresh),† 2 medium
    Apricots (dried),† 4 halves
    Banana, ½ small
    Berries: blackberries, ½ cup;
        blueberries, ½ cup
    Cherries, 10 large
    Cranberries, 1 cup
    Dates, 2 (1 cup = 12 fruit
        exchanges)
    Figs (fresh or dried), 1
    Grapes, 12
    Peach, † 1 medium
    Pear, 1 small
    Persimmon (native),† 1 medium
    Pineapple, ½ cup
    Plums, 2 medium
    Prunes, 2 medium
    Raisins, 2 tablespoons (1 cup =
        8 fruit exchanges)
    Apple cider, ⅓ cup
    Apple juice, ⅓ cup
    Grape juice, ¼ cup
    Pineapple juice, ⅓ cup
    Prune juice, ¼ cup

B.  **Vitamin-C-rich fruits and juices**
    Raspberries, ½ cup
    Strawberries, ¾ cup
    Grapefruit, ½
    Guava, ¼ medium
    Mango,† ½ small
    Cantaloupe,† ¼ small
    Honeydew, ⅛ medium
    Nectarine,† 1 small
    Orange, 1 small
    Papaya, ¾ cup
    Tangerine, 1 medium
    Grapefruit juice, ½ cup
    Orange juice, ½ cup
    Watermelon, 1 cup

†High vitamin A content

# Breads and Starchy Vegetables

Relatively high in carbohydrates, most items on this list are an excellent source of energy. Moderate reduction of high-carbohydrate foods enables one to lower total calorie load without risking loss of nutritional balance. Whenever possible, choose to retain items high in vitamins, minerals and protein and avoid only those "empty-calorie" carbohydrates which offer little more than energy. One exchange is equal to the portion size shown. Breads and cereals supply protein, thiamin, vitamin E, niacin, riboflavin, and iron and other trace minerals.

| | Amount Equal To One Exchange |
|---|---|
| **A.  Bread** | |
| Bagel | ½ |
| Dried bread crumbs | 3 tablespoons |
| English muffin | ½ small |
| French | 1 slice |
| Frankfurter roll | ½ |
| Hamburger roll | ½ |
| Italian | 1 slice |
| Plain roll | 1 |
| Pumpernickel | 1 slice |
| Raisin | 1 slice |
| Rye | 1 slice |
| Tortilla | 1, 6" |
| White | 1 slice |
| Whole wheat | 1 slice |
| **B.  Cereal** | |
| Barley (cooked) | ½ cup |
| Bran flakes | ½ cup |
| Cereal, ready to eat, unsweetened | ¾ cup |
| Cereal, puffed, unsweetened | 1 cup |
| Cornmeal (dry) | 2 tablespoons |
| Farina (cooked) | ½ cup |
| Flour* | 2 ½ tablespoons |
| Grits (cooked) | ½ cup |
| Pasta (cooked): macaroni, noodles, spaghetti | ½ cup |
| Popcorn (popped, no fat added) | 3 cups |
| Rice (cooked) | ½ cup |
| Wheat germ | ¼ cup |

*FLOUR: For recipe conversion, the following flour exchanges are useful. Use the same figures for plain, whole-wheat, rye, or other flour:

2 ½ tablespoons = 1 bread exchange
8 tablespoons = ½ cup = 3.2 bread exchanges
16 tablespoons = 1 cup = 6.4 bread exchanges

### C. Crackers

| | |
|---|---|
| Arrowroot | 3 |
| Graham, 2 ½" square | 2 |
| Matzoh, 4" x 6" | ½ |
| Oyster | 20 |
| Pretzels, 3 ½" x 1/8" | 25 |
| Rye wafers, 2" x 3 ½" | 3 |
| Saltines | 6 |
| Soda, 2 ½" square | 4 |

### D. Vegetables (cooked)

| | |
|---|---|
| Baked beans (canned) | ¼ cup |
| Corn | ⅓ cup |
| Corn on cob | 1 small |
| Dried beans | ½ cup |
| Dried lentils | ½ cup |
| Dried peas | ½ cup |
| Lima beans | ½ cup |
| Parsnips | ⅔ cup |
| Peas, green (canned or frozen) | ½ cup |
| Potato, sweet | ¼ cup |
| Potato, white | 1 small |
| Potato, mashed | ½ cup |
| Pumpkin | ¾ cup |
| Soybeans | ½ cup |
| Winter squash (acorn or butternut) | ½ cup |
| Yam | ¼ cup |

## Meat Exchanges

All three meat categories contain foods that are good sources of protein. Many of the animal-origin foods on the list also provide significant amounts of iron, zinc, and several B-complex vitamins. Group A, lean meats, is recommended for those wishing to avoid high cholesterol levels. Peanut butter, a vegetable food from List B, is high in fat, yet contains no cholesterol.

| | Amount Equal To One Exchange |
|---|---|
| **A. Lean meat** | |
| Beef: baby beef (very lean), chipped beef, chuck, flank steak, tenderloin, plate ribs, plate skirt steak, round (bottom or top), rump (all cuts), spare ribs, tripe | 1 ounce |
| Lamb: leg, rib, sirloin, loin (roast and chops), shank, shoulder | 1 ounce |
| Pork: leg (whole rump, center shank), ham (smoked center slice) | 1 ounce |

| | |
|---|---|
| Veal: leg, loin, rib, shank, shoulder, cutlets | 1 ounce |
| Poultry: chicken, turkey, Cornish hen, guinea hen, pheasant (all without skin) | 1 ounce |
| Fish: fresh, frozen, or canned salmon, tuna, mackerel | 1 ounce |
| Crab, lobster | ¼ cup |
| Clams, oysters, scallops, shrimp | 1 ounce or 5 pieces |
| Sardines (drained) | 3 |
| Cheese with less than 5% butterfat* | 1 ounce |
| Cottage cheese, dry and 2% butterfat* | ¼ cup |
| Dried beans and peas (omit one bread exchange) | ½ cup |

**B.  Medium-fat meat**

| | |
|---|---|
| Beef: ground (15% fat), corned beef (canned), ribeye, round (ground commercial) | 1 ounce |
| Pork: loin (all cuts tenderloin), shoulder arm (picnic), shoulder blade, Boston butt, Canadian bacon, boiled ham | 1 ounce |
| Variety meats: Liver, heart, kidney, sweetbreads (high in cholesterol) | 1 ounce |
| Cheese: cottage (creamed) | ¼ cup |
| Mozzarella, ricotta, farmer's cheese, Neufchatel | 1 ounce |
| Parmesan* | 3 tablespoons |
| Eggs (high in cholesterol) | 1 |
| Peanut butter (omit two extra fat exchanges) | 2 tablespoons |

**C.  High-fat meat**

| | |
|---|---|
| Beef: brisket, corned beef (brisket), ground beef (about 20% fat), hamburger (commercial), chuck (ground commercial), roast (rib), steaks (club and rib) | 1 ounce |
| Lamb: breast | 1 ounce |
| Pork: spare ribs, loin (back ribs), pork (ground), country-style ham, deviled ham** | 1 ounce |
| Veal: breast | 1 ounce |
| Poultry: capon, duck (domestic), goose | 1 ounce |
| Cheese: cheddar types* | 1 ounce |
| Cold cuts: ½" x 1/8" slice | 4 |
| Frankfurter | 1 small |

NOTE:  For each exchange used from list B, one-half fat exchange will also be used. For each exchange used from list C, one fat exchange will also be used.

*Some cheeses are high in calcium and can count toward daily calcium quotas, but they do not supply iron.

**Bacon is listed on the fat-exchange list.

## Fat Exchanges

Both animal and vegetable fats are concentrated calorie sources and should be used in moderation. Those persons wishing to avoid high cholesterol intakes should avoid saturated fats. Polyunsaturated fats have been associated with decreases in blood cholesterol for some persons.

|  | Amount equal to one exchange |
|---|---|
| **A.  Polyunsaturated fats** | |
| Margarine*: soft, tub, or stick (made with corn, cottonseed, safflower, soy, or sunflower oil) | 1 teaspoon |
| Oil: corn, cottonseed, safflower, soy, sunflower | 1 teaspoon |
| Walnuts ( ½ cup = 16 fat) | 6 small |
| Dressing: French, Italian (if made with corn, cottonseed, safflower, soy, or sunflower oil) | 1 tablespoon |
| Mayonnaise-type salad dressing (if made with corn, cottonseed, safflower, soy, or sunflower oil) | 2 teaspoons |
| Mayonnaise (if made with corn, cottonseed, safflower, soy, or sunflower oil) | 1 teaspoon |
| **B.  Monounsaturated fats** | |
| Avocado (4″ diameter) | ⅛ |
| Oil, olive or peanut | 1 teaspoon |
| Olives | 5 small |
| Almonds ( ½ cup = 15 fat) | 10 whole |
| Pecans ( ½ cup = 17 fat) | 2 large |
| Peanuts ( ½ cup = 15 fat); Spanish, | 20 whole |
| Virginia | 19 whole |
| Sesame seeds ( ½ cup = 14 fat exchanges) | 1 tablespoon |
| Other nuts | 6 small |

*For recipe conversion the following margarine or butter exchanges are useful:
⅛ stick = 1 tablespoon = 3 fat exchanges
¼ stick = ⅛ cup = 3 tablespoons = 6 fat exchanges
½ stick = ¼ cup = 4 tablespoons = 12 fat exchanges
⅔ stock = ⅓ cup = 5½ tablespoons = 16½ fat exchanges
¼ pound = 1 stick = ½ cup = 8 tablespoons = 24 fat exchanges
½ pound = 2 sticks = 1 cup = 16 tablespoons = 48 fat exchanges

| **C.  Saturated fats** | |
|---|---|
| Margarine, regular stick (made from animal fat) | 1 teaspoon |
| Butter | 1 teaspoon |
| Bacon fat | 1 teaspoon |
| Bacon, crisp-fried | 1 strip |
| Coconut oil** | 2–3 tablespoons |
| Cream, light | 2 tablespoons |
| Cream, sour | 2 tablespoons |
| Cream, heavy | 1 tablespoon |
| Cream cheese | 1 tablespoon |
| Nondairy creamers** | 5 tablespoons |
| Salt pork | 5 tablespoons |
| Lard | 1 teaspoon |

**Anything made with coconut oil (including most nondairy creamers) is high in saturated fats.

## Free Exchanges

In addition to the items included in the six exchange lists above, a number of other items may be included in daily snacks and menus without restriction. These free exchanges include certain foods and almost all spices. Overly salty items on this list, such as pickles, should be avoided by those who are attempting to restrict salt intakes.

**A.  Beverages and foods**
Coffee
Tea
Club soda
Clear broth
Clam juice
Bouillon (nonfat)
Low-cal soft drinks
Lemon
Unsweetened gelatin
Unsweetened cranberries
Unsweetened pickles

**B.  Spices and flavorings**
Salt
Pepper
Herbs
Dry mustard
Chili powder
Cacao (dry)
Red or white horseradish
Lemon and lime juice
Soy sauce
Worcestershire sauce
Dehydrated onion flakes
Pure or natural extracts (lemon, maple, vanilla)

## Prepared Foods

Several commonly used prepared foods are shown below. The indicated serving size of these foods is equal to the number and type of exchanges shown. Many items have "bread" exchanges listed which are, in reality, exchanges representing simple sugars or syrups, not breads. These items should not be counted upon to fill daily bread exchange totals. They supply energy, but none of the nutrients of breads or starchy vegetables.

| FOOD | SERVING SIZE | EXCHANGE |
|---|---|---|
| **A.  Breads** | | |
| Banana | 1 slice, 3" x 3" x ½" | 1 ½ bread, 1 fat |
| Biscuit | 1, 2" diameter | 1 bread, 1 fat |
| Corn | 1 slice, 2" x 2" x 1" | 1 bread, 1 fat |
| Corn muffin | 1, 2" diameter | 1 bread, 1 fat |
| Crackers (round butter type) | 5 | 1 bread, 1 fat |
| Croutons (no fat added) | 1 cup | 1 bread |
| Doughnuts (plain) | 1 | 1 bread, 1 fat |
| Muffin | | |
|   Plain blueberry | 1, average size | 1 bread, 1 fat |
| Pancakes | 1, 5" x ½" | 1 bread, 1 fat |

| | | |
|---|---|---|
| Raisin | 1 slice | 1 bread |
| Taco shell | | |
|     Corn, ready-to-eat | 1, 5 ½″ diameter | 1 bread, 1 fat |
|     Corn, not fried | 1, 6″ diameter | 1 bread |
|     Flour, not fried | 1, 7″ diameter | 1 bread, 1 fat |
| Waffles | 1, 5″ x ½″ | 1 bread, 1 fat |

**B.  Desserts**

| | | |
|---|---|---|
| Cake | | |
|     Angel, no icing | 1 ½″ slice | 1 bread |
|     Cupcake, no icing | 1 | 1 ½ bread, 1 fat |
|     Mix, no icing | 1 ½″ slice | 1 ¼ bread, ½ fat |
|     Pound, no icing | 1 piece, 3″ x 3″ x ½″ | 1 bread, 1 fat |
|     Sponge, no icing | 1 piece, 1 ½″ | 1 bread |
| Cookies (high in fruit, nuts, and whole grains and low in sugar) | | |
|     Fig newton | 2 average | 1 ½ bread |
|     Ginger snaps | 5 small | 1 bread |
|     Oatmeal-raisin | 2 small | 1 ½ bread |
|     Peanut butter | 2 small | 1 bread, 1 fat |
|     Chocolate chip | 2 small | 1 ½ bread |
|     Date cookies | 2 small | 1 ½ bread |
| Ice cream | ⅓ cup | 1 bread, 1 ½ fat |
| Piecrust (shell only) | | |
|     Graham-cracker | ⅛ of 9″ pie | ½ bread, 1 ½ fat |
|     Pastry | ⅛ of 9″ pie | ½ bread, 1 fat |
| Pudding (regular, cooked, and instant) | | |
|     Whole-milk | ½ cup | 1 ½ bread, ½ milk, 1 fat |
|     Skim-milk | ½ cup | 1 ½ bread, ½ milk |
| Sherbet | ¼ cup | 1 bread |
| Whipped topping | | |
|     (2% milk) | 5 tablespoons | 1 fat, ⅕ 2% milk |

**C.  Soups, sauces, snacks**

| | | |
|---|---|---|
| Cheese sauce | ¼ cup | ½ bread, ½ whole milk, 1 ½ fat |
| Gravy (made with | | |
|     flour) | 2 tablespoons | 1 fat |
| Hollandaise sauce | ¼ cup | ½ meat, 3 fat |
| Tartar sauce | 1 tablespoon | 2 fat |
| White sauce | 2 tablespoons | 1 fat |
| Corn chips | 15 | 1 bread, 2 fat |
| Potato chips | 15 | 1 bread, 2 fat |
| French fries | 8, 2″ to 3 ½″ long | 1 bread, 1 fat |
| Cheddar-cheese soup | | |
|     (diluted) | 1 cup | ¼ bread, ½ whole milk |

| | | |
|---|---|---|
| Cheddar-cheese soup (undiluted) | 1 10¾-ounce can | ¾ bread, 1 ¼ whole milk, 2 ½ fat |
| Cream-of-celery soup (diluted)* | 1 cup | ½ bread, 1 fat |
| Cream-of-celery soup (undiluted) | 1 10¾-ounce can | 1 bread, 2 ½ fat |
| Cream-of-chicken soup (diluted) | 1 cup | ½ bread, 1 fat |
| Cream-of-chicken soup (undiluted) | 1 10¾-ounce can | 1 bread, 2 ½ fat |
| Cream-of-mushroom soup (diluted) | 1 cup | ½ bread, 2 fat |
| Cream-of-mushroom soup (undiluted) | 1 10¾-ounce can | 2 bread, 4 fat |
| Tomato soup (diluted) | 1 cup | 1 bread, ½ fat |
| Tomato soup (undiluted) | 1 10¾-ounce can | 2 ½ bread, 1 ¼ fat |

*Diluted means half soup, half water.

## Simple Carbohydrates

The following items provide energy but have little nutritional value. Honey or brown sugar may be substituted for white sugar to achieve variety of flavor, but there is no nutritional advantage to such substitution. Molasses contains a significant amount of iron. The simple carbohydrate exchanges are expressed as breads, yet they should *not* be exchanged for one of the minimum number of bread exchanges recommended for each age group. They may count as additional breads beyond the minimum number of recommended bread exchanges.

| CARBOHYDRATE | EXCHANGE |
|---|---|
| Jam or jelly | 1 tablespoon = ¾ bread exchange |
| Molasses | 1 tablespoon = ½ bread exchange |
| | 1 cup = 8 bread exchanges |
| Table syrups (corn syrup, maple syrup, etc.) | 1 tablespoon = 1 bread exchange |
| | 1 cup = 8 bread exchanges |
| Sugar (white, granulated, or brown) | 1 tablespoon = ⅔ bread exchange |
| | 1 cup = 11 bread exchanges |
| Sugar (powdered) | 1 cup = 6 ½ bread exchanges |
| Honey | 1 tablespoon = ⅔ bread exchange |
| | 1 cup = 10 bread exchanges |

# Converting Recipes to Exchange Values

The number of cookbooks which include exchange values for each recipe has grown, but these books are often limited to recipes especially devised for persons with health problems such as diabetes. Normal family menus may include occasional high-carbohydrate treats not suitable for diabetics. Recipes for these treats may be easily converted to exchanges by following the instructions below. Once a recipe has been exchanged, the exchanges may be written into the cookbook or onto the recipe card to be ready for use in the future. Soon a family will build a sizeable list of exchange-notated recipes.

The conversion chart which follows gives four basic steps for converting recipes to exchange values, plus a sample recipe conversion. A table of portion equivalents for meats is included, since meat portions often cannot be conveniently weighed. Exchange values for many soups and sauces commonly used in recipes have already been given in the prepared-foods exchange list. When in doubt, make an intelligent guess based on available data.

## Portion Equivalents and Measures

3 ounces of cooked meat (3 meat exchanges) equal:
   4 ounces of lean raw meat or fish without skin or bone
   ¾ cup cooked, flaked, or diced meat, poultry or fish
   2 slices dark or light cooked turkey, 4½″ x 2″ x ¼″ each
   ½ large chicken breast, cooked (without skin)
   1 chicken leg plus thigh, cooked (without skin)
   2 lean lamb chops (cooked) 3¾″ x 2″ x ¾″
   1 lean pork chop (cooked) 3¾″ x 2″ x ⅜″
2 ounces of cooked meat (2 meat exchanges) equal:
   1 serving veal, 2½″ x 3″ x ½″ (roasted or baked)
   1 hamburger patty, 2½″ x ½″
   5 1″ cubes of stew meat (raw)

## Conversion Chart of Recipes to Exchange Values

| | Step 1 | Step 2 | Step 3 | Step 4 |
|---|---|---|---|---|
| **Instructions** | List all ingredients for the chosen recipe. | To the right of this list note the exchange value of each ingredient. | Determine the number of portions that the recipe makes and divide each exchange by that number. | Consolidate the items (as shown below) to obtain exchange values for one portion of the recipe. |
| **Sample recipe conversion** | 3 medium chicken breasts, halved and skinned | 24 meat exchanges* | ÷ 6 = 4 lean-meat exchanges | 3 fat exchanges |
| | 6 strips bacon<br>1 jar dried beef (2½ ounces)<br>½ pint sour cream (8 ounces) | 6 fat exchanges<br>2½ lean-meat exchanges<br>8 fat exchanges | ÷ 6 = 1 fat exchange<br>÷ 6 = ½ lean-meat exchange | negligible bread exchange |
| | 1 can mushroom soup (undiluted) | 2 bread, 4 fat exchanges** | ÷ 6 = ⅓ bread, ⅔ fat exchange | 4½ lean-meat exchanges |

*Since the exchange value of meats and some vegetables is based on cooked amounts, you will need to adjust amounts by assuming that 1 pound of raw meat yields ¾ pound of cooked meat. For vegetables make adjustments only if there is a marked size increase or decrease after cooking. Since exact measurements are not crucial, using the chart of portion equivalents will make determining exchange values simpler.
**Items such as canned soups can be difficult to assess, unless one consults special exchange-list supplements found in relevant publications (see bibliography in Appendix D).

# Appendix B
# Menus for Well-fed Families

# Day One

**Breakfast**
Scrambled eggs with ham bits
Cinnamon toast
Orange juice
Milk

**Lunch**
Toasted Cheese on Whole-wheat Bread*
Fruit Salad*
Apple-Oatmeal Cookies*
Milk

**Dinner**
Shrimp Creole with Rice*
Chef's Salad*
French Bread*
Banana-Grape Dessert*
Milk or tea

# Day Two

**Breakfast**
Cornmeal Pancakes* with butter and syrup
Strawberries
Milk

**Lunch**
Hearty Beef-Vegetable Soup*
Crackers
Banana
Milk

**Dinner**
Whole-wheat Herb Pizza*
Applesauce Whip*
Milk or tea

*Indicates that recipe is given in the recipe section of this book, Appendix C.

# Day Three

**Breakfast**
  Blueberry-Lemon Muffins* with margarine
  Orange juice
  Milk

**Lunch**
  Choo-Choo Train Sandwich* (peanut
butter/vegetable/fruit)
  Grape Gelatin*
  Milk

**Dinner**
  Enchiladas Verdes (Green Enchilada Casserole)*
  Red Chili Enchiladas*
  Sopapillas with Honey*
  Milk or tea

# Day Four

**Breakfast**
  Granny's Granola*
  ½ Whole-wheat English Muffin*
  South American Cocoa*

**Lunch**
  Cheddar Cheese Soup*
  Garden Sandwich*
  Spiced Fruit*
  Milk

**Dinner**
  Hamburger pattie
  Alpine Rice* (or rice with butter)
  Veggies with Hot Cheddar Dip*
  Milk or tea

*Indicates that recipe is given in the recipe section of this book, Appendix C.

# Day Five

**Breakfast**
Toasted Cheese on Whole-wheat Bread*
Fruit cup (orange, grapefruit, banana, apples)
Milk

**Lunch**
Tomato Soup
Cheese-Bran Crackers*
Celery
Pumpkin Bread*
Milk

**Dinner**
Panhandle Steak*
Texas Pintos*
Sunshine Salad*
Missie's Southern Cornbread*
Milk or tea

# Day Six

**Breakfast**
Huevos Rancheros*
Orange sections
Milk

**Lunch**
Macaroni and cheese
Veggies (raw sticks of cauliflower, broccoli, carrots, celery)
Apple
Aunt Winnie's Date Delights*
Milk

**Dinner**
Chicken-Ham Lasagne*
Green salad
Whole-wheat Bread*
Milk

*Indicates that recipe is given in the recipe section of this book, Appendix C.

# Day Seven

**Breakfast**
 Strawberry-Orange Eye-opener*
 Seven-week Bran Muffin*

**Lunch**
 Breadless Sandwich*
 Carrot Bread*
 Milk

**Dinner**
 Turkey
 Mississippi Cornbread-Oyster Dressing*
 Giblet Gravy*
 Quick Cranberry Sauce*
 Green beans
 Spicy Sweet Potatoes*
 Mac's Mandarin Orange Salad*
 Milk or tea

*Indicates that recipe is given in the recipe section of this book, Appendix C.

# Appendix C:
# Recipes, Sack-Lunch Tips,
# Fun Food Ideas

## Metrics in the Kitchen

Within the next ten years, the United States will complete a planned conversion to the metric system of measurement. This will affect every aspect of measurement, including how our recipes are written and how our oven temperatures are gauged. It will probably be a while before we are measuring everything in metrics—you don't have to throw away your measuring cups —but as time goes on you will encounter more and more metric measurements.

We are including a conversion table for your information and convenience. While the ingredients for the recipes in this section are measured the "old-fashioned" way, for all baking temperatures we have supplied the Celsius (centigrade) equivalent in parentheses.

| When you know | multiply by | to get |
|---|---|---|
| Cups | 250 | milliliters (ml) |
| Fluid ounces | 30 | milliliters (ml) |
| Dry ounces | 28 | milliliters (ml) |
| Tablespoons | 15 | milliliters (ml) |
| Teaspoons | 5 | milliliters (ml) |
| Ounces | 28 | grams (g) |
| Pounds | 0.45 | kilograms (kg) |
| Degrees Fahrenheit: Subtract 32. Multiply new number by | 0.5555 | degrees Celsius (centigrade) |

### Temperature Changes Made Easy*

| Degrees Fahrenheit | Description of Oven Temperature | Degrees Celsius (centigrade) |
|---|---|---|
| 300 | slow | 150 |
| 325 | slow | 160 |
| 350 | moderate | 175 |
| 375 | moderate | 190 |
| 400 | hot | 200 |
| 425 | hot | 220 |
| 450 | very hot | 232 |
| 475 | very hot | 246 |

*Use Celsius (centigrade) temperatures only on stoves or ovens with controls given in Celsius. Most ovens in the United States will have controls given in Fahrenheit.

# MAIN DISHES

## Chicken-Ham Lasagna

1 medium onion, diced
1 tbsp. margarine
½ cup chopped celery
1 cup frozen broccoli
1 15-ounce can tomatoes
2 cups liquid (may be chicken broth or water)
1 4-ounce can mushrooms (drained)
2 cups diced, cooked chicken
2 cups diced, cooked ham
1 ½ tsp. oregano leaves
½ tsp basil leaves
½ tsp. ground rosemary
½ pound lasagna noodles (cooked and drained)
¼ pound Gouda cheese
¼ pound Parmesan cheese
1 pound Cheddar cheese, sliced

Preheat oven to 350 degrees (175 C). Stir-fry onions in margarine until transparent. Add celery and broccoli and stir-fry 5 to 10 minutes longer. Add can of tomatoes, liquid (broth or water), mushrooms, meats, and spices. Simmer 5 to 10 minutes. Arrange cooked, drained lasagna noodles on bottom of 9 x 13-inch pan. Cover with one layer of meat-vegetable mixture. Sprinkle half the Gouda and half the Parmesan over this mixture and top with half the Cheddar slices. Repeat layers, using same order. Bake for 20 to 25 minutes or until cheese is melted and lightly browned, and casserole is bubbling.

Servings: 12
Exchanges per serving: 4 ½ meat, 1 vegetable, ½ bread, 1 ½ fat

## Chinese Egg Rolls

½ pound plain pork sausage (no spices) *or* ½ pound beef or chicken, sliced very thin
½ pound shelled, uncooked shrimp
1 to 2 tbsp. whiskey or wine
2 tsp. salt or 3 tbsp. soy sauce
1 tsp. sesame oil
1 stalk celery, sliced paper thin
2 carrots, pared and finely grated
⅓ cup thinly sliced button mushrooms
½ pound fresh, crisp bean sprouts *or* one can sprouts, drained
1 unbeaten raw egg
1 beaten egg
30 to 40 egg-roll skins*
oil for deep frying

Stir-fry pork sausage for about 2 minutes. Spoon out any excess fat. Add shrimp and stir-fry for about 1 minute longer or until shrimp turns pink. Place shrimp and sausage in a bowl and pour whiskey or wine over. Allow to sit two to three minutes. Add soy sauce or salt, and sesame oil and allow to marinate while other items are prepared.

Stir-fry celery, mushrooms, carrots, and bean sprouts for about one minute. Combine vegetables and meat and mix well. Break raw egg over mixture and mix well once more.

Place an egg roll skin on a board or plate diagonally in front of you. Dab beaten egg on all corners except the bottom one. Place two tablespoons of the vegetable/meat mixture on the lower two-thirds of the skin and begin rolling from the bottom corner. Roll to the halfway point, bring in the two sides, secure them, using the beaten egg as "glue," and complete the rolling, sticking down the top corner.

Place enough oil in a wok or other suitable frying utensil to allow egg rolls to be completely covered, and heat until one drop of water sizzles when dropped in fat (375 degrees). Fry only two rolls at a time so that every roll is evenly browned and crisp. Use chopsticks or tongs to turn egg rolls. Drain and serve hot.

Servings: 20 (2 egg rolls per serving)
Exchanges per serving: ½ meat, ½ fat, ½ bread

---

*Egg-roll skins are stocked by many supermarkets. If they aren't stocked by your supermarket, they can usually be ordered a week in advance. You will have no trouble obtaining them if your city has a Chinese supermarket.

## Enchiladas Verdes (Green Enchiladas)

1 pound ground beef
1 medium onion, chopped
¼ tsp. garlic powder
1 tbsp. flour
2 cups water
1 tsp. salt
2 4-ounce cans chopped green chili peppers
2 cups grated Cheddar cheese
12 corn tortillas (frozen or fresh-packaged)
2 cups shredded lettuce

Brown ground beef in a large skillet and drain off and reserve excess fat. Add onions and garlic powder and cook until onions are transparent. Mix flour with ⅓ cup water, then add salt and remaining water and mix well. Pour green chilies into the water-and-flour mixture and mix well. Bring mixture to a boil, stirring constantly. Add cheese and stir just until melted. Do not boil. Add meat to cheese mixture.

Preheat oven to 350 degrees (175 C). Fry 12 tortillas in ½ inch fat, approximately ½ minute per side. Drain well. Layer the tortillas and meat-cheese mixture in a 3-quart casserole dish. Place in oven until mixture begins to bubble. Do *not* cook until dry.

When ready to serve, place shredded lettuce on top of each serving of casserole. Leftovers may be placed in a covered dish in the refrigerator. Add water and reheat to serve.

Servings: 6
Exchanges per serving: 2 bread, 2 fat, 3 meat

## Huevos Rancheros

1 16-ounce can tomatoes
2 4-ounce cans green chilies
1 jalapeño pepper, if desired
8 eggs
1 cup Cheddar cheese, grated
4 flour tortillas

Place tomatoes, chilies, and jalapeño (if added zest is desired) in blender. Blend thoroughly and place in jar which can be tightly capped and refrigerated for a week. Sauce refrigerates well.

Preheat oven to 350 degrees (175 C). Place four tortillas on oven-proof plates or on cookie sheet. Cook eggs, sunny-side up, and place 2 eggs in the center of each tortilla. Pour 1/8 cup sauce over each pair of eggs. Sprinkle equal amounts of cheese over each pair of eggs, then fold tortilla edges up and turn tortillas over so that they will remain closed while baking. Place in oven for 10 to 12 minutes or until cheese is melted.

Servings: 4
Exchanges per serving: 3 meat, 1 bread

## Panhandle Steak

$1/8$ cup salad oil
1 ½ pounds round steak, ½ inch thick, cut in serving-sized pieces
1 tsp dry mustard
2 tbsp. flour
½ tsp. salt
pepper to taste
2 tsp. Worcestershire sauce
½ cup water

Heat the oil in large heavy frying pan.

Combine flour, mustard, salt, and pepper in paper bag. Shake steak pieces in flour mixture and brown in hot oil.

Push meat to one side and stir remaining flour mixture into drippings. Combine water with Worcestershire sauce and stir into flour mixture.

Simmer until thickened and bubbling, stirring constantly to prevent sticking.

Reduce heat, simmer meat in gravy (covered) for 1 to 1 ½ hours or until tender. Add additional water as needed.

Remove meat to serving platter, skim excess fat from gravy, and pour gravy over meat.

Servings: 4
Exchanges per serving: 4 ½ meat, ¼ bread, 1 ½ fat

## Red Chili Enchiladas

12 corn tortillas (frozen or fresh-packaged)
1 cup vegetable oil (approximately)
1 pound lean ground beef
1 large onion, diced
½ tsp. garlic powder
1 tsp. salt
2 cans (15 ½-ounce) enchilada sauce, *or* Enchilada Sauce recipe *below*
2 cups grated cheese

Preheat oven to 325 degrees (160 C). Fry corn tortillas in ½ inch hot oil. Drain well. Brown ground beef in skillet. Remove excess grease. Add onion, garlic powder, and salt to meat and simmer 5 minutes longer.

Dip one tortilla in Enchilada Sauce. Place layer of meat and layer of cheese on tortilla, roll tortilla, and place in 9 x 13-inch baking pan or dish. Continue adding tortillas until pan is filled. Pour remaining sauce over tortillas. Place in oven until sauce boils. Do NOT cook long enough to allow tortillas to dry out.

Servings: 6 (2 enchiladas per serving)
Exchanges per serving: 3 meat, 1 vegetable, 2 fat, 2 bread

### Enchilada Sauce

4 tbsp. ground red chili powder
½-tsp. cayenne pepper
2 tbsp. flour
1 8-ounce can tomato sauce
2 cups water

Combine all ingredients and mix well. Cook over medium heat, stirring frequently, until mixture thickens to the consistency of undiluted tomato sauce. Use as described in Red Chili Enchiladas recipe.

## Sweet and Sour Pork

3 ¾ pounds pork steak, cut in 1-inch cubes
¾ cup flour
1 tbsp. plus one tsp. ginger
½ cup salad oil
2 8 ½-ounce cans pineapple chunks, drained with syrup reserved
½ cup vinegar
½ cup soy sauce
¾ cup brown sugar
1 tbsp. Worcestershire sauce
1 tbsp. salt
¾ tsp. pepper
2 small green peppers, cut in strips
1 16-ounce can bean sprouts, drained
2 5-ounce cans water chestnuts, drained and thinly sliced
2 tbsp. chili sauce

Trim excess fat from pork. Combine half the flour and ginger in a paper bag, place three or four pieces of pork at a time in bag, and shake to coat. Heat oil in large, heavy skillet or Dutch oven. Brown pork on all sides and remove pieces to a platter as they brown.

Add water to pineapple syrup to measure 1 ¾ cups liquid, and gradually stir remaining flour/ginger mixture into water. Add vinegar, soy sauce, and Worcestershire to flour/water mixture and stir well. Pour into pork drippings and heat to boiling, stirring constantly. Boil until thickened slightly (about one minute). Stir in sugar, salt, pepper, and meat. Cover and simmer for 1 hour or until meat is tender. Stir occasionally to prevent sticking.

Add pineapple and green pepper and cook uncovered for 10 minutes. Stir in bean sprouts, water chestnuts, and chili sauce and cook for 5 minutes longer, uncovered. Serve over rice ( ½ cup rice = 1 bread exchange).

Servings: 8
Exchanges per serving: 6 meat, 2 bread, 1 fruit, 1 vegetable

# Shrimp Creole

2 tbsp. bacon drippings
2 tbsp. flour
½ cup chopped celery
1 finely chopped clove of garlic *or* ½ tsp. garlic powder
1 cup green pepper, chopped
½ cup onions, chopped
½ cup scallions, chopped
3 ½ cups tomatoes (#2 ½ can, 28 ounces)
½ cup water
1 bay leaf
¾ tsp. cayenne pepper
¾ tsp. black pepper
½ tsp. salt
1 pound shrimp, peeled and cooked
2–3 cups cooked rice

First make a roux: heat bacon drippings slowly in a large Dutch oven or an extralarge iron skillet and add flour. Stir mixture constantly over low to moderate heat to prevent burning. At any hint of scorching, clean the skillet and begin again. When mixture has turned a rich brown, authentic Creole roux is ready for the addition of other ingredients.

Add chopped celery, garlic or garlic powder, green pepper, onions, and scallions to roux. Cook until onions are nearly transparent, stirring occasionally to prevent sticking. Add tomatoes and water, stirring constantly. Add bay leaf and other spices, stirring well. Simmer one-half-hour on low heat. Add one pound peeled, cooked shrimp and simmer one-half hour longer. Serve over fluffy white rice.

Servings: 4
Exchanges per serving: 4 meat, 1 ½ fat, 3 vegetable, 2 bread (with rice)

# Whole-wheat Herb Pizza

## Crust
1 pkg. active dry yeast
½ cup warm water (110–115 degrees F.)
½ cup whole-wheat flour
1 cup white flour
½ tsp. salt
1 tbsp. cooking oil
½ tsp. oregano
⅛ tsp. garlic powder

Stir yeast into warm water in a bowl. Add flour, salt, oil, oregano, and garlic powder. Knead the mixture on a lightly floured surface until it forms a smooth ball. Place dough in a greased bowl, turn once, cover, and let rise in a warm place until doubled (about 20 minutes). Pat the dough into a 12-inch greased pizza pan, pressing dough up on sides.

While crust is rising, prepare sauce.

## Sauce
3 ½ cups tomatoes (1-pound-12-ounce can)
1 6-ounce can tomato paste
½ tsp. oregano leaves
¼ tsp. basil leaves
1 finely chopped clove garlic *or* 1 tsp. garlic powder
¼ tsp. rosemary leaves
¼ tsp. thyme
¼ tsp. cayenne pepper
¼ tsp. black pepper

Place all ingredients in blender and blend until relatively smooth. Cook in saucepan over low-to-medium heat, stirring occasionally. Allow mixture to cook until it is reduced to about one half the original volume, leaving about 2 cups of sauce. Spoon sauce over pizza crust and cover with topping, as described below.

## Topping
1 pound ground or chopped beef, pork, or chicken
1 onion, finely chopped
1 6-ounce package pepperoni, sliced
1 large green pepper, cut into thin strips
1 can green chili peppers, drained and chopped
2 4-ounce cans mushrooms, drained
1 cup finely chopped scallions
8 ounces Mozzarella cheese, sliced
½ tsp. basil leaves
½ tsp. oregano leaves
½ tsp. thyme leaves

Preheat oven to 425 degrees (220 C). Brown ground beef in skillet and drain off excess fat. Add finely chopped onion to beef and allow to cook until onion begins to turn transparent. Sprinkle ground beef-onion mixture over pizza sauce on pizza. Arrange pepperoni in a large circle 2 inches from outside edge of pizza, overlapping edges of pepperoni. Place strips of green pepper on pizza, arranging like spokes in a wheel. Sprinkle green chili peppers, mushrooms, and scallions over entire pizza. Cover pizza with slices of Mozzarella cheese. Sprinkle basil, oregano, and thyme on pizza. Place pizza in oven for 25 minutes.

Servings: 3 ( ⅓ pizza per serving)
Exchanges per serving: 3 bread, 2 vegetable, 5 meat, 4 fat

# SALADS

### Chef's Salad

½ head iceberg lettuce
1 bunch endive or escarole
1 red onion, sliced and separated into rings
2 medium tomatoes cut in wedges
8 unpeeled, sliced radishes
2 carrots, thinly sliced
2 sliced hard-cooked eggs
½ tsp. basil

Toss shredded greens with carrots, onion, tomato, and radishes in large salad bowl. Add Connie's Vinegar and Oil Dressing *(below)* and toss again lightly. Arrange eggs on top of mixture, and sprinkle basil over salad.

Servings: 4
Exchanges per serving: 1 vegetable A; 1 vegetable B; ½ vegetable C; 2 fat (if dressing is used)

### Connie's Vinegar and Oil Dressing

2 tsp. wine vinegar
2 tsp. olive oil
2 tbsp. vegetable oil
freshly ground black pepper to taste
1 garlic clove, crushed

Mix all ingredients well and pour over salad. Toss. The secret of this dressing is its freshness; it should be mixed in small quantities and used at a single meal.

Servings: Dresses one salad for four
Exchanges per serving: 2 fat

# Fruit Salad

1 16-ounce can fruit cocktail
1 large orange or tangerine
1 banana

Peel and cut fruit into bite-sized pieces. Add to fruit cocktail. Serve.

Servings: 4
Exchanges per serving: 2 fruit

# Mac's Mandarin Orange Salad

2 3-ounce packages orange-flavored gelatin
2 cups boiling water
1 pint orange sherbet
1 15½-ounce can crushed pineapple
1 small can mandarin orange sections, drained
lettuce leaves

Dissolve gelatin in boiling water and allow to cool for at least 20 minutes at room temperature. Stir in sherbert. Add pineapple and oranges and stir again. Pour into mold and refrigerate. Serve on lettuce leaves.

Servings: 12
Exchanges per serving: 1½ bread, ½ fruit

# Quick Cranberry Sauce

1 cup sugar
1 cup water
4 cups cranberries

Place sugar and water in saucepan and bring to a boil. Add cranberries and return to boiling point. Cook until cranberries burst. Chill and serve or serve warm.

Servings: 16
Exchanges per serving: ½ fruit, 1 bread

## Spiced Fruit

1 can pear halves (1-pound-14-ounce can)
1 can peach halves or quarters (1-pound-14-ounce can)
1 small jar maraschino cherries
⅓ cup brown sugar
½ cup cider vinegar
2 sticks cinnamon
2 tsp. whole cloves
1 tsp. whole allspice

Drain fruit juice into saucepan and place fruit in 1 ½-quart casserole. Add brown sugar, vinegar, cinnamon, cloves, and allspice to syrup from fruit. Boil gently for 5 minutes. Pour warm syrup over fruit and refrigerate for at least 4 hours before serving.

Servings: 8
Exchanges per serving: 2 fruit, ½ bread

## Sunshine Salad

2 cups torn fresh spinach leaves
3 cups torn leaf lettuce
2 medium oranges, segmented, with segments halved and seeds removed, *or* one can mandarin oranges
¼ cup orange juice or juice from canned mandarin oranges
¼ tsp. ginger
¼ tsp. dry mustard
1 tbsp. cornstarch

Shred spinach and lettuce and place in large bowl. Add orange segments and toss lightly. Place orange juice or liquid from mandarin oranges in a saucepan. Add ginger, mustard, and cornstarch and blend thoroughly. Cook over medium heat, stirring constantly until dressing thickens and turns clear. Cool. Pour over greens and oranges and blend well.

Servings: 4
Exchanges per serving: 2 ½ vegetable, ½ fruit

# VEGETABLES AND SIDE DISHES

## Alpine Rice

¾ cup raw brown rice
¼ cup Parmesan cheese
¼ cup grated Swiss cheese
1 tbsp. margarine
¼ cup roasted sesame seeds
¼ cup hot milk

Cook rice. Toss hot rice with cheese, margarine, and sesame seeds, stirring until cheese melts. Stir in hot milk. Serve immediately.

Servings: 4
Exchanges per serving: 1 bread, 3 fat, 1 meat

## Mississippi Cornbread-Oyster Dressing

½ pound chicken or turkey giblets (gizzard, heart, neck, liver)
4 cups water
1 large onion, finely chopped
1 ½ cups scallions, chopped
1 clove garlic, crushed
1 large green pepper, chopped
2 cups celery, finely chopped
2 tsp. salt
¼ tsp. cayenne pepper
½ tsp. black pepper
1 tsp. celery seed
1 tsp. sage
2 tbsp. margarine
2 recipes Missie's Southern cornbread (p. 292), crumbled (3 ½–4 cups)
1 cup cooked rice
3 eggs, lightly beaten
½ cup minced parsley
1 pint fresh oysters

Preheat oven to 350 degrees (175 C). Boil giblets in water and cut into fine pieces. Sauté onion, scallions, garlic, green pepper, celery, salt, cayenne pepper, black pepper, celery seed, and sage in margarine.

Crumble cornbread and mix with rice.

Add sautéed vegetables, chopped giblets, and slightly beaten eggs to cornbread mixture. Add enough liquid from giblets (2 ½ to 3 cups) to make a moist dressing. Fold in parsley and oysters and pour in a 9 x 13-inch pan. Bake for 25 to 30 minutes, or until dressing is firm, but not dry. Serve with turkey and giblet stuffing (p. 283).

Servings: 12
Exchanges per serving: 1 vegetable, 1 bread, 1 meat, 1 ½ fat

# Giblet Gravy

4 tbsp. flour
salt to taste
½ tsp. pepper
4 tbsp. turkey or chicken drippings
1 ½–2 cups water
½ pound chopped giblets (chicken or turkey liver, gizzard, heart, neck)
4 hard-cooked eggs, sliced

Brown flour, salt, and pepper in turkey drippings. Slowly add water, stirring until smooth. Continue to cook on low setting, stirring frequently, until gravy reaches desired consistency.

Add giblets and eggs and serve over Mississippi Cornbread-Oyster Dressing.

Servings: 12
Exchanges per serving: 1 fat, 1 meat

# Spicy Sweet Potatoes

6 sweet potatoes (approximately 6 cups, mashed)
2 tbsp. margarine (¼ stick)
2/3 cup evaporated milk (small can)
3 eggs, slightly beaten
¼ cup brown sugar
½ tsp. nutmeg
½ tsp. cinnamon
½ tsp. salt
¼ tsp. cloves
1 tsp. vanilla
1 cup miniature marshmallows

Preheat oven to 350 degrees (175 C). Boil sweet potatoes and remove peel. Mash thoroughly and add margarine. Add milk, eggs, sugar, spices, and vanilla, and mix well. Pour sweet-potato mixture into a large casserole and sprinkle marshmallows over the top of the potatoes. Bake for 15 to 20 minutes or until marshmallows are golden brown.

Servings: 12
Exchanges per serving: 2 ½ bread, ½ fat

# Texas Pintos

1 cup dried pinto beans
2 slices bacon
½ cup chopped onion
¼ cup chopped scallions
½ tsp. garlic powder
1 tsp. salt
Dash pepper
Dash hot-pepper sauce
1 16-ounce can tomatoes
½ cup chopped green pepper
2 tsp. sugar

Place beans in a 1½-quart casserole, cover them with water, and soak overnight. Add bacon, onion, scallions, garlic powder, salt, pepper, and hot-pepper sauce to the water and beans. Simmer beans, covered, for about two hours. Add undrained tomatoes, green pepper, and sugar. Cover and simmer for three hours more.

For quick preparation, beans may be pressure-cooked without soaking. Place beans, 2½ cups water, and all additional ingredients *except tomatoes and juice* in pressure cooker at once. Cook at 15 pounds pressure for 1 hour 20 minutes. Reduce pressure, remove lid, add tomatoes and juice and cook for 15 to 20 minutes longer. TOMATOES SHOULD NOT BE COOKED UNDER PRESSURE owing to danger of explosion.

Servings: 6
Exchanges: 1 vegetable, ⅓ fat, 2/3 bread

# Veggies with Hot Cheddar Dip

1 16-ounce can tomatoes
1 4-ounce can mild green chili peppers
1 pound Cheddar cheese or ½ pound Cheddar and ½ pound
  American cheese
Assorted vegetables—broccoli flowers, cauliflowerettes, carrot and
  celery sticks

Blend tomatoes and chilies in blender and then heat in saucepan until boiling. Add grated cheese and stir until smooth. Do not boil. Place in chafing dish and keep heated while vegetables are being dipped.

Servings: 12
Exchanges per serving: 2 meat, 2 fat, 1 vegetable for every ½ cup of vegetables eaten with dip.

# DESSERTS

## Apple Oatmeal Cookies

½ cup margarine
¾ cup brown sugar
2 eggs, lightly beaten
1 ½ cups whole-wheat flour
½ cup rolled oats
¼ cup wheat germ
½ tsp. salt
2 tsp. baking powder
½ tsp. cinnamon
1 ½ cups apples, finely chopped
1 ½ cups raisins

Preheat oven to 350 degrees (175 C). Melt margarine and cream with sugar. Beat in eggs. Combine next six ingredients and stir into creamed sugar, margarine, and eggs. Add apples and raisins and stir well. Drop cookies onto greased baking sheet and bake for 12 to 15 minutes. Cool on rack.

Servings: 20 (2 cookies per serving)
Exchanges per serving: 1 bread, 1 fat, ½ fruit

## Applesauce Whip

6 egg whites
6 tbsp. sugar
2 tbsp. lemon juice
3 cups applesauce, chilled
1 orange, sectioned
6 maraschino cherries

Whip egg whites until they are stiff and peaked. Add sugar very slowly, beating after each addition. Add lemon juice and beat one minute longer. Gently fold beaten egg whites into chilled applesauce. Garnish with orange slices and cherries. Use immediately. Do not store in refrigerator for use later. Dishes made with uncooked egg whites can not safely be stored.

Servings: 6
Exchanges per serving: 1 fruit, ½ meat, 1 bread

## Aunt Winnie's Date Delights

1 cup shortening
1 tsp. salt
1 tsp. vanilla
1 ½ cups sugar
3 eggs, beaten
3 ½ cups flour
¾ tsp. soda
5 tbsp. milk
3 cups pitted, chopped dates

Preheat oven to 350 degrees (175 C). Combine shortening, salt, and vanilla. Blend until smooth. Add sugar and cream well. Add beaten eggs and mix well. Sift flour and soda together. Add to creamed mixture alternately with milk, mixing well after each addition. Add dates and mix well. Drop walnut-sized amounts of stiff cookie dough onto sheet, leaving approximately 1 inch between cookies. Bake for 10 to 12 minutes or until lightly browned.

Servings: 30 (two cookies per serving)
Exchanges per serving: 1 ½ bread, ½ fruit, 1 ½ fat

## Banana-Grape Dessert

2 cups green seedless grapes
2 sliced bananas
½ cup 2-percent or low-fat yogurt (plain)
¼ tsp. nutmeg
¼ tsp. grated lemon peel
4 tsp. brown sugar
4 maraschino cherries

Mix all ingredients except brown sugar together in a large bowl. Spoon mixture into four individual serving dishes and chill for 1 to 2 hours. When ready to serve, sprinkle brown sugar over each serving and top with a maraschino cherry.

Servings: 4
Exchanges per serving: 2 fruit

## Blender Banana Pudding

½ cup applesauce
2 tbsp. peanut butter
1 tbsp. honey
2 bananas

Blend all ingredients and serve.

Servings: 4
Exchanges per serving: 1 fruit

# Grape Gelatin

1 ½ cups unsweetened grape juice
1 tbsp. unflavored gelatin
½ cup boiling water

Pour ¼ cup cold grape juice into flat-bottomed bowl. Sprinkle gelatin on top and allow to soften. Add boiling water and stir until gelatin has dissolved. Add remaining cold grape juice, stir well, and chill until set.

Servings: 3
Exchanges per serving: 2 fruit

# Green Apple Cake

1 ¼ cups sugar
½ cup strong coffee (instant, decaffeinated)
1 ½ cups salad oil
4 eggs, well beaten
2 cups white flour
1 cup whole-wheat flour
2 tsp. cinnamon
½ tsp. allspice
½ tsp. ground cloves
½ tsp nutmeg
1 tsp. salt
2 tsp. baking soda
3 cups finely chopped raw apples (sour and firm)
1 cup raisins (dredged in 2 tbsp. flour)

Preheat oven to 350 degrees (175 C). Mix sugar, coffee, oil and eggs. Mix next eight ingredients. Stir flour mixture into sugar mixture. Add fruit. Bake in greased and floured standard-sized bundt pan for 50 to 60 minutes.

Servings: 25
Exchanges per serving:  ½ fruit, 2 bread, 3 fat (without icing)

# Sopapillas

4 cups flour
4 tbsp. baking powder
½ tsp. salt
3 tbsp. shortening
Vegetable oil (enough for deep-fat frying)
Honey to taste

Mix flour, baking soda, and salt. Cut in shortening until dough is consistency of cornmeal. Add enough water to make a dough which holds together but is not sticky. Knead slightly, then set in covered, greased bowl to rest for 15 minutes.

Divide dough in half. Roll out thinly and cut into triangles. Drop triangles into deep, hot oil. Hold down until they puff. Turn, if browning is uneven. Drain in basket and then on paper. Serve hot, with honey.

Servings: 12
Exchanges per serving: 3 bread, 1 ½ fat (if served with honey)

## Zucchini Fruitcake

3 eggs
1 cup salad oil
2 cups brown sugar, firmly packed
1 tbsp. vanilla extract
3 cups flour
1 tbsp. cinnamon
2 tsp. allspice
1 tsp. salt
1 tsp. nutmeg
1 tsp. cloves
2 tsp. soda
½ tsp. baking powder
2 cups shredded raw zucchini
2 cups raisins
2 cups chopped walnuts
1 cup currants
2 cups coarsely chopped dried fruit (apples, pears, peaches,
   prunes, dates, apricots)
¼ cup brandy, rum, or water
8 tbsp. brandy or rum (optional)

Preheat oven to 325 degrees (160 C). Combine eggs, oil, sugar, and vanilla extract and beat well. Mix flour, spices, soda, and baking powder. Mix dry and wet ingredients with mixer. Fold in shredded zucchini.

Mix chopped dried fruits together with ¼ cup brandy, rum, or water. Cook just until liquid is absorbed and fruit is tender (about 4 to 6 minutes). Cool to room temperature, then stir into cake mixture with spoon.

Spoon batter into 2 greased and floured loaf pans (5 x 9-inch or 4 ½ x 8 ½-inch). Bake for 1 hour 10 minutes or until toothpick comes out clean.

Allow to cool on racks. If desired, spoon 4 tablespoons of rum or brandy over each loaf while warm. When completely cool, remove cakes from pans, wrap in foil, and freeze.

Servings: 34
Exchanges per serving: 1 bread, 1 fruit, 2 fat

# BREADS

## Blueberry-Lemon Muffins

1 ¾ cups flour
¼ cup sugar
2 ½ tsp. baking powder
¾ tsp. salt
¾ cup milk
1 beaten egg
⅓ cup salad oil
1 cup blueberries (if frozen, thaw first)
2 tbsp. sugar
1 tsp. grated lemon peel

Preheat oven to 400 degrees (200 C). Mix flour, ¼ cup sugar, baking powder, and salt in a large bowl, making a well in the center. Mix milk, beaten egg, and salad oil and pour all at once into well in center of dry ingredients. Stir quickly, just enough to mix well and moisten.

Toss berries, 2 tablespoons sugar, and lemon peel together and fold gently into batter. Fill twelve 2 ½-inch muffin cups two-thirds full. Bake 25 minutes.

Servings: 12
Exchanges per serving: 1 bread, 1 fat

## Carrot Bread

2 cups flour
1 tsp. salt
2 tsp. soda
2 cups sugar
2 ¼ tsp. cinnamon
1 ½ cups salad oil
4 eggs
3 cups grated carrots

Preheat oven to 350 degrees (175 C). Mix dry ingredients. Add salad oil and mix well. Add eggs one at a time, beating after each addition. Add carrots and mix well. Pour into two small loaf pans, a 9 x 13-inch pan or 18 muffin tins, greased and floured. Bake for 50 minutes or until toothpick inserted in center comes away clean. Allow to cool for 10 minutes, then remove from pans and ice if desired.

Servings: 18
Exchanges per serving: 2 bread, 4 fat, ⅓ vegetable

# Cheese-Bran Crackers

1 cup bran
1 ¼ cups white flour
¼ cup whole-wheat flour
½ cup sesame seeds
2 tbsp. Parmesan cheese
½ tsp. soda
1 tsp. salt
1 cup water

Preheat oven to 350 degrees (175 C). Mix bran, flours, sesame seeds, cheese, soda, and salt in large bowl. Add water and mix to form soft dough. Lightly sprinkle a pastry cloth with whole-wheat flour and roll out dough to a large 1/8-inch-thick rectangle. Score the dough into 2 x 4-inch rectangles, using a table knife. Place on well-greased baking sheet and bake for 10 minutes. Lower oven temperature to 300 degrees and continue baking for about 10 minutes more or until the crackers are crisp.

Servings: 20 (2 per serving)
Exchanges per serving: ½ bread, ½ fat

# Cornmeal Pancakes

1 egg
1 ¼ cups buttermilk
1 tbsp. molasses
¼ cup salad oil
¾ cup yellow cornmeal
¾ cup flour
1 tsp. salt
½ tsp. baking soda
1 tsp. baking powder

In a medium-sized bowl, beat egg and add buttermilk, molasses, and salad oil. Beat again. In a large bowl, combine cornmeal, flour, salt, baking soda, and baking powder. Add the liquid mixture to the dry mixture and stir until smooth.

Cook on hot griddle (droplets of water should skitter around on surface). Turn when pancakes start to bubble and become dry on edges.

Serve hot with margarine and molasses.

Servings: 4 (2 5-inch pancakes per serving)
Exchanges per serving: 3 fat, 3 ½ bread (1 tablespoon molasses equals ½ bread exchange)

# French Bread

7 ¼ –7 ¾ cups white flour

1 tbsp. salt
2 packages active dry yeast
2 ½ cups very warm water (120–130 degrees)
2 tbsp. cornmeal or farina
1 egg white, slightly beaten
1 tbsp. water

Mix 2 cups flour with yeast and salt in large mixing bowl. Gradually add warm water to flour and yeast. Beat with electric mixer at high speed for at least 2 minutes. Beat in 1 to 1 ½ additional cups flour. Set mixer aside and add remaining flour gradually, kneading for 8 to 10 minutes.

Form dough into a ball and place in greased, cloth-covered bowl to rise until doubled (about ½ hour). Dough has doubled when thumb pressed gently into dough leaves impression. Punch down dough. Reform ball, replace cloth, and let rise 1 ½ hours.

Divide ball of dough in half. Let rest 10 minutes. Roll each half into 8 x 14-inch rectangle. Roll rectangle tightly, like a jelly roll, beginning with long side. Sprinkle two greased cookie sheets lightly with cornmeal or farina. Place one loaf diagonally on each sheet. Make ¼-inch-deep diagonal slashes on top of each loaf at 2-inch intervals. Brush top with half of egg white-and-water mixture.

Let loaves rise uncovered in warm place for about 1 ½ hours. Place in 425-degree (220 C) oven and bake for 10 minutes. Brush loaves again with egg-white mixture and reduce oven temperature to 375 (190 C) degrees. Bake for 30 more minutes.

Servings: 24
Exchanges per serving: 2 bread

## Granny's Granola

5 cups rolled oats
1 cup raw wheat germ
1 cup dessicated coconut
½ cup chopped dates
¾ cup raisins
½ cup vegetable oil
¾ cup honey
½ cup water

Preheat oven to 225 degrees (108 C). Mix oats, wheat germ, coconut, dates, and raisins. Mix vegetable oil, honey, and water and add to cereal mixture. Spread cereal on two large cookie sheets and bake for 2 hours, stirring once or twice. Cereal should be lightly browned.

Servings: 12 (¾ cup each)
Exchanges per serving: 1 ½ bread, 1 ½ fat, ½ fruit

## Missie's Southern Cornbread

¾ cup cornmeal
½ cup flour
2 tsp. baking powder
½ tsp. salt
1 egg, beaten
½ cup milk
1 tbsp. bacon drippings

Preheat oven to 425 degrees (220 C). Mix cornmeal, flour, baking powder and salt. Add beaten egg and milk, mixing until smooth. Over medium heat, melt bacon drippings in small skillet. Stir drippings into meal mixture, pour mixture into skillet and return skillet to burner for one minute. Place skillet in oven for 10 to 12 minutes or until top begins to brown. Turn bread out onto plate immediately. Serve while hot, with butter or margarine.

Servings: 6 to 8
Exchanges per serving: 1 bread, 1 fat

## Pumpkin Bread

2 ½ cups sugar
¾ cup oil
¾ cup orange juice
4 eggs
2 cups mashed pumpkin (#2 can)
3 ½ cups flour
1 ½ tsp. salt
2 tsp. soda
1 tsp. nutmeg
1 tsp. cinnamon
2 cups raisins

Preheat oven to 350 degrees (175 C). Combine sugar, oil, and juice. Add eggs one at a time, beating after each addition. Add pumpkin and mix well. Mix flour, soda, salt, nutmeg, and cinnamon. Gradually add dry ingredients to pumpkin mixture and mix well. Fold in raisins and pour bread into three greased and floured 9 ½ x 5 ¼ x 2 ¾ -inch loaf pans. Bake for 1 hour or until toothpick inserted in bread comes out clean. Allow to cool for 10 to 15 minutes, then remove from pans, cool on rack, and wrap for freezer, if desired.

Servings: 33
Exchanges per serving: 1 ½ bread, 1 fat

# Seven-week Refrigerator Bran Muffins

2 cups bran flakes
4 cups All-Bran
2 cups boiling water
1 cup shortening
2 cups sugar
4 eggs, beaten
1 quart buttermilk
5 cups flour
5 tsp. baking soda
1 tsp. salt

Soak bran flakes and All-Bran in boiling water. Cool. Cream shortening and sugar, and add eggs and buttermilk.

Combine bran mixture with buttermilk mixture. Combine flour, soda, and salt and add to bran mixture. Store in tightly covered refrigerator bowl or large jar for as long as seven weeks.

When ready to cook, preheat oven to 400 degrees (200 C), fill greased muffin tins with batter and bake for 20 minutes.

Servings: 76
Exchanges per serving: 1 bread, 1 fat

# Whole-wheat Bread

2 packages active dry yeast
2 cups warm water (110–115 degrees)
2 cups milk
⅓ cup shortening
½ cup molasses
2 tbsp. salt
4 ½ cups whole-wheat flour
5 ¼ to 5 ½ cups white flour
2 tbsp. melted margarine

Stir yeast into warm water in large bowl. Heat milk, shortening, molasses, and salt together to about 110 degrees. Add to yeast. Beat in 3 cups of whole-wheat flour. Mix remaining whole-wheat flour with white flour and add as much of this mixture as possible while beating with mixer. Then add the remainder while kneading. Knead at least 8 to 10 minutes.

Place dough in large greased bowl, cover and let rise in warm place (85 degrees F) until doubled (about 1 ½ hours). Divide dough into three equal portions. Allow dough to rest 10 minutes before shaping. Shape loaves and place in three greased 9 ½ x 5 ¼ x 2 ¾ -inch bread pans. Brush tops with melted margarine. Cover and let rise in warm place until doubled (about 1 hour). Preheat oven to 375 degrees (190 C) and bake for about 45 minutes.

Servings: 48
Exchanges per serving: 1 bread

## Whole-wheat English Muffins

1 package active dry yeast
¼ cup warm water (105–115 degrees)
3 tbsp. margarine
1 tbsp. sugar
1 ½ tsp. salt
1 ⅔ cups milk, scalded
2 ⅓ cups whole-wheat flour
2 ⅓ cups white flour
margarine
½ cup cornmeal

Dissolve yeast in warm water in large bowl and let stand for 5 to 7 minutes. Add margarine, sugar, and salt to scalded milk. Cool to lukewarm and add to dissolved yeast. Mix whole-wheat and white flour, then stir flours into milk mixture. Dough will not be of kneading consistency. Beat for 2 minutes with spoon. Cover. Let rise until double (about 1 hour).

Place dough on well-floured surface and roll out to ½-inch thick. Use floured 3-inch cutter to cut 20 to 24 muffins. Arrange muffins on floured surface and cover. Let rest for 30 minutes. Heat griddle over medium heat. Grease by passing end of stick of margarine over hot surface. Sprinkle surface lightly with cornmeal. Carefully lift muffins to griddle with spatula. Cook for 10 to 12 minutes over medium heat. Turn with spatula. Cook for 15 to 20 minutes longer. Split muffins horizontally with a fork before serving. Serve hot. For later use, split muffins may be frozen and toasted before use.

Servings: 2 dozen 3-inch muffins, ½ muffin per serving
Exchanges per serving: 1 bread

# SANDWICHES, SOUPS, AND SNACKS

## Banana Shake

½ banana
1 cup milk
1 tbsp. wheat germ
Ice (2 or 3 cubes)

Combine all ingredients and blend at high speed until ice is smooth and shake is thick.

Servings: 1
Exchanges per serving: 1 fruit, 1 milk, 2 fat

## Banana Teething Popsicles

1 package unflavored gelatin
½ cup hot water
1 large banana

Float gelatin in hot water. Mash banana well and add to gelatin mixture. Mix well, pour thick mixture into plastic popsicle molds. Freeze.

Servings: 4
Exchanges per serving: ½ fruit

## Breadless Sandwich

2 thick (1-ounce) slices Cheddar or Swiss cheese
2 slices luncheon meat or thin-sliced ham
Endive, dark green lettuce, or spinach leaves

Place 1 slice of cheese on saucer. Alternate meat and lettuce on top of cheese. Top with second slice of cheese. If desired, place cheese, meat, and lettuce together and roll. Secure with toothpick. Repeat to form second roll.

Servings: 1
Exchanges per serving: Cheddar variety: 4 meat, 4 fat; Swiss variety: 4 meat, 3 fat

## Cheddar Cheese Soup

1 onion, sliced
1 cup celery, diced
2 tbsp. margarine
¼ cup flour
½ tsp. dry mustard
1 tsp. Worcester sauce
½ tsp. garlic salt
2 bouillon cubes
2 cups water
1 carrot, diced
4 cups milk

8 ounces sharp Cheddar cheese, shredded
Salt and pepper to taste
Parsley sprig

Sauté onion and celery in margarine until transparent. Blend in next four ingredients. Add bouillon cubes, water, and carrot. Bring to a boil, reduce heat, and simmer for 15 minutes. Add milk and heat almost to boiling. Add cheese, stir until melted, but do not boil. Season to taste. Garnish with parsley sprig.

Servings: 6 (one cup each)
Exchanges per serving: 1 meat, 1 milk, 1 vegetable, 2 fat

## Cheddar-Chili Sandwiches

½ pound Cheddar cheese, grated
1 4-ounce can green chili peppers
2 tbsp. mayonnaise
Rye bread (8 slices)

Mix cheese, chili peppers, and mayonnaise. Spread on bread and serve or freeze for later use.

Servings: 4
Exchanges per serving: 2 meat, 2½ fat, 2 bread

## Choo-Choo-Train Sandwich

2 slices whole-grain bread
5 tbsp. peanut butter
½ banana
5 seedless grapes
3 celery sticks
1 carrot
1 tbsp. raisins

Cut bread in halves, spread each half with peanut butter, and arrange halves in sequence on tray with ¼- to ½-inch space between each piece. Cut banana into rounds and arrange rounds as wheels on train cars. Add one round in front of lead car to serve as base of light. Load rear car with cargo of four grapes. Place fifth grape on top of banana round which serves as base for headlight. Place celery sticks between cars to serve as hitches. Load car near grapes with shredded carrot bits. Load next car with raisins. Place top inch of carrot stick on lead car to serve as smokestack. This is more impressive if fresh carrot with greenery attached is used. Invite children to choose a car and enjoy lunch.

Servings: 2
Exchanges per serving: 1 fruit, 1 bread, 1 meat, 1½ fat, ½ vegetable

# Citrus Popsicles

¼ cup honey
2 cups water
3 oranges
3 lemons
2 bananas

Place honey and water over low heat and simmer until honey dissolves well. Allow to cool for 15 minutes. Squeeze juice from oranges and lemons. Peel and mash bananas. Place fruit juices and mashed banana in honey mixture and mix well. Pour into ice trays. Allow to soft-freeze, then insert about a third of a plastic straw into each cube. Allow to freeze hard. Popsicles may be popped from tray and stored in plastic bag.

Servings: 12
Exchanges per serving: 1 fruit, ½ bread

# Frozen Banana Popsicles

4 bananas
4 stiff plastic straws or 4 popsicle sticks
4 sandwich baggies or clear plastic wrap

Peel bananas. Insert straw or stick lengthwise, leaving 2-inch handle exposed. Wrap banana end in baggie or plastic wrap. Freeze. Serve frozen. CAUTION: Do not use metal spoon for popsicle handle, since cold metal will adhere to moist lips and cause freezer burn! Bananas may also be frozen without sticks and sliced for serving as quick dessert for the family.

Servings: 4
Exchanges per serving: 2 fruit

# Garden Sandwich

1 slice whole-wheat bread
½ tsp. margarine
1 tbsp. peanut butter
2 slices tomato
1 thick (1-ounce) slice Cheddar or Swiss cheese
1 tsp. sesame seeds
1 tsp. roasted soy beans
½ cup alfalfa sprouts

Spread bread with margarine, then with peanut butter. Top with tomato slices and thick slice of cheese. Place under broiler until cheese melts. Top with sesame seeds, soy beans, and alfalfa sprouts.

Servings: 1
Exchanges per serving: 1 bread, 1 ½ fat, 1 vegetable, ½ meat. (If Swiss cheese is used and margarine is omitted, reduce fat exchanges to 1.)

# Hearty Vegetable-Beef Soup

1 cup chopped onion
1 ½ cloves garlic, crushed
2 tbsp. margarine
1 pound boneless stew meat, well trimmed
2 cups canned tomatoes with juice
1 cup cut green beans
½ cup whole-kernel corn
½ cup chopped cabbage
½ cup chopped celery
½ cup diced beets
½ cup diced potatoes
½ cup diced yellow or zucchini squash
½ cup beet greens or spinach, chopped
1 bay leaf
½ tsp. thyme
¼ tsp. black pepper
⅛ tsp. cayenne pepper
3 to 4 cups water
½ cup barley
¼ tsp. parsley

Sauté onion and garlic in margarine in large Dutch oven. Add stew meat and brown lightly. Add all vegetables and spices except parsley and barley. Add water. Simmer, covered, for 20 minutes. Add barley and parsley and simmer 40 minutes longer. Add salt to taste.

Servings: 4 or 5 (2 cups each)
Exchanges per serving: 4 vegetables, 4 meat, 1 fat

# Pat-a-Pizza

8 ounces tomato paste
Dash of salt
⅛ tsp. thyme
⅛ tsp. oregano
⅛ tsp. basil
⅛ tsp. rosemary
6 Whole-wheat English Muffins (p. 294)
½ cup chopped onions
1 4-ounce can mushrooms
½ cup diced green pepper
½ pound Cheddar cheese, sliced
½ cup Parmesan cheese, grated

Preheat oven to 450 degrees (232 C). Mix tomato paste, salt, spices. Spread on muffin halves and arrange halves on cookie sheet. Arrange layers

of meat and vegetables on muffins and top arrangement with cheeses. Bake
15 to 20 minutes.

Servings: 12
Exchanges per serving: 1 bread, 1 ½ meat, 1 fat, ½ vegetable

## South American Cocoa

¼ cup water
3 tbsp. cocoa
2 tbsp. sugar
2 cups milk
1 tsp. vanilla extract

Bring water to boil in saucepan. Mix cocoa and sugar in a cup and add
mixture to boiling water. Stir until blended well. Reduce heat to simmer and
slowly pour milk into saucepan. Stir over low heat until milk reaches desired
temperature. Do not boil. Remove from heat and stir in vanilla. Serve hot.

Servings: 2
Exchanges per serving: 1 bread, 1 milk, 4 fat

## Strawberry-Orange Eye-opener

1 cup orange juice
1 egg
18–20 fresh strawberries
⅔ cup nonfat dry milk
1 cup 2-percent milk
2 tsp. honey

Place all ingredients in blender and blend until mixture is smooth, reserv-
ing two strawberries. Pour into glasses and garnish each serving with a fresh
strawberry. Serve immediately.

Servings: 2
Exchanges per serving: 2 ½ fruit, 1 ½ milk, ½ meat

## Supershake

1 medium peach, washed, peeled and quartered
1 egg
½ cup cold low-fat milk
⅛ tsp. vanilla extract
1 small scoop vanilla ice-milk

Place peaches, egg, vanilla flavoring, and milk into blender container.
Cover and blend 30 seconds. Add ice-milk and blend 15 seconds longer.

Servings: 1
Exchanges per serving: ½ milk, 1 fruit, ½ bread, ½ fat, 1 meat

# BASIC BABY FOOD RECIPES*

## Baby Egg Yolk

1 cooked egg yolk
1 tbsp. liquid baby formula

Purée yolk with liquid formula until smooth. (Use whites in salads, casseroles, or sandwiches for other family members but do not feed egg whites to baby.)

## Baby Fruits (Cooked)

½ cup cooked fruit
2 tsp. liquid from fruit

Remove any skin or seeds. Place fruit and liquid in food mill or blender and blend to desired degree of smoothness. Store in clean container.

## Baby Fruits (Raw)

¾ cup raw fruit
1 tsp. fruit juice
1 tsp. lemon juice water (1 quart of water mixed with 1 tbsp. lemon juice)

Remove skin and seeds from fruit. Place fruit in food mill or blender and blend to desired degree of smoothness. If fruit does not liquefy easily, add another teaspoon of lemon juice water. This water helps prevent darkening of raw fruits. Store in clean container.

## Baby Meat

½ cup cooked meat, cut in small pieces
3 tbsp. formula or liquid from meat

Cut away any fat from meat and remove fat from liquid before using liquid in baby food. Place meat and liquid in blender and blend to desired degree of smoothness. Store in clean container.
NOTE: Avoid using meats high in nitrates and nitrites such as luncheon meats, processed hams, bacon, and frankfurters.

## Baby Vegetables (Cooked)

½ cup cooked vegetables
2 tbsp. formula or liquid from vegetables

Cut or tear cooked vegetables into chunks. Place vegetables and liquid in food mill or blender and blend to desired degree of smoothness. Store in clean container.

*Meats, fruits, and vegetables may be prepared in larger quantities and frozen for use later. See Chapter 5 for details.

# Sack-Lunch Tips

Since the noon meal may provide one-third of a day's total calories, sack lunches should be varied enough to provide adequate nutrients. A typical sack lunch might include Green Chili Cheese Sandwiches on Rye, carrot sticks, an apple, a cookie, and milk. This meal provides a protein food, dairy products, two vegetables, a fruit, and two breads (rye and cookie). By varying the breads, spreads, and fillings used in sandwiches, you can provide adequate nutrition in a form which does not become monotonous to the children who open a sack lunch each noontime. Tips on spread and filling variations and on freezing and packing follow.

By varying the beverage in each day's lunch, a parent can add still more variety to the lunch. If milk is available in the cafeteria or in vending machines, children should plan to purchase it at school, thus avoiding the problem of keeping it cool. If no thermos is available and milk is to be sent to school, ice cubes of milk should be frozen the night before and included in the foil-wrapped jar in which the milk is carried. Small cans of fruit juice are now available with easy-opening tabs, and these make excellent lunch drinks. Hot soup may be carried in a thermos in place of a conventional beverage.

## Spreading Tips

1. Spread margarine, butter, peanut butter, or cheese spread to the edges of the bread to avoid moisture from salad-type fillings making bread soggy.
2. Do not use melted butter or margarine, since melted spreads will soak into the bread.
3. Avoid using mayonnaise or salad dressing for sandwiches which will be frozen, since these spreads tend to separate when frozen.
4. Spreads will go on frozen bread slices more easily.

## Special Spreads

Melt ½ cup butter or margarine. Add:

3 tablespoons orange juice and 1 teaspoon orange rind for *Orange Butter*
½ teaspoon basil and 1 tablespoon grated lemon rind
   for *Lemon-Herb Butter*
1 teaspoon curry powder and ½ teaspoon salt for *East India Butter*
2 tablespoons prepared mustard for *Magic Mustard Butter*
¼ cup grated Parmesan and 1 teaspoon Worcestershire for *Parmesan Butter*

Place in a covered jar or bowl in the refrigerator to become firm.

# Fancy Fillings

*Peanut butter with*
Shredded carrots
Sliced apple or pear
Diced celery
Lettuce leaves
Cabbage
Honey, jam, or jelly
Raisins
Orange juice and rind
Applesauce
Crisp bacon (chopped) and raw apple slices
Banana

*Cream cheese with*
Honey and grated orange rind
Chopped nuts, crisp bacon
Pickle relish
Crushed pineapple
Raisins
Diced celery
Shredded carrot
Chopped, cooked, diced apricots or prunes
Dried beef
Chopped dates or figs
Diced olives

*Grated Cheddar cheese with*
Pimiento
Green chilies, chopped
Chopped celery and applesauce
Crushed pineapple and chopped bell peppers

# Freezer-Fresh Fillings

1. Freeze all meat sandwiches for safety. They will remain cool all morning and be ready to be eaten at lunch. Use an insulated lunchbox if the box will be in a hot locker or parked car.
2. Make up a week's sandwiches on the weekend. Wrap, label, and freeze them. Sandwiches will keep two to four weeks in the freezer. Do not use the refrigerator freezer compartment unless that compartment stays at zero degrees Fahrenheit or colder.
3. Do not freeze crisp or watery vegetables (lettuce, celery, tomatoes, cucumbers, carrots, etc.), egg whites, mayonnaise or salad dressing, jelly.

## Wrapping and Packing

1. Keep lettuce, tomato, and other such items in separate foil or plastic packets to be added to the sandwich just before it is eaten.
2. Wash and dry fruits and vegetables and wrap them in plastic to keep them fresh.
3. Pack plenty of napkins.
4. Wrap sandwiches individually if filling is different, so that flavors won't mix.
5. Pack heavy items on the bottom, light items on top.
6. Pack a small surprise in the lunch bag occasionally—a new pencil, a cartoon or joke, a note to say "I love you" or "Enjoy this day," a stick of sugarless gum.

# Fun Food Ideas

Funny-face franks: Cut out a round cheese sandwich with a cookie or biscuit cutter. Around each side attach half a wiener, split lengthwise, with toothpicks. Brush bread and franks with melted butter. Make face on bread with catsup. Bake on greased cookie sheet at 400 degrees for 5 minutes.

Raisin face on cooked cereal or pudding

Chocolate chip face on pudding

Pancakes shaped like animals (children have great imaginations)

Sandwiches cut out in interesting shapes with cookie cutters

Slip foods such as cheese or meat onto pretzel sticks

Spread peanut butter or cheese spread on a cabbage leaf and let children make a "jelly roll"

Apple slice spread with peanut butter with an animal cracker on top

Salad that looks like a bunny:
  Body: ½ pear is body, narrow end is head
  Eyes: 2 raisins
  Nose: cinnamon candy
  Ears: 2 blanched almonds
  Tail: cottage cheese ball

Salad that looks like Raggedy Ann:
  Body: ½ peach
  Arms and legs: celery sticks
  Head: large marshmallow
  Eyes, nose, shoes, and buttons: raisins
  Mouth: cut cherry
  Hair: shredded cheese
  Skirt: leaf of lettuce

Salad that looks like a rocket:
  Launch pad: 1 slice pineapple
  Rocket: ½ peeled banana standing in center of pineapple slice

Nosecone: ½ cherry attached to top of banana with a toothpick

Soup with a face made of oyster crackers or croutons.

Muffins with jam inside.

Meatloaf shaped like a football, basketball, or baseball with celery strips for strings.

Meatloaf cooked in muffin tins with cheese bits for face (put cheese on at the end of cooking time).

Fruit kabob: push a straw through chunks of fruit; use with punch or fruit juice.

Branded pancakes: place a backward letter made from pancake batter on the grill—when it has browned, pour enough batter for a regular pancake over it. Turn both layers together.

Ready-to-eat-cereal face: make face in ready-to-eat cereal with ½ peach or pear and raisins or piece of banana with raisin features; apple slices make good ears or mouth.

Curly carrot or celery sticks; radish roses.

Hamburger faces: on top of bun, place sliced green olives for eyes, cheese triangles for nose, and catsup or pimiento for mouth.

Potato boat: make slice in one side of baked potato, put piece of cheese (large triangle) on toothpick and place at one end of slice for sail. People may be placed in the boat by adding mushrooms, carrot chunks, or green beans.

Dips made of cottage cheese or yogurt may help to make the raw vegetables disappear.

Sandwich boat: hot-dog bun (unsliced) with filling in a slit in the top (egg salad or meat); a triangle cheese slice on a toothpick forms the sail.

Picnics in the house or outside provide variety in meals.

# Appendix D: Bibliography

Most of the books and articles that follow were included in this list because they offer broad coverage of various general aspects of nutrition, birth through teen years. The first section contains titles relevant to nutrition for all age groups, whereas the last three sections list titles dealing with the nutrition-related problems of infants, children, and adolescents, respectively. In all three sections, references of special interest to vegetarians are marked with an asterisk.

For extensive reading on prenatal nutrition see *Pregnancy and Nutrition,* National Nutrition Education Clearing House, Society for Nutrition Education, 2140 Shattuck Avenue, Suite 1110, Berkeley, California 94704 ($3.00 per copy). For personal help with prenatal nutrition·or any other aspect of prenatal care, contact International Childbirth Education Association (ICEA), Box 5852, Milwaukee, Wisconsin 53220 or the American Society for Psychoprophylaxis in Obstetrics (ASPO), 7 West 96 Street, New York, New York 10025. These organizations will be glad to provide information on childbirth education instructors in your area.

Those interested in going more deeply into the subject or in finding out more about specific problems and issues may wish to consult the complete, detailed, and comprehensive bibliography used by the authors in writing this book. Containing over 750 references, many of them highly technical articles from professional journals, this chapter-by-chapter bibliography may be obtained from the authors on request. Write: Peavy/Pagenkopf, 521 South Sixth Avenue, Bozeman, Montana 59715. Send $3.00 plus $1.00 for postage and handling.

## General Readings

Abraham, Sidney; Margaret D. Carroll; Connie M. Dresser; and Clifford L. Johnson. "Dietary Intake of Persons 1–74 Years of Age in the United States." *Advance Data* 6 (1977): 30.

Barnes, R. H. "Nutrition and Man's Intellect and Behavior." *Federation Proceedings* 30 (1971): 1429.

Cinnamon, Pamela, and M. A. Swanson. *Everything You Always Wanted to Know (But Were Unable to Find out) about Exchange Values for Foods.* Moscow, Idaho: University Cities Diabetes Education Program, 1973.

Deutsch, Ronald. *Realities in Nutrition.* Palo Alto, Calif.: Bull Publishing Company, 1976.

*Erhard, Darla. "The New Vegetarians: Part One—Vegetarianism and Its Medical Consequences." *Nutrition Today* 8 (Nov–Dec 1973): 4.

*———— . "The New Vegetarians: Part Two—The Zen Macrobiotic Movement and other Cults Based on Vegetarianism." *Nutrition Today* 9 (Jan–Feb 1974): 20.

*Ewald, Ellen B. *Recipes for a Small Planet*. New York: Ballantine Books, 1973.

*Exchange Lists for Meal Planning*. American Diabetes Association, and American Dietetic Association, 1976.

Fomon, Samuel J. *Nutritional Disorders of Children*. Rockville, Md.: Public Health Service, U.S. Department of Health, Education and Welfare, 1976.

———— and Thomas A. Anderson, eds. *Practices of Low-Income Families in Feeding Infants and Small Children with Particular Attention to Cultural Subgroups*. Rockville, Md.: U.S. Department of Health, Education and Welfare, Maternal and Child Health Service, 1972.

Gifft, Helen H.; Marjorie B. Washbon; and Gail G. Harrison. *Nutrition, Behavior, and Change*. Englewood Cliffs, N.J.: Prentice-Hall, 1972.

Gussow, Joan Dye. *The Feeding Web: Issues in Nutritional Ecology*. Palo Alto, Calif.: Bull Publishing Company, 1978.

Hamill, P.V.V.; T. A. Drizd; C. L. Johnson; R. B. Reed; A. F. Roche. *NCHS Growth Curves for Children, Birth–18 Years*. National Center for Health Statistics Publication, Series 11, Number 165, November, 1977.

Huenemann, Ruth L.; Mary C. Hampton; Albert R. Behnke; Leona R. Shapiro; and Barbara W. Mitchell. *Teenage Nutrition and Physique*. Springfield, Ill.: Charles C. Thomas, 1974.

Kallen, D.J., ed. *Nutrition, Development, and Social Behavior* (NH#73–242). Rockville, Md.: National Institute of Health, U.S. Department of Health, Education and Welfare, 1973.

Labuza, Theodore. *Food for Thought*. Westport, Conn.: Avi Publishing Company, 1974.

*Lappé, Frances Moore. *Diet for a Small Planet*. New York: Ballantine Books, 1971.

Masters, Donald D., and Howard Lewis. "The Sour Side of Sugar." *Journal of American Society for Preventive Dentistry*. (Jan–Feb 1975): 23.

Mayer, Jean. *Human Nutrition: Its Physiological, Medical, and Social Aspects*. Springfield, Ill.: Charles C. Thomas, 1972.

————. *Overweight—Causes, Cost and Control*. Englewood Cliffs, N.J.: Prentice-Hall, 1968.

————, ed. *U.S. Nutritional Policy in the Seventies.* San Francisco: W. H. Freeman, 1973.

National Academy of Science, Food and Nutrition Board. "The Relationship of Nutrition to Brain Development and Behavior." *Nutrition Today* 9 (1974): 12.

National Center for Health Statistics. *The Health of Children—1970* (PHS#2121). Rockville, Md.: Public Health Service, U.S. Department of Health, Education and Welfare.

National Research Council, Food and Nutrition Board. *Recommended Dietary Allowances.* 9th ed. Washington, D.C.: National Academy of Science, 1980.

Nelson, Waldo E. *Textbook of Pediatrics.* Philadelphia: W. B. Saunders, 1969.

Nizel, Abraham. *The Science of Nutrition and Its Application in Clinical Dentistry,* 2nd ed. Philadelphia: W. B. Saunders, 1966.

Parkins, Frederick. "Prescribing Fluoride Supplements For Home Use." In *Fluorides: An Update for Dental Practitioners.* New York: American Academy of Pedodontics, Medcom, 1976.

Pipes, Peggy. *Nutrition in Infancy and Childhood.* St. Louis: Mosby, 1977.

Read, M. S. "Malnutrition, Hunger and Behavior: Malnutrition and Learning." *Journal of American Dietetic Association* 63 (1973): 379.

*Robertson, Laurel; Carol Flinders; and Godfrey Bronwen. *Laurel's Kitchen.* Berkeley, Calif.: Nilgiri Press, 1976.

Robinson, Corinne. *Fundamentals of Normal Nutrition.* London: Collier-Macmillan, 1978.

Scrimshaw, N. S., and J. E. Gordon, eds. *Malnutrition, Learning, and Behavior.* Cambridge, Mass.: MIT, 1968.

Sherman, Mikie. *Feeding the Sick Child* (NIH#77-795). Rockville, Md.: National Institute of Health, U.S. Department of Health, Education and Welfare, 1977.

*Smith, Elizabeth B. "A guide to Good Eating the Vegetarian Way," *Journal of Nutrition Education* 7 (1975): 109.

*A Sourcebook on Food Practices with Emphasis on Children and Adolescents.* Chicago: National Dairy Council, 1968.

Spock, Dr. Benjamin. *Baby and Child Care.* New York: Pocket Books, 1973.

Stare, Frederick, and Margaret McWilliams. *Living Nutrition.* New York: Wiley, 1973.

Sweeney, Edward A., ed. *The Food That Stays: An Update on Nutrition, Diet, Sugar, and Caries.* New York: Medcom, 1977.

U.S. Congress, Senate, Committee on Nutrition and Human Needs, *Dietary Goals for the United States,* 95th Congress, 1st Session. January 14, 1977: p. 75.

U.S., Department of Health, Education and Welfare. *The Health of Children—1970.* Prepared for the National Center of Health Statistics, Public Health Service Publication 2121.

U.S. Department of Health, Education and Welfare. *Ten-State Nutrition Survey 1968–1970.* (HSM 72–8134). Atlanta: U.S. Department of Health, Education and Welfare.

White, Phillip L., and Nancy Selvey. *Let's Talk About Food.* Acton, Mass.: Publishing Sciences Group, 1974.

Williams, Sue Rodwell. *Nutrition and Diet Therapy.* St. Louis: Mosby, 1977.

Winick, Myron, *Childhood Obesity.* New York: Wiley, 1975.

———. *Malnutrition and Brain Development.* New York: Oxford, 1976.

———. *Nutrition and Cancer.* New York: Wiley, 1977.

# Infancy—
# Birth to Eighteen Months

American Academy of Pediatrics, Committee on Nutrition. "Iron Supplementation for Infants." *Pediatrics* 58 (1976): 765.

Brewer, Gail Sforza, and Tom Brewer. *What Every Pregnant Woman Should Know: The Truth about Diets and Drugs in Pregnancy.* New York: Random House, 1977.

California Department of Health. *Nutrition During Pregnancy and Lactation.* Sacramento: California Department of Health, 1975.

Castle, Sue. *The Complete Guide to Preparing Baby Foods at Home.* New York: Doubleday, 1973.

Ewy, Donna, and Roger Ewy. *Preparation for Breastfeeding.* New York: Doubleday, 1975.

Fomon, Samuel J., ed. *Infant Nutrition.* 2d ed. Philadelphia: W. B. Saunders, 1974.

Fomon, Samuel J.; L. J. Filer; T. A. Anderson; E. E. Ziegler. "Recommendations for Feeding Normal Infants." *Pediatrics* 63 (1979): 52–59.

Hambraeus, Leif. "Proprietary Milk Versus Human Breast Milk in Infant Feeding: A Critical Appraisal from the Nutritional Point of View." *Pediatric Clinics of North America* 24 (Feb 1977): 17.

"Iron Absorption from Breast Milk or Cow's Milk." *Nutrition Reviews* 35 (1977): 203.

Jackson, Robert L. "Long-term Consequences of Suboptimal Nutritional Practices in Early Life: Some Important Benefits of Breast Feeding." *Pediatric Clinics of North America* 24 (1977): 17.

Jakobsson, Irene, and Tor Lindberg. "Cows' Milk As a Cause of Infantile Colic in Breast-fed Infants." *Lancet* 2 (August 26, 1978): 437–39.

Jelliffe, D. B., and Jelliffe, E.F.P. *Human Milk in the Modern World.* London: Oxford, 1976.

Kenda, Margaret, and Phyllis Williams. *The Natural Baby Food Cookbook.* New York: Avon, 1973.

Klaus, Marshall H., and John H. Kennell. *Maternal-Infant Bonding.* St. Louis: C. V. Mosby, 1976.

La Leche League International. *The Womanly Art of Breast-Feeding.* Franklin Park, Ill.: La Leche League, 1963. (For extensive information on all aspects of breast-feeding, write to La Leche League International, Inc., 9616 Minneapolis Avenue, Franklin Park, Illinois 60131.)

McMillan, J. A.; S. A. Landaw; and F. A. Oski. "Iron Sufficiency in Breast-fed Infants and the Availability of Iron from Human Milk." *Pediatrics* 58 (1976): 686.

Nizel, Abraham E. " 'Nursing Bottle Syndrome': Rampant Dental Caries in Young Children." *Nutrition News* 38 (Feb 1975): 1.

*Peavy, Linda S. "Breastfeeding Your Baby." *Vegetarian Times* 22 (1977): 27.

———. *Have a Healthy Baby: A Guide to Prenatal Nutrition and Nutrition for Nursing Mothers.* New York: Drake Division, Sterling Publishers, Inc, 1977.

Pryor, Karen. *Nursing Your Baby.* New York: Pocket Books, 1973.

Saarinen, U. M. "Need for Iron Supplementation in Infants on Prolonged Breast Feeding." *Journal of Pediatrics* 93 (1978): 177.

Turner, Mary D., and James Turner. *Making Your Own Baby Food.* New York: Workman, 1977.

Woodruff, Calvin W. "Iron Deficiency in Infancy and Childhood." *Pediatric Clinics of North America* 24 (1977): 85.

Worthington, Bonnie; Joyce Vermeersch; and Sue Rodwell Williams. *Nutrition in Pregnancy and Lactation.* St. Louis: C. V. Mosby, 1977.

# Childhood—
# Eighteen Months to Ten Years

The National Dairy Council (111 North Canal Street, Chicago, Illinois 60606) and the National Livestock and Meat Board (36 South Wabash Avenue, Chicago, Illinois 60603) both have available several excellent publications for childhood nutrition education. Price lists are available upon request. Local U.S. Extension Service nutritionists can provide several pamphlets for children interested in nutrition.

*A Complete Summary of the Iowa Breakfast Studies.* Chicago: Cereal Institute, 1976.

Crook, William G. "Food Allergy—the Great Masquerader." *Pediatric Clinics of North America* 22 (1975): 227.

Ellison, Virginia H. *The Pooh Cookbook.* New York: Dutton, 1969.

Expert Panel on Food Safety and Nutrition and Committee on Public Information. *Diet and Hyperactivity: Any Connection?* Chicago: Institute of Food Technologists, 1976.

MaKinen, K. K. "The Role of Sucrose and Other Sugars in the Development of Dental Caries: A Review." *International Dentistry Journal* 22 (1972): 363.

McClenahan, Mary, and Ida Jaqua. *Cool Cooking for Kids: Recipes and Nutrition for Preschoolers.* Belmont, Calif.: Fearon, 1976.

Moore, Eva. *The Lucky Cookbook.* Englewood Cliffs, N.J.: Scholastic Book Service, 1970.

National Research Council, Committee on Nutrition of Mother and Preschool Child, Food and Nutrition Board. "Summary of a Workshop: Fetal and Infant Nutrition and Susceptibility to Obesity." *Nutrition Reviews* 36 (1978): 122.

Nizel, Abraham E. "Preventing Dental Caries: The Nutritional Factors." *Pediatric Clinics of North America* 24 (1977): 141.

Palmer, Sushma; Judith L. Rapoport; and Patricia O. Quinn. "Food Additives and Hyperactivity." *Clinical Pediatrics* 14 (Oct 1975): 956.

Read, M.S. "Malnutrition, Hunger and Behavior: School Feeding Programs and Behavior." *Journal of American Dietetic Association* 63 (1973): 386.

*Vyhmeister, Irma B.; U. D. Register; and Lydia M. Sonnenberg. "Safe Vegetarian Diets for Children." *Pediatric Clinics of North America* 24 (1977): 203.

Walker, Sydney, III. "Drugging the American Child: We're Too Cavalier about Hyperactivity." *Psychology Today* 8 (Dec 1974): 43.

# Adolescence—
# Eleven to Nineteen Years

Bruch, Hilde. "Anorexia Nervosa." *Nutrition Today* 13 (1978): 14.

Bogert, Jean; George Briggs; and Doris H. Calloway. *Nutrition and Physical Fitness.* Philadelphia: W. B. Saunders, 1973.

Hodges, R.E. "Nutrition and 'The Pill.' " *Journal of American Dietetic Association* 59 (1971): 212.

Meyer, Eleanore E., and Charlotte G. Neumann. "Management of the Obese Adolescent." *Pediatric Clinics of North America* 24 (1977): 123.

McKigney, John I., and Hamish N. Munro. *Nutrient Requirements in Adolescence* (NIH#76–77). Rockville, Md.: National Institute of Health, U.S. Department of Health, Education and Welfare. 1976.

National Research Council, Committee on Maternal Nutrition, Food and Nutrition Board. *Maternal Nutrition and the Course of Pregnancy: Summary Report.* Reprinted by U.S. Department of Health, Education and Welfare, 1970.

*Nutrition for Athletes: A Handbook for Coaches.* Washington, D.C.: American Association for Health, Physical Education and Recreation, 1971.

*Nutrition in Maternal Health Care.* Chicago: American College of Obstetricians and Gynecologists, Committee on Nutrition, 1974.

Smith, Nathan J. *Food for Sport.* Palo Alto, Calif.: Bull Publishing, 1976.

Winick, Myron. *Nutritional Disorders of American Women.* New York: Wiley, 1977.

Zackler, J., and W. Brandstadt. *The Teenage Pregnant Girl.* Springfield, Ill.: Charles C. Thomas, 1975.

# INDEX

Absorption. *See also* Malabsorption
 of calcium, 45
 of fats, 87–88
 of iron, 43, 83, 88, 118
 of protein, 51
 of zinc, 46
Acceptance of Various Solids, 77
Acne, 224
ACT (Action for Children's Television), 143
Activity Required to Expend Calories, 217–18
Actometers, 104
Additives, food, 1
 in analogs, 93
 in baby foods, 89–91
 in enriched foods, 114
 hyperactivity and, 174, 176
 in juices, 116
 sugar as, 113
Adenosine triphosphate (ATP), 235
Advertising, 88, 139–40, 142–44, 167, 222
Age-Related Willingness to Try New Foods, 120
Alcohol, use of, during
 lactation, 56
 pregnancy, 228
 training and competition, 237
Alcoholism, teen, 229
Allergic responses, 98
Allergies
 complexion problems and, 224
 emotional and physical problems and, 176, 177–78, 223
 hyperactivity and, 174, 176
 in infancy, 62, 63, 83, 89, 97–98, 103
 milk-related, 51, 60, 67, 69, 71, 164
 obesity and, 103
American Academy of Pediatrics, 49, 50, 90, 117, 163
American Academy of Pedodontics, 46
American College of Obstetrics & Gynecology, 228
American Diabetes Association, 8
American Dietetic Association, 8
American Heart Association, 14, 17, 115, 161, 198
American Medical Association, 189

American Newspaper Publishers Association, 142
American Public Health Association, 50
Amino acids, 16, 43
 metabolism errors of, 67
Amphetamines, 174–75
Amylase (enzyme), 90
Analogs, 93, 164
Anemia, 2, 59
 effects on behavior and, 117
 iron deficiency, 3, 87, 117, 203–204
 macrocytic, 45, 226
 megaloblastic, 21, 45, 87, 202
 pernicious, 87, 149, 150, 164, 202
*Anorexia nervosa,* 212–13
Antibodies in breast milk, 50
Appetite
 drug stimulation of, 147
 psychological aspects of, 119, 165, 168–69
 as reliable guide to sound nutrition, 12, 32, 36, 154, 194
 variations in, 12, 108, 121
Appetite control mechanism, 36–37, 52, 53, 63, 73, 82, 88, 96, 108
Appetite loss
 alcohol use and, 229
 dieting and, 221
 drug use and, 175, 229
 excessive protein intake and, 231
 illness and, 148
 vitamin and mineral deficiencies and, 119
Arachiodonic acid (fatty acid), 43
Ascorbic acid. *See* Vitamin C
Asthma, food, 98
Atherosclerosis, 76, 114, 161, 198
Athletes and diet, 6, 179–81, 220, 221, 230–38

Baby foods. *See also* Formula
 commercially prepared
  additives and preservatives in, 81, 89–91
  cereals, 80, 88–89
  storage of, 78–79, 89
 home prepared, 81, 91–93
  storage of, 78–79

Bacteria
  caries-causing, 100, 131, 135, 137
  food contamination and, 47, 61, 62,
    78–79, 90
  resistance to, of breast-fed babies, 50–
    51
Behavior modification, 6, 150
*Beikost,* 88
Beriberi, 45
Bile acids, 43, 114
Bile salts, 15
Biotin (water soluble vitamin), 18, 23
Blood clots, 44, 226
Blood pressure. *See* Hypertension
Blood sugar levels, 13
  breakfast-skipping and, 209
  hyperactivity and, 174
  hypoglycemia and, 178–79
  vitamin C megadoses and, 163
Body fat, 74, 220, 234
  "puppy fat," 198, 210
Body types, 210–11
Bone development, 180
  amino acids and, 16
  calcium and, 164, 202
  drug use and, 175
  vitamin A and, 6
  vitamin D and, 44
Bottle-feeding. *See also* Formula
  bonding and, 64–66
  breast-feeding vs., 47–54
  formula preparation for, 58–62
  growth spurt during, 76
  "nursing bottle syndrome" and, 84,
    99–100
  overfeeding and, 37, 52, 62, 73
  psychological aspects of, 64–67
  weaning, 85
Botulism, infant, 69, 83–84
Bowel movements, 72, 161, 237
Brain development, 33
  cholesterol intake and, 14
  fatty acid intake and, 43
  malnutrition and, 2, 16
  protein intake and, 16, 112
Breakfast, 142, 186
  -skipping, 186, 208–209
Breast-feeding
  advantages of, 47–54
  appetite control mechanism and, 36–37
  bonding and, 51–52, 64–65
  bottle-feeding vs., 47–54
  bowel movements and, 72
  colic and, 69–72
  deficiency symptoms and, 94
  fears about, 54–58
  growth spurt during, 74, 76
  illness and, 47–48, 51, 99
  immunities given through, 43, 50–51
  "nursing bottle syndrome" and, 99,
    101–102
  optimum nutrition and, 34, 58
  psychological aspects of, 64–67
  schedules and, 85
  supplements and, 43–44, 46, 79
  weaning, 15, 77, 87

"Bronze diabetes," 204
Brucellosis, 222

Cafeteria meals, 181–84, 239
Calcium (mineral), 25
  deficiencies, 3, 25, 45, 174
  enamel formation and, 45, 134
  in fad diets, 221
  in fast-foods diets, 238
  food sources, 25, 60, 128, 164
  functions, 25
  hyperactivity and, 174
  needs during:
    adolescence, 9n, 200, 201, 208
    elementary school years, 157, 161,
      163
    infancy, 36
    lactation, 57, 201
    pregnancy, 201
    preschool years, 109
  in soy-based milk, 60, 164
  supplements, 149, 164, 202
  toxicity, 25
  in vegetarian diets, 60, 117, 149, 164,
    202
Calorie Distributions in Infant Milk, 42
Calorie expenditure, 12, 80, 104, 219,
    231–32
  activity and, 216, 217–18
  obesity and, 214–215
Calorie intake, 12, 18
  adolescence, 194, 195, 198, 200
  elementary school years, 156, 157, 158,
    160, 162, 164
  fad diets and, 219–21
  infancy, 35, 36
  lactation, 57, 195
  obesity and, 104, 214–15
  pregnancy, 195, 228
  preschool years, 108, 109, 114
  sources of, 13–15, 42, 76, 78, 167, 231–
    32
  training and competition, 180,
    231–32
  in vegetarian diets, 161
  in weight control diets, 145, 146, 214–
    15, 239
Calories, balance of intake and
  expenditure, 10, 12, 80, 104, 219,
    231–32
Calories, "empty," 140, 203, 208, 229
Cancer, 14, 55, 132
Carbohydrate loading, 236–37
Carbohydrate Percentage of Various
  Infant Foods, 78
Carbohydrates
  caries and, 100, 136
  energy source, 13
  in fad diets, 220
  hypoglycemia and, 179
  in infant's diet
    breast milk, 42, 43, 50, 78
    formula milk, 42, 50, 78
    skim milk, 42, 77
    solid foods, 77, 78
  metabolic problems and, 67

Carbohydrates *(continued)*
   in preschooler's diet, 109, 113–14, 140
   in recovery diet, 99
   in snacks, 136, 140
   in training and competition, 230, 235,
      236–37
   types of, 13–14, 32, 51, 114, 161, 199
Carcinogens, 90, 137
Cardiovascular system, 233
Caries, dental
   in adolescents, 224
   causes of, 131–32, 134–37
      "nursing bottle syndrome," 85, 99,
         100, 101-102, 131
      snacks and sweets, 134–35, 140, 199
   in elementary school children, 169
   fluoridation of water and, 132–34, 169
   history of, 129–31, 130
Cariogens, 99, 101, 135, 137
Casein (protein), 43, 59
Cavities. *See* Caries, dental
Cereals
   breakfast food, 140, 141, 142
   food group, 9, 138
   in infant diet, 77, 80, 83, 93
   snack, 138, 168
Charren, Peggy (ACT), 143
Chewing, 92, 126, 131, 137
Chewing gum, 137
Chloride (mineral), 26
Cholesterol
   in breast and formula milk, 43
   excessive intake of, 1, 9n, 74, 198–99
   functions of, 14–15
   levels in preschoolers, 114–15
   reduced intake of, 14, 161, 199
   in snack foods, 136, 138n
   in training diets, 231, 234
   in vegetarian diets, 149, 221
Chromium (trace element), 31
*Clostridium botulinum,* 83–84
Cobalt (trace element), 29
Colic, infant, 68–72
College meals, 239
Colostrum, 50, 64
Commercials, 139–40, 142–44, 167
Complementary Protein Guide, 17
Computer analyses of dietary intake
      records, 241, 244, 246, 248, 250
Constipation, 58, 72, 178
Consumer education, 143–44, 167
Contraceptives and diet, 56–57, 225–27
Convulsions, 45
Cooking and children, 151–52, 184, 239
Copper (trace element), 29, 46
Coulehan, J.L., 163
Cup, as infant utensil, 85, 87, 95
Cyanocobalamin. *See* Vitamin $B_{12}$

Dairy products. *See also* Milk, cow's
   snacks, 138–39
   sources of:
      calcium, 9n, 161, 163, 202
      non-heme iron, 118
      vitamin $B_{12}$, 164, 202
   in vegetarian diets, 149, 164, 202
DDT (ecological toxicant), 56

Deficiencies, nutrient, 54, 94, 200, 202
   fatty acid, 15
   mineral, 24, 119, 176, 200, 202
   protein, 15–16
   vitamin, 24, 119, 176, 200, 202
Deficiency disorders. *See* Anemia;
      Hyperactivity; Goiter; Kwashiorkor;
      Marasmus; Wernicke-Korsakoff's
      Syndrome
Dehydration
   excessive protein intake and, 231
   fad diets and, 221
   heat exhaustion and, 181
   infant diarrhea and, 72, 99
   training diets and, 233, 235
Dental hygiene, 100, 102, 131
Dentine, 100, 132
Depression, 203, 226, 229
Diabetes, 8, 179
   "bronze," 204
Diarrhea
   excessive protein intake and, 231
   fat deprivation and, 15, 115, 161
   in infancy, 47–48, 72, 99
Diet
   acne and, 224
   "of affluence," 199
   constipation and, 58, 72, 178
   diabetes and, 179
   fad, 13, 180, 210, 219-21
   high-carbohydrate, 236–37
   high-protein, 179, 230
   hypoglycemia and, 179
   inadequate, 2, 194
   low-carbohydrate, 220, 236
   low-cholesterol, 114–15
   during pregnancy and lactation, 57–58,
      227–28
   during recovery from illness, 148–49
   during training and competition, 6,
      179–81, 228-36
Diet alterations, 219–23
   fad weight-loss, 219–21
   group membership weight-loss, 219
   health foods and, 222–23
   liquid formula, 221, 237
   meal-skipping, 221
   natural foods and, 222–23
   organically grown foods and, 222–23
   restriction, 220
   starvation, 221
*Diet for a Small Planet* (Lappé), 16
Dietary Intake Records, 240–41, 243,
      244–45, 247, 249
Digestion
   of carbohydrates, 13
   colic and, 68
   immature system of infant and, 33, 68,
      76, 83
   of proteins, 16
   psychological aspects of, 125, 168–69
   during training and competition, 237
Disliked foods, 96, 124, 126, 128
Disliked Foods by Categories, 128
Diuretics, 180, 212, 233
Drug use
   for appetite stimulation, 147

Drug use *(continued)*
  for colic, 68–69
  for hyperactivity, 173–75, 177
  during lactation, 56–57
  during pregnancy, 228–29
  during training and competition, 234–35
Dyslexia, 174

Eating habits, 14, 67
  in adolescence, 207, 209–10, 239
  behavior modification and, 6, 105, 150, 173
  fad diets and, 219–21
  family influence and, 1, 85, 113–14, 251
  obesity and, 145, 171
  overeating, 77, 214
  preventive dental care and, 132, 134
  supplementation in poor, 115
Ectomorph, 210–11
Electrolyte balance
  disturbance of, 180–81
  restoration of, 72, 99
Electrolytic iron, 80
Enamel
  damage to, in caries, 131, 132, 134
  formation of, 45, 134
Endocrine activity, 191
Endomorph, 210–11
Energy, 11–13
  expenditure, 216, 217–18
  needs of:
    adolescents, 195
    athletes, 180, 231–33, 235–37
    elementary school children, 157
    infants, 36
    preschoolers, 109, 113
  sources, 13, 15, 114, 161, 199, 208, 220, 231–32
Energy Expenditure for Selected Recreational Activities, 216
Enriched foods. *See also* Fortified foods
  breads and flours, 114
  formula, 43–46, 60, 79
  milk, 222
Environmental factors in growth and development, 2, 5
Enzyme deficiency, 67, 164
Enzymes, 16
  in breast milk, 43
  food contamination and, 90
  tooth decay and, 132
Estrogen (hormone), 226
Exchange plan, 7–8, 9, 96, 154–55, 171, 179, 187, 199
  *See also* Family Guide to Minimum Exchanges Chart
Exercise
  *anorexia nervosa* and 212
  as energy expenditure, 12–13, 216, 217–18
  obesity
    adolescent, 214–16, 218–19
    childhood, 145–47, 172–73
    infantile, 104–105
Extension Service. *See* United States Department of Agriculture

Fad diets, 13, 180, 219–21
  *See also* Diet alterations
Family Guide to Minimum Exchanges Chart, 9
Fast Foods, 238–39
Fat(s)
  absorption of, 87–88
  cancer and, 14
  in child's diet, 109, 164
  cholesterol intake and, 14, 114–15
  content of infant foods, 42, 50, 76–77, 91
  deprivation of, 115, 161
  dietary reduction of, 14, 17, 198–99
  in fad diets, 220
  in fast-foods diets, 238
  as food group, 8, 9
    saturated, 14, 164, 220
  in training diet, 234, 235
    unsaturated, 9n
  in vegetarian diets, 149, 164, 198
Fat cell number theory, 4, 52–53, 103, 145–46, 170–71
Fat soluble vitamins (A, D, E, K), 14–15, 19–20
Fatty acid deprivation, 15
Fatty acids, 43, 44
Favorite Foods by Categories, 127
Feingold, Dr. Ben, 176
Feinstein, Susan, 184
Ferrous sulfate, 80
Fetal alcohol syndrome, 228
Fiber (dietary), 1, 8, 13, 18, 161, 199
  cancer and, 14
  iron absorption and, 118
  in vegetarian regimen, 149, 164
  whole grain foods and, 114
Fingernail growth, 225
Flexibility, 106
Fluid intake
  dental hygiene and, 135
  heat exhaustion and, 181
  during illness, 148–49
  during lactation, 58
  during training and competition, 233, 237
  vegetarian diets and, 149, 164
Fluoridation of water, 132–34
Fluoride (trace element), 29
  deficiencies, 29
  food sources, 29
  functions, 29
  supplements, 46–47, 132, 134, 169
  topical application, 131, 134
  toxicity, 29
Folacin (water soluble vitamin), 21
  deficiencies, 21, 45, 226
  food sources, 9n, 21
  functions, 21
  needs during:
    adolescence, 201
    elementary school years, 157
    infancy, 36
    lactation, 58, 201
    oral contraceptive use, 226–27
    pregnancy, 201, 227
    preschool years, 109

Folacin *(continued)*
  supplements, 45, 87, 226–27
  toxicity, 21
  vitamin B₁₂ deficiency and, 150
Folic acid. *See* Folacin
Fomon, Dr. Samuel, 33, 35, 42, 77, 114
Food exchanges. *See* Exchange plan;
    Family Guide to Minimum
    Exchanges Chart
Food groups, 7–8, 9, 105, 138, 200, 233
Food jags, 97, 123–24
Food preparation. *See also* Formula
    preparation
  additives and, 80–81, 90–91
  child participation in, 137, 151–52, 168,
    184
  contamination and, 78–79, 89–90
  of infant foods, 89, 93
  nutrient loss during, 27, 32
  for travel, 89
  of vegetables, 127
Foods, introduction of
  allergies and, 63, 88, 98
  psychological aspects of, 94–95, 119–
    20, 124, 150
  solids in infant diet, 62–64, 88
  weight gain and, 103
Football, 180–81, 230, 234
Force-feeding
  during childhood, 108, 119, 120
  during infancy, 27, 52, 62, 82, 94, 96,
    103, 104
  infantile obesity and, 73
Foreman, Carol Tucker, 162
Formula, milk, 58–61
  calories in, 42
  contaminants in, 56
  first commercial, 47
  fortified, 43–46, 79
    nutrient content of, 42–47, 50
    carbohydrates, 42, 78
    fats, 42
    minerals, 34, 45–57
    protein, 42, 43
    vitamins, 43–45
  other foods and, 63
  overfeeding, 37, 52, 62
  supplementation with, 77
  water content of, 35
  weaning, 87
Formula preparation
  commercial, 58–62
  home-prepared, 58–59, 60
Fortified foods, 11, 24, 140
  formulas, 43–46, 60, 79
  iron in, 46, 79, 83, 204
  in vegetarian diets, 164
  vitamin B₁₂ in, 164
  vitamin C in, 116
  vitamin D in, 222
Fructose (carbohydrate), 67, 113, 136
Fruits
  carbodydrate content of, 78
  caries formation and, 131, 132
  as food group, 8, 9
  introduction of, to infant diet, 77, 126
  as snacks, 138–39, 168

Gas-forming foods
  colic and, 68, 69, 70–71
  in training and competition, 237
  in vegetarian diets, 93
Gastrointestinal disorders, 61, 62, 72, 79,
    87
Gastrointestinal tract, 62
Gelatin, 224–25
Gerrard, Dr. John, 51
Glass and Fleisch, 140
Glucose (carbohydrate), 113, 136, 236
  level in hypoglycemia, 178–79
Glucose intolerance, 4, 74
Glucose tolerance test, 179
Glycogen stores, 234, 236
Goiter, 2
Grains in protein complementarity, 17, 93
Growth charts
  adolescents, 196, 197
  elementary school-age, 158, 159
  infants, 38–41
  preschool-age, 110–115
Growth patterns
  during adolescence, 191–94, 206–207,
    234
  decrease in growth rate, 108, 147
  drug use and, 175
  during elementary school years, 157–60
  fad diets and, 180
  growth spurt
    during adolescence, 160, 192
    infancy, 74, 76
    preschool years, 121
  hormone treatments and, 234
  during infancy, 37–41, 81
  during preschool years, 112
  protein needs and, 15
  zinc deficiency and, 119
*Guide for Nutra Lunches and Natural
    Foods* (Sloan), 183
Guidelines for Healthful Snacks, 138–39
Gum. *See* Chewing gum
Gussow, Joan Dye, 140


Hair growth, 224
Hall, Dr. Barbara, 53
Hallucinogens, 56, 228, 229
Health foods, 135, 223
*Health of Children, The* (HEW), 2
Heart disease
  fats and, 198–99
  fatty acids and, 14
  low-cholesterol diet and, 14, 43, 114–15
  mineral balance and, 46
  vegetarian diet and, 165
Heart failure, 68, 181
Heat exhaustion, 180–81, 235
Height norms. *See also* Growth charts
  for adolescents, 192–94
  calcium deficiency and, 3
  for elementary school children, 160
  for infants, 37–41, 88
  for preschoolers, 112
Heme iron, 118
Hemochromatosis ("bronze diabetes"),
    204

Hemoglobin, 117, 203
Hemorrhage
  immature digestive tract and, 59, 76, 87
  postpartum, 53
  vitamin C dependency and, 45
  vitamin K, in prevention of, 44
Hemorrhagic disease, 44
High-protein diet, 179, 230
Histidine (amino acid), 16
History of Incidence of Dental Caries, 130
Honey
  caries and, 101
  in infant botulism, 69, 83–84
  in infant diet, 80
  as natural food, 222
Hormonal change
  during drug use, 175
  during lactation, 52, 53, 56
Hormones,
  cholesterol and, 14–15, 43
  development of, 14–15, 114, 191
  use of:
    in acne treatment, 224
    in training diets, 234–35
"Hundred Days Party," 72
Hyperactivity, 3–4, 173–77
  allergies and, 176, 223
  *anorexia nervosa* and, 212
  causes of, 174
  deficiencies and, 174
  diagnosis of, 173, 174
  drug therapy in, 173, 174–76, 177
  glucose intolerance and, 4
  restrictive diet in, 176
  symptoms of, 173
  vitamin therapy in, 176–77
Hypercholesterolemia, 115, 164
Hyperkinetic. *See* Hyperactivity
Hypertension, 46, 80
Hypoglycemia, 178–79
  diagnosis of, 179
  diet for, 179
  hyperactivity and, 174

Illness
  in bottle- and breast-fed infants, 47–48,
    50–51
  colds and vitamin C therapy, 162–63
  growth patterns and, 112, 160
  inadequate diet and, 194
  obesity and, 102–103
  psychosomatic, 223
  recovery diet, 87, 148–49
Immunological properties of breast milk,
    43, 50–51
Infant foods. *See* Baby food; *Beikost;*
    Formula, milk; Milk
Influence of prenatal nutrition, 2, 47,
    227–28
Influence on diet patterns
  of culture, 2
  of family, 1–2, 113–14, 147
  of parents, 105, 107–108, 124, 156, 251
  of peers, 156, 165, 194
  of television, 5, 139–40, 142–44
Insecticides, 56
Insulin (hormone), 179

Intrauterine device (IUD), 57, 225, 227
Iodine (trace element), 27, 28
  deficiencies, 28, 203
  food sources, 28
  functions, 28
  needs during:
    adolescence, 201
    elementary school years, 157
    infancy, 36
    lactation, 58, 201
    pregnancy, 201
    preschool years, 109
  toxicity, 28
  in vegetarian diets, 24, 150
Iron (trace element), 24, 27, 28
  absorption of, 79, 80, 83, 88, 118
  in breast and formula milk, 46, 50, 79
  deficiencies, 3, 28, 117, 118–19, 164,
    203–204
  in fast-foods diets, 238
  food sources, 28, 204–205
  functions, 28
  heme and non-heme iron, 118
  needs during:
    adolescence, 200, 201
    contraceptive use, 226–27
    elementary school years, 157, 163
    infancy, 36
    lactation, 201
    menstruation, 3, 232
    pregnancy, 3, 201, 227
    preschool years, 109
  supplements, 3, 45–46, 50, 79–80, 203–
    204
  toxicity, 28, 115
  in vegetarian diets, 161
Isoleucine (amino acid), 16

Juices
  in infant diet, 89
  as snack food, 168
  vitamin C in orange, 116
Junk food, 6, 161, 162, 169, 222

Ketones, 220
Ketosis, 13, 220, 221
Kidney function
  growth patterns and, 160
  heat exhaustion and, 181
  megadoses of vitamin C and, 163
  metabolic errors and, 67
  protein overload and, 15, 59
  rapid weight loss and, 234
Kilocalorie, 12
Klaus and Kennell, 65
Knittle, Dr. Jerome, 170
Kokoh, 60
Kwashiorkor, 15–16

Labels and nutrient content, 24, 27, 91,
    222
Lactalbumin (protein), 43
Lactation. *See also* Breast-feeding
  breast cancer and, 55
  contraceptive use during, 56–57
  "let-down" reflex in, 34, 34n, 49, 65

Lactation *(continued)*
  nutritional needs during, 12, 53, 57–58,
    201
Lactoferrin (protein), 50, 79
Lactose (carbohydrate), 43, 101, 113
  intolerance, 67, 99
Lactovegetarian. *See* Vegetarian diets
Lacto-ovo vegetarian. *See* Vegetarian
  diets
La Leche League International, 55, 70
Lappe, Frances (*Diet for a Small Planet*),
  16
Laxatives, 178, 212, 233
Lead poisoning, 56, 62
  in hyperactivity, 174
Legumes in protein complementarity, 17,
  93
"Let-down" reflex, 34, 34n, 49, 53, 65
Leucine (amino acid), 16
Leukocytes, 50
Linoleic acid (fatty acid), 15, 43
Lipase (enzyme), 43
Lipids. *See* Fat(s)
Liquid meals
  in training diets, 237
  in weight loss diets, 220, 221
Liver function, 15, 179, 236
Low-carbohydrate diets, 179, 220, 236
Low-cholesterol diets, 114–15
Lunch
  sack, 187
  school lunch programs, 181–84
Lymph, 16
Lymphocytes, 50
Lysine (amino acid), 16

Macrobiotic diet, 149, 221
Magnesium (mineral), 25
  deficiencies, 25
  food sources, 25
  functions, 25
  loss in fad diets, 221
  needs during:
    adolescence, 201
    elementary school years, 157
    infancy, 36
    lactation, 201
    pregnancy, 201
    preschool years, 109
  toxicity, 25
Malabsorption, 10, 194
Malnutrition, 2–3, 5
  brain development and, 2
  deficiency disorders and, 2–3, 15
  obesity and, 13
Manganese (trace element), 29
Marasmus, 2, 15
*Maternal Nutrition and the Course of
  Pregnancy* (NRC), 228
Mayer, Dr. Jean, 54, 98, 113, 115, 140
Meal patterns. *See also* Eating habits;
  in adolescence, 207–209
  in infancy, 73–75, 85, 106
  in preschool years, 123, 154
Mealtimes
  infants and, 82, 85–86, 94–97
  psychological aspects of, 82, 86, 97,
    119–26, 129

snack foods for, 138–39
  toddlers and, 119–29
Meats
  in elementary-school child's diet, 161
  as a food group, 8, 9
  in infant's diet, 77, 78, 79
  in preschooler's diet, 127, 128
  as snack food, 138
Megadoses, vitamins and minerals, 24,
    115, 223, 232
  hyperactivity and, 176–77
  iron, 204
  vitamin A, 176–77, 224
  vitamin C, 45, 162–63, 232
Menadione (vitamin K), 20
Menstruation
  contraceptive use and, 227
  iron depletion during, 3, 203, 232
  lactation and, 57
  onset of, 191–92, 193
Mesomorph, 210–11
Metabolism, 12, 13, 15
  of carbohydrates, 175
  of cholesterol, 43
  of fats, 220
  of vitamin $B_{12}$, 226
Metabolism errors, 67
Methemoglobinemia, 35, 78
Methionine (amino acid), 16
Milk. *See also* milk entries below
  allergies, 51, 60, 67, 69, 164
  anti-milk movement, 163–64
  as a food group, 9
Milk, almond, 60
Milk, breast
  calories in, 42–43
  contaminants in, 56
  drugs in, 56–57
  immunological properties of, 50–51
  iron absorption and, 79, 80
  nutrient content of, 34, 42, 43–46, 50,
    76–77
    carbohydrates, 42–43
    fats, 42–43
    minerals, 34, 45–46, 79
    protein, 42–43
    vitamins, 43–45
  in recovery diet, 87
  supplements with, 44, 46–47, 77, 79
  tooth decay and, 100–102
  water content of, 35
Milk, cow's
  evaporated, 56, 59
  formula
    constipation and, 72
    digestive problems and, 60, 69
    fortified, 43–46, 79
    nutrient content of, 42–47, 50
    carbohydrates, 42, 78
    fats, 42
    minerals, 34, 45–47
    protein, 42, 43
    vitamins, 43–45
  skim
    calories in, 42
    in infant diet, 43, 76–77, 88
    in low-cholesterol diet, 114
    nutrient content of, 42

Milk, cow's *(continued)*
  two-percent (low fat)
    calories in, 42
    in child's diet, 104
    in infant's diet, 42, 88
    in low-cholesterol diet, 114
    nutrient content of, 42
  whole
    in adolescent's diet, 202
    allergies and, 51, 60, 71, 174
    in elementary-school child's diet, 163–64
    hyperactivity and, 174
    in infant's diet, 59, 76, 88
    nutrient content of, 42–46
      carbohydrates, 42, 43
      fats, 42–43
      minerals, 45–46
      protein, 42, 43
      vitamins, 43–44
    pathogens in, 47
    in preschooler's diet, 113, 116
    as snack food, 168, 186
    in vegetarian diets, 164
    weaning to, 87
Milk, formula. *See* Formula, milk
Milk, goat's, 45, 59, 87
Milk, human. *See* Milk, breast
Milk, soy-based, 33, 43, 59
  calories in, 42
  fortified, 45
  inadequacies, of, 60, 164
  lactose intolerance and, 67
  nutrient content of, 42, 49
  in recovery diet, 99
  in vegetarian diets, 60, 149, 164
Minerals, 24–31
  content of breast and formula milk, 45–46
  deficiencies in hyperactivity, 174, 176
  in fast-foods diet, 238
  needs during:
    adolescence, 200, 202–204
    elementary school years, 163–64
    infancy, 45–46, 79–81
    lactation, 58, 200, 228
    pregnancy, 200, 228
    preschool years, 115–19
    training and competition, 232, 234
  in snack foods, 136–37
Minimum exchanges chart, 8, 9, 10, 27, 32, 124, 154
Molybdenum (trace element), 30
Monolaurin, 102
Monosodium glutamate, 89
Mortality rates
  *anorexia nervosa* and, 212
  in infancy, 48, 227
Mottling in enamel formation, 46, 133, 134
Multivitamins
  balanced diet and, 5, 18, 96, 115, 162
  for bottle- and breast-fed infants, 77
  during contraceptive use, 226–27
  containing fluoride, 134
  health-food diets and, 223
Muscle development, 180, 191
  iron and, 203

protein and, 16, 112, 198, 231
  weight gain and, 233, 234
Muscle energy, 235

National Academy of Science, 10
National Heart and Lung Institute, 8
National Institute of Health, 8
National March of Dimes Foundation, 228
National Research Council (NRC), 12, 24, 118, 228
National School Lunch Act, 182
Natural food diet, 221
Nausea, 221, 227
Necrotizing enterocolitis, 50
Niacin (water soluble vitamin), 21
  content of breast and formula milk, 45
  deficiencies, 21, 229
  food sources, 21
  functions, 21
  needs during:
    adolescence, 201
    elementary school years, 157
    infancy, 36
    lactation, 58, 201
    pregnancy, 201
    preschool years, 109
  toxicity, 21
Nickel (trace element), 31
Nicotinic acid. *See* Niacin
Night vision, 6
Nitrates, 78–79, 89
Nitrites, 35, 78–79, 89
Nizel, Dr. Abraham, 132, 139n, 169
Non-heme iron, 118
Nora, a case history, 188–91, 239–40
  Computer Analysis of diet, 250
  Dietary Intake Record, 249
Nursing. *See* Breast-feeding;
  "Nursing bottle syndrome," 84–85, 99–102, 131
Nutra Natural Lunch, 183, 184
Nutrient absorption. *See* Absorption.
Nutrient balance in diet, 7, 8, 18, 53, 57, 89, 96, 119, 121, 148, 162, 163, 178, 180, 210, 214, 224, 225, 231, 239
Nutrient loss
  enriched foods and, 114
  food preparation and, 27, 32, 91–92
  orange juice storage and, 116
Nutrition, optimum
  balanced diet and, 1, 32, 89
  breast-feeding and, 33, 58
  dental health and, 169
  family influence and, 107, 154
  RDAs and, 10, 11
Nutrition education
  family and, 1, 5, 6, 107, 184–86, 190
  pregnant adolescent and, 227
  preschooler and, 105, 144, 150, 152, 153
  school and, 165, 172, 183
  teens and, 222
  television and, 5, 142
Nutritional patterns.
  in adolescence, 190–91
  family influences on, 1–2, 107–108
Nuts and seeds in protein
  complementarity, 17, 93

Obesity
  during adolescence, 4, 208-209, 210-19,
    229, 238
  allergies and, 103
  behavior modification in treatment of,
    171-73
  during elementary school years, 169-73
  exercise and, 13, 144-47, 172, 214-19
  fat-cell-number theory of, 4, 52-53,
    103, 145-46, 170-71
  during infancy, 73, 102-105
    breast- and bottle-fed babies, 81
    infant formula preparation and, 59,
      77
    milk intake and, 164
    nursing mother and, 53-54
    overfeeding and, 36, 52, 62
    predisposition towards, 4, 147, 170
  during pregnancy, 227
  during preschool years, 144-47
  weight control and, 105, 146, 171,
    218-19, 229
Oral contraceptive agent. See "Pill"
Organically grown food diets, 222-23
Overeating
  causes, 170
  "clean plate syndrome" in, 96, 120, 171
  obesity and, 40, 144, 170, 214, 215
  use of skim milk and, 76
Overfeeding, 40, 103-104, 170
  See also Force-feeding
Oxytocin (hormone), 34n, 53

Pantothenic acid (water soluble vitamin),
    18, 23
  deficiencies, 23, 229
  food sources, 23
  functions, 23
Parental influence on diet and nutrition,
    105, 107-108, 124, 156, 251
Parker, Dr. Richard, 136
Parkins, Dr. Frederick, 46
Parties and holidays, 151, 166, 184, 185-
    86, 239
Pathogens, 47, 50
Pauling, Dr. Linus, 162
Peckos, Penelope, 214
Peer influence on diet and nutrition, 156,
    165, 194
Phenylalanine (amino acid), 16
Phenylketonuria (PKU), 67
Phosphocreatine (PC), 235
Phosphorus (mineral), 25
  content in breast and formula milk, 45
  deficiencies, 25
  food sources, 25
  functions, 25
  needs during:
    adolescence, 200, 201
    elementary school years, 157
    infancy, 36
    lactation, 201
    pregnancy, 201
    preschool years, 109, 116
  tooth development and, 134
  toxicity, 25
Pica, 226
Pickwickian Syndrome, 171

"Pill," the (oral contraceptive agent)
  effect on teen nutrition and, 226-27
  use of, during lactation, 57
Plaque, dental, 132, 134, 136
Plasma, 16, 181
Poisoning. See also Toxicity
  carbon monoxide, 174
  iron, 204
  lead, 174
  vitamin and mineral, 44
Portions, children's, 9n, 96, 120, 121
Potassium (mineral), 26
  deficiencies, 26
  depletion of, during:
    athletic activity, 180, 232
    fad dieting, 221
  food sources, 26
  functions, 26
  toxicity, 26, 68
Potassium chloride, 68
Pregnancy, 227-29
  folacin deficiency during, 226
  iron supplements during, 3
  during lactation, 57
  megadoses of vitamin C during, 45
  nutritional needs during, 200, 201
Premature infants
  bonding and, 65
  calorie needs of, 36
  iron needs of, 45-46, 80, 117
  vitamin E needs of, 44
Prenatal dietary influences, 2, 47, 227-29
Preservatives, 79, 89, 221
Preventive dental care, 100, 132, 133-34,
    169
Prolactin (hormone), 52, 56
Protein. See also High-protein diet
  deficiencies, 15-16
  in fast-foods diets, 238
  food sources, 16, 42, 43, 161, 164, 198,
    199
  functions, 13, 15-16
  in infant diet, 42, 43, 50, 77, 91
  needs during:
    adolescence, 195, 208
    athletic training, 231, 234
    elementary school years, 157, 161
    infancy, 36
    lactation, 57, 58, 195
    pregnancy, 195, 228
    preschool years, 109, 112-13
  overload, 15, 60
  pre-digested, 60, 237
  in snack foods, 135
  in vegetarian diets, 16-17, 113, 149-50,
    161
  vitamin $B_6$ and, 45
Protein complementarity, 16, 17, 93, 113,
    149-50, 198
Pyridoxine. See Vitamin $B_6$
Pubescence, 191
  pre-, 191, 200
  post-, 191

RDAs (Recommended Dietary
    Allowances)
  during adolescence, 194, 195, 201, 208,
    238

RDAs *(continued)*
during athletic training, 231, 232
calories, 12–13
defined, 10–11, 27
during elementary school years, 157, 176, 182, 187, 189
food labeling of, 24, 27
during infancy, 34, 36, 76, 88, 94
during lactation, 195, 201
minerals, 24, 27, 116–18, 162, 163, 200, 202–204
during pregnancy, 195, 201, 228
during preschool years, 108, 109, 119
protein, 17, 113, 161, 198
vitamins, 18, 115–16, 162, 200
Ready-to-use formula, 59, 61–62
Recipe Conversion Chart, 9n
Recipes (Appendix C), 271, 304
*Recommended Dietary Allowances,* 1980 (NRC), 10, 18, 118
Retardation
drug use and, 175, 228
fetal alcohol syndrome and, 228
malnutrition and, 2, 3, 33
metabolism errors and, 67
protein deficiency, 15–16, 60
vegetarian diet and, 60, 149
zinc deficiency, 3
Riboflavin (water soluble vitamin), 22
content of breast and formula milk, 45, 60
deficiencies, 22
in fast-foods diets, 238
food sources, 22
functions, 22
needs during:
adolescence, 201, 202
contraceptive use, 226
elementary school years, 157
infancy, 36
lactation, 57–58, 201
pregnancy, 201
preschool years, 109
in snack foods, 208
toxicity, 22
Richards, Ellen, 182
Rickets, 2, 149
Risk Factors in Childhood Obesity, 170
Roughage, 114

Sack lunches, 187
*See also* Appendix C
Salicylates, 176
Saliva, 62–63
caries development and, 99, 132, 135, 137
food contamination and, 90
Salmonella, 50
Salt. *See also* Sodium
heat exhaustion and, 181
infant foods and, 46, 80–81, 89, 91, 92
intake
hypertension and, 46, 80
during training and competition, 232
vegetarian diets and, 24
iodine in, 24, 150, 203
in snack foods, 136

Sanitation, 47, 51, 61
*See also* Sterilization
Schedules. *See also* Meal patterns
during infancy, 73, 76, 85, 106
during preschool years, 154
television interference with, 167
School lunch programs, 181–84
Scurvy, 45
Seascape, 214
Seasonings, 80–81, 89, 91, 92, 136
Selenium (trace element), 30
Self-feeding, 94, 95
Sensory approach to foods, 97, 126–27, 153
Sensory Approach to Learning about Foods, 153
Sexual maturation
body fat and, 198, 210
growth rates and, 192–93, 225
puberty, 191
zinc deficiency and, 3
Shalita, Alan, 224
Shigella, 50
Silicon (trace element), 31
Skin, 6, 223–24
Skin-fold test, 112, 213
Sloan, Sara, 183, 184
Snacks
breakfast cereals as, 140
energy source, 8, 187, 208
guidelines for, 138–39
habits in eating, 105, 121, 127, 134, 136, 154, 167, 168
infants and, 73
nutrient content of, 12, 136, 168
school performance and, 186
sweets as, 105, 132, 135–36, 162
toddlers and, 106
vending machines, 161–62, 169
Sodium (mineral), 26.
nitrate and nitrite, 89
content of breast and formula milk, 46
deficiencies, 26
in fast-foods diets, 238
food sources, 26
functions, 26
in snacks, 136
toxicity, 26
in training diets, 232
Solid foods in infant diet
acceptance of, 77
allergies from, 63, 88
introduction of, 62–63, 82, 83, 88, 98, 103
cereal, 80, 83
fruit, 77, 83
meat, 83
vegetables, 78, 83
Sorbitol, 137
Sources of Iron, 204–205
Spices, 93
Spock, Dr. Benjamin, 85
"Spoiling," 74–75
Spoon-feeding, 63, 80, 82, 89, 95
Staphlococci, 50–51
Starch
in baby foods, 90, 91
in breast milk, 51

Starch *(continued)*
  as complex carbohydrate, 13
  as energy source, 113
Sterilization and food preparation, 61, 78
Steroids (hormones), 234
*Streptococcus mutans,* 131–32, 137
Sucrose (Carbohydrate)
  in baby foods, 78, 90
  as energy source, 113
  tooth decay and, 101, 102, 131, 132, 134, 136
Sudden Infant Death Syndrome (SIDS), 69, 84
Sugar. *See also* Sucrose
  in baby foods, 80, 91
  in cereal, 140, 141, 142
  forms of, 222
  as simple carbohydrate, 13, 113, 199
  tooth decay and, 131, 132, 134–35, 162, 199, 224
Supplements:
  protein, 231
  vitamin and mineral. *See also* specific vitamins and minerals
    balanced diet and, 18, 162
    contraceptive use and, 226–27
    deficiency symptoms and, 10–11, 24, 147
    fad diets and, 221, 223
    hyperactivity and, 176
    infancy and, 43–44, 58, 69
    meeting RDAs and, 11
    toxicity of, 10, 18, 27, 69, 220–21
Sweets, 113
  breakfast cereals as, 140
  desserts and parties and, 105, 150, 151, 166
  junk food, 105, 167, 199
  snacks, 167, 168
  television advertising of, 142–43
  tooth decay and, 113, 132, 134–36, 137, 162, 169, 199
Syringelike infant feeder, 63, 80, 89

Table food for infants, 92, 94
Table manners, 95, 121–23, 125–26, 166, 168
Teen mothers, 227–29
Teething, 84
Television influences
  on food choices, 5, 139–44, 167
  on meal patterns, 124–25, 167
Thiamin (water soluble vitamin), 22
  content of breast and formula milk, 45
  deficiencies, 22, 229
  in fast-foods diets, 238
  food sources, 9n, 22
  functions, 22
  needs during:
    adolescence, 201, 208
    elementary school years, 157
    infancy, 36
    lactation, 57–58, 201
    pregnancy, 201
    preschool years, 109
  toxicity, 22
Threonine (amino acid), 16

Thyroid activity, 203
Tin (trace element), 31
Tobacco, 229
Tofu, 93
Tooth decay. *See also* Caries, dental
  factors in, 134–35
  fluoride supplementation and, 132–34
  history of incidence of, 129–31, 130
  "nursing bottle syndrome" and, 99–100
Tooth development, 117, 134, 164, 202
Toothpaste with fluoride, 134
Total Sugar Content of Commercial Breakfast Cereals, 141
Toxic effects of drugs, 68, 229
Toxic effects of nutrient supplements, 10, 18, 27, 220–21
Toxicants
  botulinal, 83–84
  ecological, 56, 62, 174
Trace elements, 11, 24, 27, 28–31, 96, 161, 162, 226
  *See also* Chromium; Cobalt; Copper; Fluoride; Iodine; Iron; Manganese; Molybdenum; Nickel; Selenium; Silicon; Tin; Vanadium; Zinc
Training and competition, diet during, 179–81, 230–38
Travel and nutrition, 89, 185
Triceps skin-fold test, 112, 213
Triglyceride, 199
Tryptophan (amino acid), 16
Tuberculosis, 222
Typhoid fever, 50
Typical Vegetarian Menu for Ages 18–36 Months, 155

United States Department of Agriculture, 7
  Extension Service, 5, 115, 127
  Food and Consumer Services, 162
  Food Intake Survey, 200, 202, 203
  WIC (Women, Infants, and Children) Program, 5, 115, 228
United States Department of Health, Education, and Welfare, 2
  Public Health Service, 8
United States Senate Report on Dietary Goals, 143
Utensils in infant feeding, 61, 63, 80, 85, 87, 89, 95

Vacation foods. *See* Travel and nutrition
Valine (amino acid), 16
Vanadium (trace element), 31
Variety in diet, 7, 8, 89, 93, 106, 124, 157
Vegan. *See* Vegetarian diets
Vegetable Preparation Tips, 127
Vegetables
  carbohydrate content of, 78
  food group, 9
  introduction of, to infant diet, 78, 88
  preparation of, 126, 127
  in protein complementarity, 17, 164
  snack food, 137, 138, 168
Vegetarian diets, 221
  calcium content of, 117, 164, 202
  fat content of, 198

Vegetarian diets *(continued)*
  infancy and, 60, 93
  lactation and, 58
  lacto-, 117
  lacto-ovo, 45, 149, 164
  preschool years and, 149–50, 155, 161
  protein complementarity in, 16, 17, 113, 198
  supplements with, 24, 202
  vegan, 16, 45, 60, 117, 149, 164, 226
  vitamin $B_{12}$ deficiency and, 45, 149–50, 164, 202, 226
  Zen Macrobiotic, 149, 221
Vending machines and snacks, 162
Vitamin(s), 1, 8, 18, 19–23, 24, 58, 89
  in breakfast foods, 140
  deficiency in hyperactivity, 176
  loss of, in rapid weight loss, 234
  supplements, 10–11, 115
  therapy in alcoholism, 229
  in vegetables, 137
Vitamin A (fat soluble vitamin), 19
  deficiencies, 19
  fast-foods diets and, 238
  food sources, 9n, 19, 71
  functions, 6, 19
  needs during:
    adolescence, 200, 201, 202
    athletic training, 232
    contraceptive use, 226
    elementary school years, 157
    infancy, 36
    lactation, 57–58, 201
    pregnancy, 201, 227
    preschool years, 109, 115–16
  snack foods and, 208
  supplements, 43–44
  tooth development and, 134
  toxicity, 18, 19, 43–44, 115, 176–77, 224, 232
Vitamin B-complex (water soluble vitamins), 18.
  training diet and, 232
  vegetarian diets and, 232
Vitamin $B_1$. *See* Thiamin
Vitamin $B_2$. *See* Riboflavin
*Vitamin $B_3$. See* Niacin
Vitamin $B_6$ (pyridoxine) (water soluble vitamin), 22
  content of breast and formula milk, 45
  deficiencies, 22, 226–27, 229
  food sources, 22
  functions, 22
  needs during:
    adolescence, 201
    contraceptive use, 226–27
    elementary school years, 157
    infancy, 36
    lactation, 58, 201
    pregnancy, 201, 227
    preschool years, 109
  toxicity, 22
Vitamin $B_9$. *See* Folacin
Vitamin $B_{12}$ (cyanocobalamin) (water soluble vitamin), 23
  content of breast and formula milk, 45
  cobalt and, 29

  deficiencies, 23, 149–50, 164, 202, 226
  food sources, 23
  functions, 23
  needs during:
    adolescence, 201
    elementary school years, 157
    infancy, 36
    lactation, 201
    pregnancy, 201, 227
    preschool years, 109
    training and competition, 232
  soy-based formula and, 60
  supplements, 164
  toxicity, 23
  vegetarian diet and, 45, 149–50, 164, 202, 226
Vitamin C (water soluble vitamin), 21
  content of breast and formula milk, 44, 59
  deficiencies, 21, 44
  fad diets and, 220
  Fast-foods diets and, 238
  food sources, 21, 71, 89, 116
  functions, 21
  iron absorption and, 118
  megadoses of, 45, 162–63
  needs during:
    adolescence, 201, 202, 208
    contraceptive use, 226
    elementary school years, 157
    infancy, 36
    lactation, 57–58, 201
    pregnancy, 201, 227
    preschool years, 109, 115–16
    training and competition, 232
  tooth development and, 134
  toxicity, 18, 21
Vitamin D (fat soluble vitamin), 19
  additive in milk, 222
  content of breast and formula milk, 44, 50
  deficiencies, 19
  food sources, 19
  functions, 19, 44
  needs during:
    adolescence, 201
    elementary school years, 157
    infancy, 36
    lactation, 201
    pregnancy, 201
    preschool years, 109
    training and competition, 232
  supplements, 44
  toxicity, 18, 19, 44, 115, 232
Vitamin E (fat soluble vitamin), 19
  deficiencies, 19
  food sources, 19
  functions, 19
  needs during:
    adolescence, 201
    elementary school years, 157
    infancy, 36
    of premature infant, 44, 80
    lactation, 57–58, 201
    pregnancy, 201
    preschool years, 157
    training and competition, 232

Vitamin E *(continued)*
    toxicity, 19
Vitamin K (fat soluble vitamin), 20
    deficiencies, 20
    food sources, 20, 44
    functions, 20
    needs of neonatal infant, 44
    toxicity, 18, 20

Walker, Dr. Sidney III, 177
Water, fluoridation of, 46, 132–34
Water in infant diet, 35, 104
Water soluble vitamins, 21–23
Weaning, 15, 53–54, 77, 85, 87
Weight, "making," 233
Weight control, 105, 146, 171–72, 218–21,
    229
Weight loss, 180, 211–12, 218, 219–21
Weight loss diets. *See* Diet alterations
Weight norms.
    for adolescents, 192–94
    for elementary school children, 160
    for infants, 37–41, 88
    for preschoolers, 112
Wernicke-Korsakoff's syndrome, 229
Whole grain foods, 27, 58, 93, 114, 161,
    199, 222

WIC (Women, Infants, and Children)
    Program, 5, 115, 228
World Health Organization (WHO), 50,
    90
Working mothers and breast-feeding, 54–
    55
Wrestling, 233–34

Xylitol, 137

Zen Macrobiotic diet, 149, 221
Zinc (mineral), 27, 29
    -binding ligand (zbl), 46
    content of breast and formula milk, 34
    -to-copper ratio, 46
    deficiencies, 29, 119, 226
    food sources, 29
    functions, 29
    needs during:
        adolescence, 201
        elementary school years, 157
        infancy, 36
        lactation, 57–58, 201
        pregnancy, 201
        preschool years, 109, 116
    toxicity, 29